Drug Interactions in Psychiatry

SECOND EDITION

Drug Interactions in Psychiatry

SECOND EDITION
Edited by

DOMENIC A. CIRAULO, M.D.
Professor of Psychiatry
Lecturer, Department of Pharmacology and Experimental Therapeutics
Tufts University School of Medicine
Chief, Psychiatry Service
Veterans Affairs Medical Center
Boston, Massachusetts

RICHARD I. SHADER, M.D.
Professor of Pharmacology and Experimental Therapeutics
Tufts University School of Medicine
Boston, Massachusetts

DAVID J. GREENBLATT, M.D.
Professor and Chairman
Department of Pharmacology and Experimental Therapeutics
Professor of Psychiatry, Medicine, and Anesthesia
Tufts University School of Medicine
Chief, Division of Clinical Pharmacology
New England Medical Center Hospital
Boston, Massachusetts

WAYNE L. CREELMAN, M.D.
Associate Clinical Professor of Psychiatry
State University of New York at Buffalo
Psychiatrist-in-Chief and Medical Director
BryLin Hospitals
Buffalo, New York

Editor: David C. Retford
Managing Editor: Kathleen Courtney Millet
Production Coordinator: Barbara J. Felton
Copy Editor: Carol Zimmerman
Designer: Dan Pfisterer
Illustration Planner: Ray Lowman

Copyright © 1995
Williams & Wilkins
351 West Camden Street
Baltimore, Maryland 21201 USA

Printed in the United States of America

First Edition 1989

Library of Congress Cataloging in Publication Data
Drug interactions in psychiatry / edited by Domenic A. Ciraulo . . . [et al.].—2nd ed.
   p. cm.
  Includes bibliographical references and index.
  ISBN 0-683-01944-9 (pbk.)
  1. Psychotropic drugs—Side effects.   2. Drug interactions.
I. Ciraulo, Domenic A.
  [DNLM: 1. Psychotropic Drugs—pharmacology.   2. Drug Interactions.
QV 77.2 D789 1995]
RM315,D792 1995
615'.788–dc20
DNLM/DLC
for Library of Congress   95-11652
                                                      CIP

                                 95   96   97   98   99
              1   2   3   4   5   6   7   8   9   10

PREFACE

It was an odd coincidence that the trial of Zion vs. New York Hospital was in its final stages in the winter of 1995 as we edited the first few chapters of this second edition. It was a highly publicized case centering around the medical care given to Libby Zion, a young woman who presented to the hospital with agitation and fever, who later had hyperpyrexia and died. Her family was suing her physicians and the New York Hospital for malpractice. Among the many issues in that case was the possible drug-drug interaction of a 25-mg dose of meperidine (Demerol®) (administered to treat rigors) with phenelzine (Nardil®) and/or haloperidol (Haldol®). The defense contended that chlorpheniramine, diazepam, oxycodone, and cocaine were also involved, but the plaintiff's attorney argued against the role of these other drugs in her death. The plaintiff alleged, among other things, that the physicians were guilty of malpractice because they administered meperidine to a patient who had taken a monoamine oxidase inhibitor antidepressant, a practice that was considered dangerous and had been contraindicated by the manufacturers' information in the *Physicians Desk Reference* since the 1960s. As I viewed the entire trial, trying to put myself in the jurors' place, it seemed that the only incontrovertible fact was that meperidine was administered to Libby Zion while she had been taking phenelzine. The jury saw it that way too—finding all but one of the physicians involved in the case guilty of malpractice.

I could imagine the jury wondering why doctors at a leading academic hospital did not know the basic information about a drug they were administering to a patient, even though defense experts testified that they too were unaware in 1984 of the interaction of meperidine and phenelzine. I think I would have a hard time, if I were a lay person, believing that assertion from the defense expert. But as a physician who had a similar experience, I can attest to the fact that many of us found out about the interaction almost by accident. For me it was in 1977 when I was a chief resident; one of the residents I was supervising had a patient taking phenelzine who was scheduled for elective surgery, and he questioned me about possible drug interactions. Fortunately, we did look at the *Physicians Desk Reference* and standard textbooks, which cautioned against combined use. We were puzzled though, when a computer literature search yielded no original reports of the interaction. That literature search, combined with the belief of many clinical psychopharmacologists that the hazards of MAOIs had been exaggerated, led to us to question whether this was another instance of MAOI hysteria. I discussed the case with my supervisor (a co-editor of this book [R.I.S.]) who suggested that I run the search again using "pethidine" (to identify the British literature), "iproniazid," and "pargyline" as key words. That second search, of course, provided several studies in animals and case reports in humans documenting a serious and possibly fatal interaction.

That experience left me with the feeling that it really should be easier to find documentation of drug interactions in psychopharmacology. The purpose of the first edition of this book was to assist clinicians in rapid identification and avoidance of drug-drug interactions. From the wonderful feedback that we have received from colleagues and students, the first edition appears to have fulfilled that mission. If you liked the first edition, you will like the second one even more.

This edition contains entirely revised and updated chapters, as well as the inclusion of two new chapters, one on drug interactions in electroconvulsive therapy and the other on β-adrenergic blocker drug interactions. A new section on selective serotonin reuptake inhibitors has also been included.

We have expanded the number of contributors to this edition. The revised chapter on antipsychotics has been written by two experts in that area, Ross Baldessarini, M.D., and Donald Goff, M.D., both of Harvard Medical School. Charles Welch, M.D., also of Harvard Medical School, is an authority on electroconvulsive therapy (ECT) and has contributed a chapter on drug interactions that are important in ECT. John Ratey, M.D., at Medfield State Hospital in Medfield, Massachusetts, and Kathleen McNaughton, who have done extensive clinical research in the use of β-adrenergic blockers in psychiatry, discuss clinically relevant interactions with this class of medications.

We have also included Ofra Sarid-Segal, M.D., of Tufts University School of Medicine and Director of the Lithium Clinic at the Department of Veterans Affairs Outpatient Clinic (DVAOPC), to assist in the revision of the lithium chapter. Richard O'Sullivan, M.D., of Massachusetts General Hospital, DVAOPC, and Harvard Medical School, assisted with the revision of the antidepressant chapter. John Greene, Ph.D., Director of the Drug Dependence Treatment Program at the DVAOPC, has contributed updated material relevant to chemical dependence. We believe that the addition of these clinical experts enhances the interpretations of the reported drug interactions and provides the best possible guidance for clinicians. We hope that by keeping the standard tripartite analysis of drug interactions and maintaining uniformity of style the work retains its cohesiveness.

Our clinical work and teaching lead us to believe that there is a continuing need for a reference book on drug interactions in psychiatry. Although computer databases of drug interactions are excellent resources that provide a quick assessment of possible interactions, even the best of them lack detailed analyses or comprehensive clinical recommendations. The other major source of information on drug interactions derives from standard textbooks that cover drug interactions in all areas of medicine. Although these texts provide incredibly extensive lists of references on drug interactions, we find all too often that the clinical recommendations in psychopharmacology reflect unfamiliarity with patient care.

The Second Edition of *Drug Interactions in Psychiatry* attempts to critically analyze drug interactions of importance to psychiatrists, nurses, pharmacists, and mental health professionals who prescribe and dispense psychotropic medication or practice psychotherapy with patients taking these medications. We have tried to keep it as current as possible by adding important drug interactions during the editing process. The inevitable delays to publication, however, may have resulted in the omission of some very recent interactions. Updates on drug interactions will be published regularly in the *Journal of Clinical Psychopharmacology* to supplement the material in this text.

The editors would like to thank David Retford, Katey Millet, Barbara Felton, and the rest of the staff at Williams & Wilkins for their help in the editing of this second edition. Special thanks are also due to Janet Pace for her expert word processing skills and her equanimity under the stress of deadlines.

Most of all, we would like to thank our families for their support and encouragement, and for the sacrifices that they made in support of this work.

Domenic A. Ciraulo, M.D.

CONTRIBUTORS

ROSS J. BALDESSARINI, M.D.
Professor of Psychiatry (Neuroscience)
Harvard Medical School
Boston, Massachusetts
Director, Laboratories for Psychiatric
Research
Director, Bipolar & Psychotic Disorders
Program
McLean Hospital
Belmont, Massachusetts

JAMIE G. BARNHILL, Ph.D.
Assistant Professor of Pharmaceutics
University of New Mexico College of
Pharmacy
Chief, Biopharmaceutics/
Pharmacokinetics Laboratory
Cooperative Studies Program Clinical
Research Pharmacy Coordinating
Center
Veterans Affairs Medical Center
Albuquerque, New Mexico

ANN MARIE CIRAULO, R.N.
Research Nurse
Department of Pharmacology and
Experimental Therapeutics
Tufts University School of Medicine
Psychiatry Service
Veterans Affairs Medical Center
Boston, Massachusetts

DOMENIC A. CIRAULO, M.D.
Professor of Psychiatry
Lecturer, Department of Pharmacology
and Experimental Therapeutics
Tufts University School of Medicine
Chief, Psychiatry Service
Veterans Affairs Medical Center
Boston, Massachusetts

WAYNE L. CREELMAN, M.D.
Associate Clinical Professor of
Psychiatry
State University of New York at Buffalo
Psychiatrist-in-Chief and Medical
Director
BryLin Hospitals
Buffalo, New York

DONALD C. GOFF, M.D.
Assistant Professor of Psychiatry
Harvard Medical School
Erich Lindemann Mental Health Center
Massachusetts General Hospital
Veterans Affairs Medical Center
Boston, Massachusetts

DAVID J. GREENBLATT, M.D.
Professor and Chairman
Department of Pharmacology and
Experimental Therapeutics
Professor of Psychiatry, Medicine, and
Anesthesia
Tufts University School of Medicine
Co-Chief, Division of Clinical
Pharmacology
New England Medical Center Hospital
Boston, Massachusetts

JOHN A. GREENE, Ph.D.
Assistant Professor of Psychiatry
(Psychology)
Tufts University School of Medicine
Clinical Instructor in Psychiatry
Harvard Medical School
Veterans Affairs Medical Center
Boston, Massachusetts

KATHLEEN L. MACNAUGHTON, B.A.
Ph.D. Candidate
Department of Clinical and Health
  Psychology
Florida State University College of
  Health Related Professions
Gainesville, Florida

RICHARD L. O'SULLIVAN, M.D.
Instructor in Psychiatry
Harvard Medical School
Clinical Assistant in Psychiatry
Massachusetts General Hospital
Staff Psychiatrist
Veterans Affairs Medical Center
Boston, Massachusetts

JOHN RATEY, M.D.
Assistant Professor of Psychiatry
Harvard Medical School
Medfield State Hospital
Medfield, Massachusetts

BRIAN F. SANDS, M.D.
Assistant Professor of Psychiatry
Tufts University Medical School
Director of Psychopharmacology
Substance Abuse Treatment Programs
Veterans Affairs Medical Center
Boston, Massachusetts

OFRA SARID-SEGAL, M.D.
Assistant Professor of Psychiatry
Tufts University School of Medicine
Psychiatry Service
Veterans Affairs Medical Center
Boston, Massachusetts

RICHARD I. SHADER, M.D.
Professor of Pharmacology and
  Experimental Therapeutics
Tufts University School of Medicine
Boston, Massachusetts

MICHAEL SLATTERY, M.D.
Sleep Disorder Center
Beth Israel Hospital
Boston, Massachusetts

CHARLES A. WELCH, M.D.
Instructor in Psychiatry
Harvard Medical School
Director of Somatic Therapies
  Consultation Service
Massachusetts General Hospital
Boston, Massachusetts

CONTENTS

8. INTERACTIONS OF IMPORTANCE IN CHEMICAL
   DEPENDENCE 356

JAMIE G. BARNHILL, ANN MARIE CIRAULO, DOMENIC A. CIRAULO, and
JOHN A. GREENE

1

Basic Concepts

DOMENIC A. CIRAULO, RICHARD I. SHADER,
DAVID J. GREENBLATT, and JAMIE G. BARNHILL

Drug interactions can be grouped into two principal subdivisions: pharmacokinetic and pharmacodynamic (or pharmacologic). These subgroups serve to focus attention on possible sites of interaction as a drug moves from the site of administration and absorption to its site of action. Pharmacokinetic processes are those that include transport to and from the receptor site and consist of absorption, distribution in body tissue, plasma protein binding, metabolism, and excretion. Pharmacodynamic interactions occur at biologically active sites. A basic understanding of the biologic and physiochemical processes involved in drug absorption, disposition, and action aids in the understanding of the mechanisms of drug interactions.

ABSORPTION

Normal drug absorption after oral administration begins with the delivery of active drug to the gastrointestinal mucosa—the barrier that separates the gastrointestinal lumen from the systemic circulation. The availability of the drug depends on the physical properties of the preparation (which affect disintegration and dissolution times), the integrity of the gut wall, and on metabolism, which may occur in the gut lumen and/or wall. Some substances may cause a drug to precipitate out of solution or can physically adsorb (irreversibly bind onto) a drug, thus decreasing its systemic availability. Charcoal, antacids, and kaolin-pectin may absorb some drugs. Cholesterol-lowering agents, such as cholestyramine, may bind drugs. Iron may decrease the antibacterial efficacy of tetracycline by chelation.

Enzymatic reactions may also lead to drug interactions during the

1

process of absorption. The interaction between monoamine oxidase inhibitors and tyramine-containing foodstuffs is due to the inhibition of the intestinal enzyme monoamine oxidase allowing higher than usual amounts of tyramine, an indirect sympathomimetic, to reach the systemic circulation.

If a drug interaction during absorption results in decreased serum concentrations for drugs with a relatively narrow therapeutic range (e.g. lithium), clinical effects may be compromised. Interactions may also result in an increase in the amount of drug absorbed. Lithium levels may be increased dramatically by concurrent marijuana use and may result in toxicity. This effect may be due to the anticholinergic activity of marijuana, which slows gut motility to allow increased duration of contact of the ion with the absorptive surface of the intestine (see Chap. 4). Food may interact with lithium in a similar manner.

More commonly, absorptive interactions result in a delay in the rate of absorption rather than a decrease in the amount absorbed. The graphic representation of drug concentration is expressed as the area under the curve of plasma level plotted against time on semi-logarithmic paper. The area under the curve represents the total amount of drug absorbed (or the extent of absorption) and, although this can be altered by drug interactions, it is more often the rate of absorption that is affected. Changes in the rate of absorption are most often characterized by a change in the time (T_{max}) required to reach maximum plasma concentrations. A decrease in the rate of absorption will cause an increase in the T_{max}. There will also be a change in the slope of the initial ascending portion of the concentration-versus-time curve. Altered drug absorption is of importance primarily for drugs that are given as a single dose on an intermittent basis, and it may be of particular clinical significance with benzodiazepine treatment of anxiety states. Results of studies (Greenblatt et al. 1977) have shown that a single 25-mg dose of chlordiazepoxide has a different subjective effect depending on whether it is administered with water or antacid, the latter agent decreasing the rate of absorption. Subjects report feeling more "spaced out" when chlordiazepoxide is given in conjunction with water only. The areas-under-the-curves and total amount of drug absorbed were the same in both conditions; however, the rate of absorption was greater when the drug was administered with water. When drugs are given on a chronic basis, the effect on rate of absorption is usually not clinically significant.

It is well recognized that tablet composition and dissolution characteristics may influence rate and amount of drug absorbed. Tablet dissolution can be affected by drug interactions. Elevation of gastric pH (e.g. with antacids) above the pKa of chlordiazepoxide (4.8) may reduce the dissolution rate of the drug by increasing concentrations of the poorly water-soluble non-ionized base. The ability of food to increase the amount while slowing the rate of absorbed diazepam may be due to greater tablet dissolution in the nonfasting state.

Changes in the total amount of drug absorbed can also be caused by metabolism of the drug in the gut lumen or precipitation of the drug in the gut. *In vitro* studies have suggested that caffeine may cause several antipsychotic agents to form insoluble precipitates, although the clinical implications of this phenomenon are not significant. Although gut metabolism of chlorpromazine occurs in the rat, it has not been directly demonstrated in humans (*see* Chap. 3).

In typical clinical practice, drug interactions occurring at sites of absorption are of concern primarily for substances administered via the oral route. Nevertheless, it is theoretically possible to apply some of the following considerations to simultaneous administration of more than one substance intravenously or intramuscularly.

Drug interactions that occur during absorption from the gastrointestinal tract can result in a change in the rate of absorption and/or in the amount of drug absorbed. Altered serum concentrations, delayed onset of drug action, prolonged effects, or altered subjective response can occur on the basis of alteration in the absorptive process alone. Events that combine to make up the normal process of absorption (e.g. dissolution of the tablet or capsule, passage from the stomach to the site of absorption in the small intestine) are all potential focuses of drug interactions.

DRUG DISPOSITION

The term "drug disposition" refers to the biologic processes occurring after a drug enters the systemic circulation. It may be conceptualized as involving three distinct entities: (1) distribution, (2) metabolism, and (3) excretion.

Drugs are distributed to the tissues by the systemic circulation. Entrance into the central nervous system requires penetration of the blood-brain barrier. Highly perfused tissues (brain, heart, liver, and kidney) show rapid blood-tissue equilibration of drugs. Following this initial transfer, the drug is redistributed to tissues with lower blood flow but higher drug affinity such as adipose tissue. An example of this process is the rapid onset of anesthesia after intravenous injection of thiopental. The duration of action of thiopental is short, however, because it is rapidly and extensively redistributed into the muscle and fat. Single-dose effects of benzodiazepines are more influenced by distribution factors than by elimination half-life. In fact, the effect of a single dose of lorazepam may last longer than that of diazepam despite the latter drug's longer half-life (Arendt et al. 1983). This is due to the greater lipid solubility and more extensive distribution of diazepam. Although not uncommon in general medical practice (e.g. penicillin-probenecid, quinacrine-pamaquine), drug interactions occurring as a result of tissue distribution alterations are not well studied in psychopharmacology. Aging appears to produce tissue distribution alterations attributable to changes in body composition (decreased total body water and lean body mass, increased body fat). Elderly patients appear to be more sensitive to the effects of diazepam, which may be the result of prolonged elimination half-life resulting from an increased volume of distribution (Klotz et al. 1975), as well as pharmacodynamic factors.

Protein-binding alterations may produce another type of distributional interaction. Drug binding in plasma is to albumin, which constitutes about one-half of the total plasma proteins, α_1-acid glycoprotein, and lipoproteins. The fraction of the drug that is bound is dependent on the concentration of the protein, the number of binding sites on the protein, and an equilibrium association constant. The bound portion of the drug is considered pharmacologically inactive, while the "free" or unbound portion is responsible for pharmacologic effect.

Drugs that are extensively bound (greater than 90% of total drug in plasma) present a particular problem for drug interactions. Because the unbound fraction is small, slight changes may produce a marked clinical effect. For example, with amitriptyline, which is 95% protein-bound (Borga et al. 1969), if another drug is given that displaces 5% of the bound amitriptyline, the free portion (and thus active drug) would double from 5% to 10%, whereas with phenobarbital, which is only 51% protein bound (Benet and Sheiner 1985), a displacement of 5% of the bound drug would increase the amount of free drug from 51% to 56%, which is a negligible increase.

Although not well studied, protein-binding interactions do not appear to be of major clinical importance in psychopharmacology. This type of interaction is important only for drugs that are given intravenously, metabolized primarily by the liver, and have a high hepatic extraction ratio. The usual result of displacement of orally administered drugs is that more free drug is present, *both* at receptors and hepatocytes, resulting in no net change. Transient toxicity may result if the displaced drug has a low therapeutic index.

DRUG METABOLISM

Metabolism refers to the biotransformation of a drug, usually by an enzyme-mediated reaction, to another chemical form. There are two major types of metabolic reactions: (1) phase I reactions, which include oxidation, reduction, hydrolysis reactions; and (2) phase II reactions, which include conjugation and acetylation reactions. Most drugs undergo several types of biotransformations. The metabolism of psychotropic agents may involve many steps and produce a number of intermediate metabolites that can have varying pharmacologic activities. Some metabolites are more potent than their parent compounds.

Phase I Reactions. Phase I reactions will yield intermediate metabolites that can then undergo phase II reactions to become highly polar, water-soluble metabolites. Hydroxylation and dealkylation reactions are the primary oxidative phase I reactions, with nitro reduction being the most prevalent of the reduction reactions.

Hydroxylation reactions involve the addition of a hydroxyl group to either an aromatic or nonaromatic molecular substituent (Fig. 1.1). A list of psychotropic agents that undergo hydroxylation is presented in Table 1.1.

Among the most common phase I reactions are dealkylations,

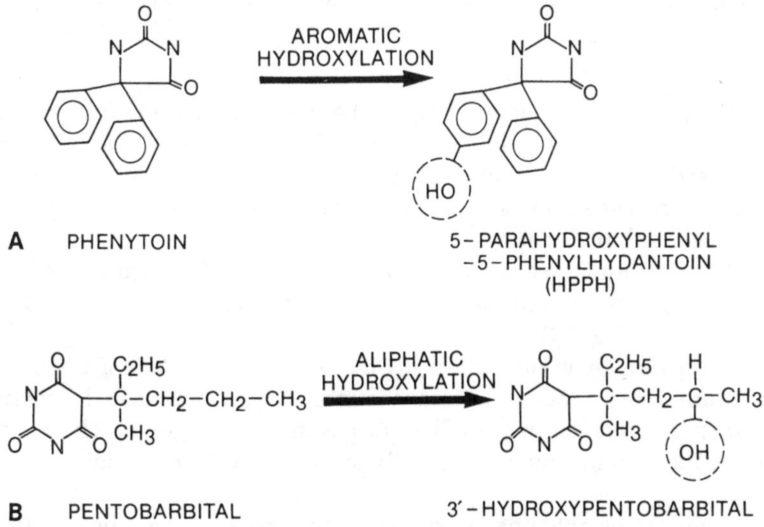

Figure 1.1. Examples of hydroxylation reactions. A, Transformation of phenytoin to HPPH by aromatic hydroxylation. B, Transformation of pentobarbital to 3'-hydroxypentobarbital by aliphatic hydroxylation. (From Greenblatt DJ, Shader RI 1985, p. 23.)

Table 1.1.
A Partial List of Psychotropic Agents That Are Known to Undergo Hydroxylation Reactions in Humans

Alprazolam
Barbiturates
Carbamazepine
Desipramine
Desmethyldiazepam
Glutethimide
Imipramine
Midazolam
Phenytoin
Propranolol
Triazolam

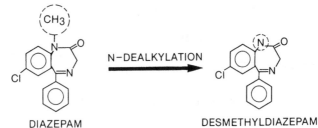

DIAZEPAM   DESMETHYLDIAZEPAM

Figure 1.2. An example of a dealkylation reaction. This represents the demethylation of diazepam to desmethyldiazepam. (From Greenblatt DJ, Shader RI 1985, p. 25.)

which may involve, for instance, the removal of a methyl or ethyl group from the drug molecule (Fig. 1.2). This group is ordinarily removed from an attachment at an oxygen, nitrogen, or sulphur atom. A list of some psychotropic agents that undergo dealkylation is presented in Table 1.2.

A less common oxidative reaction involves sulfide oxidation. This serves as a metabolic pathway for the antipsychotic agent, chlorpromazine (Fig. 1.3).

Reduction reactions, often involving the conversion of nitro substituents to amino groups, are another type of phase I reaction responsible for the metabolism of psychotropic agents. The benzodiazepine, clonazepam, is initially metabolized by this reaction (Fig. 1.4).

Another possible phase I reaction involves hydrolysis or the cleaving of a drug molecule by the addition of a water molecule. The analgesic, aspirin, undergoes hydrolysis as part of its total metabolism.

Table 1.2.
A Partial List of Psychtropic Agents That Are Known to Undergo Dealkylation Reactions in Humans

Amitriptyline
Chlordiazepoxide
Codeine
Diazepam
Flurazepam
Fluoxetine
Imipramine
Meperidine
Methamphetamine
Prazepam
Sertraline

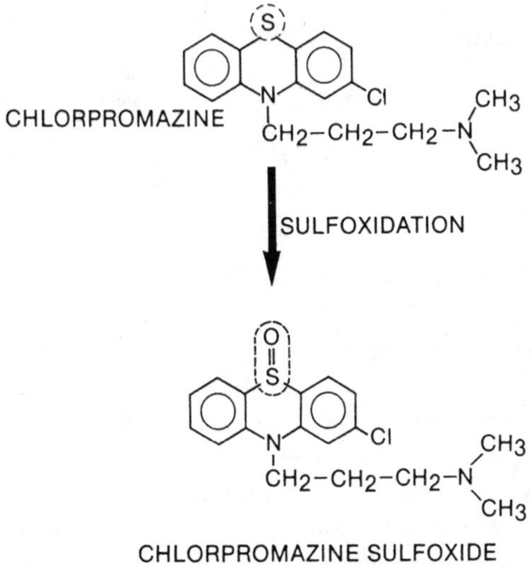

CHLORPROMAZINE

SULFOXIDATION

CHLORPROMAZINE SULFOXIDE

Figure 1.3. Transformation of chlorpromazine to chlorpromazine sulfoxide by sulfoxidation. (From Greenblatt DJ, Shader RI 1985, p. 25.)

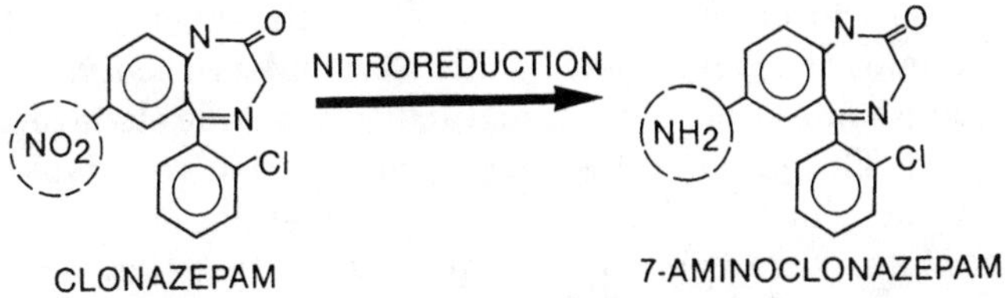

NITROREDUCTION

CLONAZEPAM

7-AMINOCLONAZEPAM

Figure 1.4. An example of a nitroreduction reaction. This represents the transformation of clonazepam to 7-aminoclonazepam. (From Greenblatt DJ, Shader RI 1985, p. 26.)

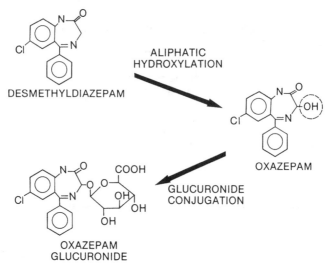

Figure 1.5. An example of sequential phase I and phase II biotransformation reactions. Desmethyldiazepam is initially biotransformed by the phase I reaction of aliphatic hydroxylation, yielding the pharmacologically active product oxazepam. Oxazepam is then transformed by the phase II reaction of glucuronide conjugation, yielding the pharmacologically inactive metabolite oxazepam glucuronide. (From Greenblatt DJ, Shader RI 1985, p. 27.)

Phase II Reactions. Phase II reactions include conjugation reactions (primarily glucuronide and sulfate) and acetylation reactions. These reactions yield the water-soluble metabolites that can easily be excreted from the body by the kidney. Many drugs that must undergo hepatic biotransformation before renal excretion will undergo both phase I and phase II metabolism (Fig. 1.5). However, many drugs require only phase II metabolism prior to excretion (Fig. 1.6). Examples of psychotropic agents metabolized only by phase II conjugative reactions include lorazepam, oxazepam, temazepam, and morphine. The glucuronide or sulfate conjugate produced by phase II metabolism is always pharmacologically inactive.

Another group of important phase II reactions involves acetylation or the addition of an acetyl group on the drug molecule (Fig. 1.7). Examples of psychotropic agents that undergo acetylation reactions during some stage of their metabolism include clonazepam and nitrazepam. The products formed by acetylation reactions may or may not be pharmacologically active. Acetylation involves the enzyme, N-acetyltransferase. The quantity of this enzyme is under genetic control and demonstrates a distinct polymorphism. Results

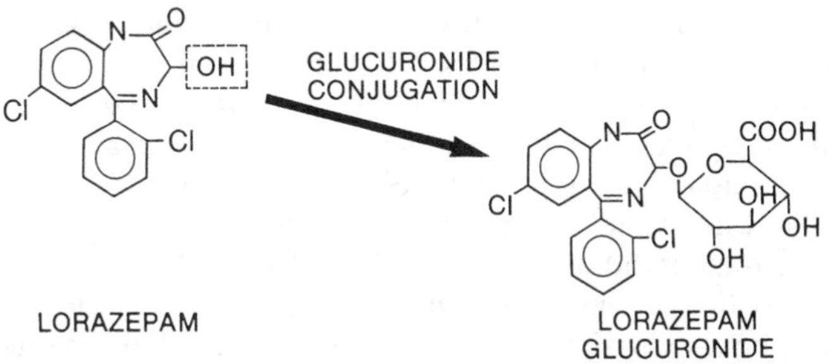

Figure 1.6. An example of glucuronide conjugation. This represents the biotransformation of lorazepam to lorazepam glucuronide. (From Greenblatt DJ, Shader RI 1985, p. 27.)

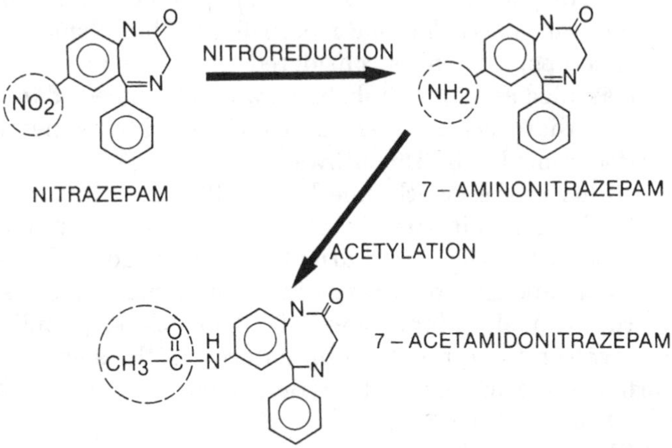

Figure 1.7. An example of an acetylation reaction. This represents the acetylation of the nitrazepam intermediate, 7-aminonitrazepam. (From Greenblatt DJ, Shader RI 1985, p. 29.)

of acetylation capacity tests have shown that humans cluster into groups of "slow" and "rapid" acetylators. Rapid acetylators are the predominant group and standardized dosages for psychotropic agents that undergo acetylation are designed for these individuals. Slow acetylators would be expected to be more sensitive to these drugs and would require dosage adjustments, as is sometimes the case when clonazepam is prescribed.

Acetylation reactions are not, however, the only reactions that rely on identifiable enzyme systems or demonstrate genetic control. The metabolism of drugs in the human body is under the control of the cytochrome P450 enzymes, located primarily, though not exclusively, in the liver hepatocytes (Murray 1992, Nelson et al. 1993). Many distinct subfamilies of the P450 enzymes have been identified. Each has a relative specificity for certain drugs and each is subject to genetic control. Many of the subfamilies of human cytochrome P450 are important to the metabolism of psychotropic agents (Brosen 1990, Cholerton et al. 1992, Murray 1992).

Cytochrome P450-2D6 is one such subfamily. It is responsible for the metabolic conversion (by phase I mechanisms) of desipramine, nortriptyline, clomipramine, perphenazine, thioridazine, and codeine. P450-2D6 is also responsible for the metabolism of other nonpsychotropic agents such as encainide, metoprolol, and dextromethorphan. Studies have demonstrated that cytochrome P450-2D6 exhibits genetic polymorphism. The majority of individuals in North America are considered "normal metabolizers," but a small fraction (5–10% of the population) is considered to be "slow metabolizers." Persons classified as slow metabolizers would be expected to require lower and perhaps less frequent doses of medications metabolized by the cytochrome P450-2D6 pathway.

The activity of the cytochrome P450-2D6 subfamily can also be inhibited. The coadministration of a drug that can inhibit cytochrome P450-2D6 with another drug that is dependent on this pathway for its metabolism could result in elevated plasma levels of the latter. Drugs capable of inhibiting P450-2D6 include quinidine, and the selective serotonin reuptake inhibitors (SSRIs) such as fluoxetine, norfluoxetine, and paroxetine (Bergstrom et al. 1992, Brosen et al. 1993, Otton et al. 1993).

The SSRIs also inhibit the cytochrome P450-3A subfamily (Ciraulo and Shader 1990). This subfamily is responsible for the metabolic conversion of the benzodiazepines triazolam, alprazolam, and midazolam. The cytochrome P450-3A subfamily also contributes to the metabolism of the tricyclic antidepressants imipramine and amitriptyline. Other inhibitors of this subfamily include ketoconazole, erythromycin, and cimetidine. The ability of fluvoxamine to inhibit 1A2 may lead to theophylline toxicity.

Other cytochrome P450 pathways can also be induced or stimulated. The cytochrome P450-2E1 subfamily may be induced by repeated ethanol ingestion. Unlike enzyme inhibition reactions, which can occur immediately after exposure to the inhibiting drug or chemical, enzyme induction reactions do not occur for some time after exposure to the inducer. The process of enzyme induction can take days or even weeks to become evident. Removal of the inducing agent will also cause a slow return to the preinduction state.

Both enzyme inhibition and induction reactions are of greatest concern with narrow therapeutic index drugs. It is only in this case that the possibility of toxic plasma levels or ineffective plasma levels can occur. This relationship is graphically represented in Figures 1.8 and 1.9 for drugs with narrow and wide therapeutic indices. Table 1.3 presents a list of drugs known to either stimulate or inhibit hepatic metabolism. Table 1.4 lists the cytochrome P450 isoenzymes that are involved in the metabolism of some commonly prescribed drugs.

Very simply, interactions via the metabolic route involve enzyme induction or inhibition, resulting in decreased or increased plasma levels, respectively. Definite enzyme inducers are barbiturates, glutethimide, and alcohol. Drugs that are affected by coadministration of enzyme inducers undergo more rapid metabolism, which results in diminished clinical effect. This can be reversed several days to

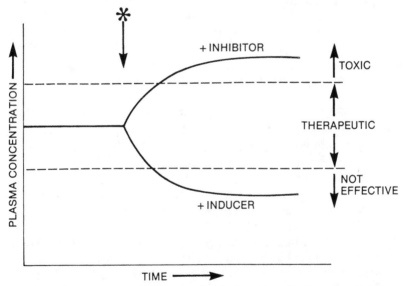

Figure 1.8. Consequences of a pharmacokinetic drug interaction for a drug that has a narrow therapeutic index. It is assumed that the drug is administered at a constant daily dose long enough for the steady-state to be reached, and the steady-state plasma concentration is assumed to be in the therapeutic range. At the vertical arrow with the asterisk (*) above, either an enzyme inducer or an enzyme inhibitor is co-administered. The inducer causes an increase in clearance, causing the plasma concentration to fall. Conversely, the inhibitor would cause a decrease in clearance, causing the plasma concentration to rise. Since the therapeutic range of the drug is narrow, the interaction with the inhibitor would cause toxicity, and the interaction with the inducer would cause loss of effectiveness. (From Greenblatt DJ, Shader RI 1985, p. 116.)

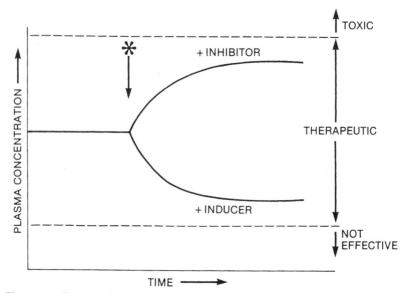

Figure 1.9. The pharmacokinetics situation is identical to that in Figure 1.8. In this case, the therapeutic index of the drug in question is wide. The same drug interactions and changes in plasma concentration as those in Figure 1.8 are of less clinical consequence this time, since the alteration in plasma concentration is not sufficient to cause toxicity or ineffectiveness. (From Greenblatt DJ, Shader RI 1985, p. 117.)

several weeks after the enzyme inducer is stopped. Cigarette smoking and chronic alcoholism induce the metabolism of imipramine, causing lower plasma levels (*see* Chap. 2). In light of research relating depression outcome to a minimum therapeutic plasma level, this may prove to have important clinical implications.

The clinical effects of enzyme induction can be managed by careful adjustment of dosage and monitoring of blood levels of drugs known to be affected by inducing agents. If possible, a noninducing drug should be substituted. For example, phenobarbital can decrease the anticoagulant effect of warfarin (Sellers and Koch-Weser 1970), and in some cases the clinician may wish to substitute a benzodiazepine for the barbiturate.

There have been many metabolic inhibition reactions reported. Typically, these interactions lead to increased serum levels and toxicity, such as is the case with disulfiram inhibiting the metabolism of phenytoin (*see* Chap. 6). Disulfiram can also prolong the half-life and reduce the clearance of chlordiazepoxide and imipramine by interfering with demethylation (*see* Chaps. 2 and 5). For patients taking disulfiram, the short or intermediate-acting benzodiazepines (e.g. oxazepam, lorazepam), which require only glucuronide forma-

Table 1.3.
A Partial List of Drugs That Are Known to Stimulate or Impair the Metabolism of Other Drugs[a]

Drugs Reported to Stimulate Metabolism
Barbiturates
Carbamazepine
Ethanol
Glutethimide
Phenytoin
Primidone
Rifampin

Drugs Reported to Impair Metabolism

Allopurinol	Methylphenidate
Antifungals (ketaconazole, miconazole, itraconazole)	Metronidazole
	Omeprazole
Chloramphenicol	Phenylbutazone
Cimetidine	Propranolol
Ciprofloxacin	Propoxyphene
Cotrimoxazole	Quinidine
Diltiazem	Selective serotonergic reuptake
Disulfiram	inhibitors (fluoxetine, paroxetine,
Estrogens	sertraline, fluvoxamine)
Ethanol (acute)	Tricyclic antidepressants
Isoniazid	Verapamil
Macrolide antibiotics (erythromycin and others)	

[a]Modified from Greenblatt DJ, Shader R, 1985.

tion prior to elimination, may be more predictable drugs to use (MacLeod et al. 1978, Sellers et al. 1980).

Metabolic inhibition may also influence individual pathways of biotransformation. Methylphenidate, for example, competes with imipramine for hydroxylation, while not affecting demethylation (*see* Chap. 2). A differential effect on particular metabolic pathways can influence whether a toxic or active metabolite is produced. In the case of imipramine-perphenazine, some metabolites (imipramine, desipramine) are increased, while the hydroxy metabolites, which may be active and cardiotoxic, are decreased.

DRUG EXCRETION

Renal excretion of drugs can be an important mechanism by which interactions occur. For this to be the case, the drug or active metabolite must be appreciably eliminated by the kidney. The three components of urinary excretion—glomerular filtration, tubular reabsorption, and active tubular secretion—may all be focuses of drug interactions.

Table 1.4.
Drugs Metabolized by Cytochrome P450

Drugs Metabolized by 3A4

Antiarrhythmic Agents
Amiodarone (Cordarone®)
Lidocaine (also 2C19 and 2D6)
Quinidine
Propafenone (Rythmol®) (see 2D6)
Disopyramide (Norpace®)

Calcium Channel Blockers
Diltiazem (Cardizem®)
Verapamil (Calan®) (also 1A2)
Nifedipine (Procardia®)

Opioid Analgesics
Alfentanil (Alfenta®)
Codeine (mainly 2D6)
Dextromethorphan (also 2D6)

Hormones/Steroids
Tamoxifen (Nolvadex®)
Testosterone
Cortisol
Progesterone
Ethinyl Estradiol

Antineoplastic
Paclitaxel (Taxol®)

Antihistamines
Terfenadine (Seldane®)
Astemizole (Hismanal®)
Loratadine (Claritin®)

Antimicrobial Agents
Erythromycin
Clarithromycin (Biaxin®)
Troleandomycin (Tao®)
Dapsone

Immunosuppressant Agents
Cyclosporine (Sandimmune®)
Tacrolimus (Prograf®)

Antiulcer (proton pump inhibiting) Agents
Omeprazole (Prilosec®) (also possibly 2C)

Drugs Metabolized by the CYP 2C
S-Mephenytoin (Mesantoin®) (2C19)
Phenytoin (Dilantin®) (2C9)
Tolbutamide (2C9)
S-Warfarin (Coumadin®) (2C9)
Ibuprofen (2C9)
Diclofenac (Voltaren®)
Naproxen (2C9)

Drugs Metabolized by CYP 1A2
Caffeine (also 2E1 and 3A4)
Theophylline
Aminophylline

Drugs Metabolized by CYP 2D6
Propranolol (Inderal®) (and possibly 2C19)
Metoprolol
Timolol
Mexiletine (Mexitil®)
Propafenone (Rythmol®) (also CYP 3A4 and CYP 1A2)
Codeine (also CYP 3A4)
Dextromethorphan (also CYP 3A4)

Glomerular filtration involves the passage of protein-free filtrate through the glomeruli. The glomerular capillaries allow free drug to pass, but protein-bound drugs are restricted; thus, alterations in the degree of protein binding may lead to drug interactions. Chloral derivatives have the potential to act in this manner.

Following filtration, drugs may undergo reabsorption in the renal tubules. Lipid-soluble drugs, such as a number of psychoactive agents, are extensively reabsorbed and alterations in urinary pH can result in significant drug interactions. An increase in urinary pH by an alkalizing agent such as sodium bicarbonate or acetazolamide may enhance the excretion of lithium or tranylcypromine, while urinary acidifiers (e.g. ammonium chloride, ascorbic acid, or methenamine mandelate) may enhance the excretion of imipramine, amitriptyline, or amphetamines. On the other hand, increasing the urinary pH will cause a prolonged half-life of drugs that are weak bases. For example, the half-life of amphetamine is doubled when urinary pH is increased from 5 to 8. As a general rule, increased urinary pH will impair elimination of weak bases and enhance excretion of weak acids, while decreased pH will have the opposite effect.

A drug such as lithium, which is not metabolized and requires adequate renal function for elimination, is especially susceptible to excretion interactions. Serum lithium levels increase when lithium is given with thiazide diuretics because of tubular reabsorption of lithium along with compensatory sodium reabsorption. Other drugs such as aminophylline, urea, and mannitol may all enhance renal excretion of lithium. Antidepressants and antipsychotics are eliminated mainly by hepatic metabolism, rendering excretion interactions clinically insignificant.

PHARMACODYNAMIC INTERACTIONS

Pharmacodynamic interactions occur when two or more drugs act at the same or interrelated receptor sites. The result may be additive, synergistic, or antagonistic. Potentiation of central nervous system sedation, which occurs when such agents as ethanol, antipsychotics, sedative-hypnotics, or anticonvulsants are taken concurrently, is perhaps the most common example of additive or synergistic effects of drug interactions. Antagonistic receptor site interactions result in decreased therapeutic effect. Levodopa may antagonize the antipsychotic action of neuroleptics, while the latter agents block the antiparkinson effects of levodopa (Hunter et al. 1970). The effect of increased dopamine at the receptor site due to levodopa can be decreased by the ability of neuroleptics to block the postsynaptic dopamine receptor. Benzodiazepines may also antagonize levodopa in a similar manner, not by blocking receptors, but by acting with γ-aminobutyric acid (GABA), a neurotransmitter that inhibits the dopaminergic system antagonist. The clinical relevance of these interactions is discussed elsewhere in this volume.

SUMMARY

Drug interactions can be understood as involving a limited number of mechanisms that constitute the normal process of drug absorption, disposition, and receptor site action. Although a drug interaction may occur by more than one of these mechanisms, an understanding of the site of interaction is essential for rational drug treatment and is a convenient way of classifying the multitude of drug interactions that affect the prescribing of psychoactive drugs.

INTRODUCTION TO PHARMACOKINETICS

Pharmacokinetics is the mathematical analysis of the process of drug absorption, distribution, metabolism, and excretion. The application of these principles to therapeutics is termed "clinical pharmacokinetics." In this section, we will outline the basic principles of pharmacokinetics and their application to pharmacotherapy with psychotropic agents. This section is intended as an introduction, and the reader is referred to one of the many textbooks in this field for a more complete discussion of pharmacokinetic principles (Bochner et al. 1983, Greenblatt and Shader 1985, Rowland and Tozer 1980, Wagner 1975).

Compartments

The concept of compartments is often difficult for physicians to understand, perhaps because most tend to think in anatomical and physiologic, rather than mathematical, terms. In pharmacokinetics the term "compartment" is a mathematical abstraction. When a drug is administered, it behaves as though the body is composed of one, two, or several compartments.

The single compartment model serves as the easiest model for conceptual purposes. For a single compartment model (Fig. 1.10), distribution of the drug is rapid and relatively uniform, because the whole body is viewed as a single large container. Graphs of plasma level versus time after oral and intravenous administration appear in Figure 1.11. Intravenous dosing is followed by instantaneous mix-

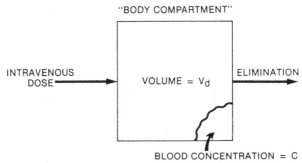

Figure 1.10. Schematic representation of the one-compartment model. (From Greenblatt DJ, Shader RI 1985.)

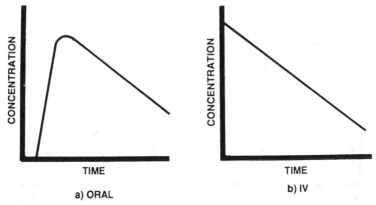

Figure 1.11. Plasma level versus time after oral (*a*) and intravenous (*b*) drug administration for a one-compartment model.

ing within the compartment and then declining levels within that compartment.

Perhaps a more useful concept is the two-compartment model, which takes into account that a declining plasma level is due to (1) distribution from plasma into tissues and (2) elimination. In this case the compartments are divided into a "central" compartment consisting of blood and highly vascular tissues and a compartment of low vascularity such as adipose tissue. If elimination of a drug is limited by hepatic blood flow (as in congestive heart failure) or if single-dose effects are important (e.g. anti-anxiety effect of benzodiazepines), the distributional phase influences clinical activity. In the case of benzodiazepines, it coincides with the termination of a single-dose clinical effect. The schematic representation of a two-compartment model (Fig. 1.12) and the plasma level time curves are

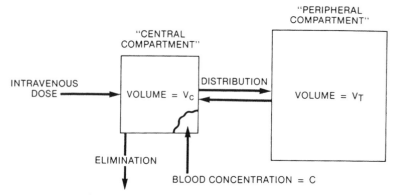

Figure 1.12. Schematic representation of the two-compartment model. (From Greenblatt DJ, Shader RI 1985.)

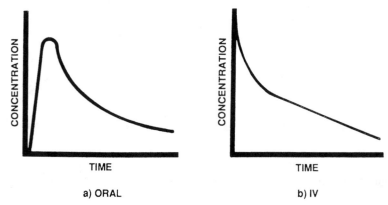

Figure 1.13. Plasma level versus time after oral (*a*) and intravenous (*b*) drug administration for a two-compartment model.

shown in Figure 1.13. In some cases more complicated multicompartment models are necessary to adequately describe disposition kinetics.

Absorption

The process of absorption requires the movement of drug molecules through cell membranes and involves the process of passive diffusion, filtration, passive facilitated diffusion, and active transport (Benet and Sheiner 1985). Diffusion is the process by which drug molecules move from an area of high to low concentration. It is often called "passive" because there is no energy expenditure required. The rate of diffusion is dependent on: (1) surface area of the membrane (the larger the area over which the substance can diffuse, the more rapid is the process); (2) the concentration difference between the two sides (the greater the difference, the more rapid is diffusion); and (3) a permeability constant (which is a characteristic of both the membrane and the drug). For most psychoactive drugs, which are highly lipid soluble, the permeability constant is high, making the diffusion rapid.

Filtration refers to the passage of drugs through channels as a result of osmotic or hydrostatic differences across membranes. The flow of water carries with it water-soluble molecules that are small enough to pass through the channels (the sizes of which vary depending on the specific body membrane).

Carrier-mediated transport consists of passive-facilitated diffusion and active transport. Passive-facilitated diffusion describes a process by which a substance moves across a concentration gradient more rapidly than could occur by diffusion alone, although no energy input is required. Examples of this system are the transport of glucose into the erythrocyte and the passage of vitamin B_{12} across the gastrointestinal epithelium.

Active transport is a carrier-mediated system characterized by specificity, saturability, competitive inhibition, movement against a concentration gradient, and an energy requirement. Active transport occurs in renal, biliary, and central nervous system secretion of drugs.

pH Partition Hypothesis

Only the un-ionized, nonpolar form of the drug passes through membranes and at equilibrium, the concentration of un-ionized drug is equal on both sides of the membrane. The degree to which a drug exists in its un-ionized form has implications for gastrointestinal absorption and secretion, and renal excretion of drugs. Because the pH is variable in both gastric fluid and urine, alterations could affect the proportion of drug present in the un-ionized (and thus diffusible) state.

The degree of ionization is determined by the pH at the site and the pKa of the drug. The pKa is a number which indicates the pH at which 50% of the drug is un-ionized. The formulae are indicated below:

For acids,

$$pH = pKa + \log \left[\frac{\text{ionized concentration}}{\text{unionized concentration}} \right]$$

For bases,

$$pH = pKa + \log \left[\frac{\text{un-ionized concentration}}{\text{ionized concentration}} \right]$$

Since log 1 = 0, the pKa is the pH at which the un-ionized and ionized concentrations are equal. Very weak acids (pKa > 7.5) are un-ionized at virtually all physiologic pH values. Acids with a pKa from 2.5 to 7.5 will show variations in the un-ionized fraction with pH fluctuations. Those with a pKa of less than 2.5 will have an un-ionized fraction so low that absorption is slow even under acidic conditions. For bases with a pKa between 5 and 11, there is pH-dependent absorption; only very weak bases (pKa < 5) will have absorption independent of pH.

Under clinical conditions, absorption is more rapid in the small intestine despite pH conditions because the surface area and blood flow are greatest here. Thus absorption is influenced more often by alterations in gastric emptying than by pH. If emptying is delayed, onset of drug action is impaired.

Other factors that influence the amount of drug reaching the systemic circulation after oral administration include: (1) gut metabolism (e.g. chlorpromazine can be metabolized in the gut to an inactive compound); (2) chemical reactions (e.g. clorazepate undergoes acid hydrolysis in the gut to form desmethyldiazepam); (3) hepatic extraction (after an oral dose between 30 and 70% of an antidepressant may be metabolized in the liver before the drug reaches the systemic circulation); and (4) tablet dissolution.

Absorption Kinetics

Absorption is usually a first-order process, although occasionally it follows zero-order kinetics. Graphic representations of the two processes as depicted on both standard and semi-logarithmic axes are shown in Figure 1.14. In a zero-order process there is a constant rate of absorption independent of the amount absorbed. In a first-order process the fractional rate of absorption is constant and the amount remaining to be absorbed declines exponentially.

A typical plasma concentration versus time (semi-log, two-compartment model, oral dose) is shown in Figure 1.15. At *point I,* the dose is ingested. After the lag time (t_o) elapses, the drug begins to appear in the systemic circulation (*point II*). Plasma concentrations rise until the rate of drug entry into blood equals the rate of removal by distribution and elimination, at which time the peak plasma level

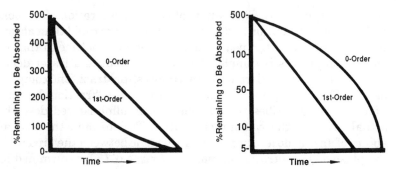

Figure 1.14. Graphic representation of first-order and zero-order kinetics plotted on regular and semilogarithmic axes.

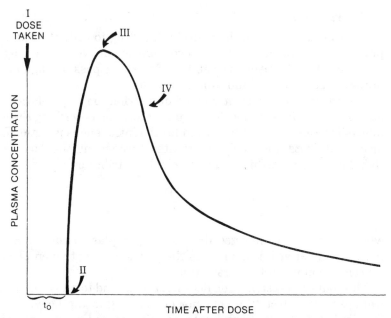

Figure 1.15. A typical plasma concentration curve following oral drug administration (the concentration axis is linear). At *point I*, the dose is ingested. After the lag time (t_0) elapses, the drug begins to appear in the systemic circulation (*point II*). Plasma concentrations rise until the rate of drug entry into blood equals the rate of removal by distribution and elimination, at which time the peak plasma level is reached (*point III*). Thereafter, plasma concentrations fall (*point IV*) because distribution and elimination are more rapid than absorption. Attainment of the peak concentration does not mean that the absorption process is complete; it continues, but at a continuously declining rate as the drug is removed from the gastrointestinal tract. (From Greenblatt DJ, Shader RI 1985.)

is reached (*point III*). Thereafter, plasma concentrations fall (*point IV*) because distribution and elimination are more rapid than absorption. Attainment of the peak concentration does not mean that the absorption process is complete; it continues, but to a lesser degree as the drug is removed from the gastrointestinal tract. The completeness of drug absorption is sometimes called the "fractional absorption" (*f*) and describes the fraction of the administered dose that actually reaches the systemic circulation. To determine the bioavailability of an oral dose, comparisons are made between the area under the plasma concentration versus time curve (*AUC*) determined following both an oral and intravenous administration of the drug and corrected for the dose administered by each route.

$$f = \frac{AUC_{oral} \times Dose_{IV}}{AUC_{IV} \times Dose_{oral}}$$

Distribution

Distribution refers to the transfer of a drug to body tissues. The process is dependent upon: (1) perfusion (the delivery of a drug to the tissues), (2) diffusion (the ability of a drug to pass through membranes), and (3) tissue and protein binding.

The concept of apparent volume of distribution (V_d) reflects the extent of drug distribution. The simplest formula describing the volume of distribution is that written for the intravenous injection of a drug that instantaneously distributes throughout the body and therefore does not exhibit an appreciable distribution phase:

$$V_d = \frac{D}{C_o}$$

where D = dose of injected drug and C_o = plasma concentration immediately after injection. C_o is the y axis intercept when plasma concentration is plotted versus time.

The volume of distribution does not correspond to an actual physical space. It reflects the behavior of the drug in the body, how it distributes, and how much binding to tissues and plasma proteins occurs. To illustrate the influence of tissue binding on V_d, consider the following example. If 100 units of a drug are added to 1 liter of fluid that contains tissue which binds 99 of the units, only 1 unit of drug remains to distribute in the 1000 ml (a concentration of 1 unit/ liter). Remembering the formula $V_d = \dfrac{D}{C_o}$ then

V_d = 100 units/1 unit/1 liter

V_d = 100 liters (which is larger than the actual volume of fluid).

Because the vast majority of drugs do exhibit appreciable distribution phases, the simple equation above does not properly reflect the volume of distribution. The actual measurement of V_d after an intravenous bolus dose of a drug that exhibits a distribution phase is based on the plasma concentration versus time curve (Fig. 1.16). Figure 1.16 represents a plasma concentration curve, using a semi-logarithmic concentration axis, following intravenous injection of a drug. C_o is the peak concentration in plasma reached just at the end of the injection (point I). B is the zero-time intercept of the terminal elimination phase of the plasma concentration curve when extrapolated back to time 0. Point II represents the distribution phase while point III marks the termination of the distribution phase. The distributional phase corresponds to an early rapid decline in plasma concentration. This decline does not reflect drug loss from the body, but movement of the drug within body tissues. Point IV indicates the elimination phase where drug disappearance is determined mainly by elimination rather than distribution, although distribution to and from the central compartment obviously continues to take place. By extrapolating the straight line of the elimination phase back to time 0 (B), V_d can be approximated by the following equation:

$$V_d = \frac{D}{B}$$

This approximation makes intuitive sense, because it uses an estimate of what the concentration would have been at time 0 if the time necessary for distribution were ignored.

The volume of distribution is often determined by the following equation:

$$V_d = \frac{\text{Clearance}}{\beta}$$

where β represents the slope of the terminal (elimination) phase. This leads us to a discussion of the pharmacokinetics of elimination and clearance.

Elimination

The elimination phase can be described by the elimination half-life. Elimination half-life (or $t_{1/2\beta}$) refers to the time required for the

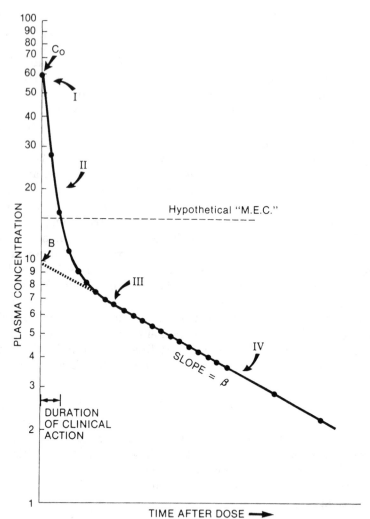

Figure 1.16. Schematic plasma concentration curve, using a semilogarithmic concentration axis, following rapid intravenous injection of a hypothetical drug. C_0 is the peak concentration in plasma (or in the "central compartment") reached just at the end of the injection. B is the zero-time intercept of the elimination phase of the plasma concentration curve when extrapolated back to time 0. *I, II, III,* and *IV* represent the four stages of the plasma concentration curve, as explained in the text. Note that the initial precipitous decline in plasma concentration between *points I and III*—attributable mainly to drug distribution—may be sufficient to terminate clinical activity if the plasma level falls below some minimum effective concentration (*M.E.C.*). (From Greenblatt DJ, Shader RI 1985.)

plasma concentration of the drug to be reduced by one-half. The concept of half-life has meaning only for drugs that are eliminated by first-order kinetics (which means the rate of elimination is proportional to the amount of drug in the body). This concept has important clinical implications in that steady-state is reached in 4 to 5 half-lives and almost all drug (97%) is out of the body in a time equal to 5 half-lives after the drug is stopped. A drug's half-life of elimination is calculated from the following relationship:

$$t_{1/2\beta} = \frac{0.693}{\beta}$$

where β represents the slope of the concentration curve during the elimination phase. Hence, for alprazolam, with an average $\beta = 0.07$ hours $^{-1}$, the terminal elimination half-life is 10 hours.

Elimination processes, similar to absorptive processes, can be described as zero-order (a constant amount eliminated independent of plasma concentration) or, more commonly, first order (the fractional rate of elimination being constant).

The most useful pharmacokinetic parameter for the evaluation of drug elimination is clearance, which relates the concentration of the drug to the rate of drug elimination. It can be related to the organ of elimination, so that one may speak of hepatic clearance, renal clearance, or total clearance (the sum of the individual organ clearances).

The overall efficiency of drug removal from the body can be characterized by clearance. Clearance is expressed in the dimensions of volume per unit time, representing the volume of blood or plasma that is cleared of drug in a given time period. High values of clearance indicate efficient and generally rapid drug removal, whereas low clearance values indicate slow and less efficient drug removal.

Clearance can be related to a variety of other parameters and the formulae for calculating it follow:

$$clearance = \beta \times V_d$$
$$clearance = \frac{Dose}{AUC}$$

APPLICATION OF PHARMACOKINETICS TO CLINICAL PSYCHIATRY

The impact of pharmacokinetics in psychiatry has primarily been in the clinical use of plasma (or serum) levels of psychotropic drugs.

Table 1.5.
Factors Known to Influence the Pharmacokinetics of Psychotropic Agents[a]

Patient Characteristics	Disease States
Age	Liver disease (cirrhosis, hepatitis)
Gender	Renal disease
Total body weight	Congestive heart failure
Body habitus	Infection
Smoking habits	Fever
Alcohol consumption	Shock
Other coingested drugs	Severe burns

[a]Modified from Greenblatt DJ, Shader RI, 1985.

The usefulness of plasma drug concentrations depends on proper sample collection and storage, valid and reproducible analytic methods, rapid analysis (so that the levels may be used to aid in clinical decision-making), and the existence of established guidelines for subtherapeutic, therapeutic, and toxic drug levels. Additionally, there must be an appreciation for the many patient variables that can alter the pharmacokinetics of psychotropic agents (Table 1.5).

At the present time, only assays for lithium and anticonvulsants meet these criteria, although therapeutic levels for the use of anticonvulsants in mood disorders is not established. There are also a number of studies identifying therapeutic levels of tricyclic antidepressants and alprazolam.

The following guidelines for plasma level monitoring of psychotropic drugs have been suggested (Shader and Greenblatt 1979):

1. For drugs with a narrow therapeutic range such that toxic concentrations are only slightly greater than therapeutic levels (e.g. lithium).
2. For drugs with a "therapeutic window" such that high and low levels are ineffective. An example is nortriptyline, where levels below 49 ng/ml or above 150 ng/ml are associated with a poor response.
3. When drug toxicity may be confused with the disease being treated. This may occur during the course of antidepressant therapy, for example. Often, dry mouth, constipation, and lethargy can be symptoms of depression as well as adverse effects of tricyclic antidepressants.
4. For drugs such as barbiturates that induce their own metabolism resulting in declining plasma levels with prolonged treatment.
5. For drugs with unpredictable bioavailability due either to

absorption from oral or intramuscular studies or marked first-pass metabolism. Diazepam, chlordiazepoxide, and phenytoin are all poorly absorbed after intramuscular injection. Tricyclic antidepressants are subjected to extensive and variable first pass metabolism by the liver.

6. For drugs whose activity is dependent upon parent compound and metabolites (e.g. several antidepressants, neuroleptics, and antianxiety agents).

7. For maintenance treatment when a minimum effective level is required for prophylaxis (e.g. lithium).

8. To evaluate drug interactions. Drug levels, rates of absorption and elimination, or protein binding may be affected by concomitant administration of other drugs. For drugs with a narrow therapeutic index or a therapeutic window, monitoring of levels may be helpful.

9. In instances where altered absorption is suspected (e.g. as a result of genetic factors, surgery, disease, etc.).

10. For treatment of special populations or high-risk patients. For example, cigarette smokers or recently detoxified alcoholics are known to be rapid metabolizers and achieve lower levels of imipramine and its active metabolites than control populations. Elderly patients may have higher plasma levels of tricyclic antidepressants than young patients given equivalent doses.

11. Evaluation of compliance.

12. Assessment of nonresponsive patients. (Do they have adequate plasma levels?)

13. For emergency management of drug overdose.

14. Prediction of dose needed to achieve a therapeutic level at steady state. Following a single 600-mg dose of lithium, a 24-hour serum lithium level can be used to determine the dosage that will be required to achieve a steady-state serum level between 0.6 and 1.2 mEq/liter. Similar nomograms are available for some tricyclic antidepressants, although therapeutic levels for these drugs are less well established.

REFERENCES

Arendt RM et al.: In vitro correlates of benzodiazepine cerebrospinal fluid uptake, pharmacodynamic action, and peripheral distribution. J Pharmacol Exp Ther 227: 95, 1983.

Benet L, Sheiner LB: Design and optimization of dosage regimens: pharmacokinetic data. In: Gilman AG, Goodman LS, Rall TW, Murad F (eds.): *The Pharmacological Basis of Therapeutics*, New York, Macmillan, 1985, pp. 1663–1733.

Bergstrom RF et al.: Quantification and mechanism of the fluoxetine and tricyclic antidepressant interaction. Clin Pharmacol Ther 51: 239–248, 1992.

Bochner F et al.: *Handbook of Clinical Pharmacology*, 2nd ed., Boston, Little, Brown, 1983.

Borga O et al.: Plasma protein binding of tricyclic antidepressants in man. Biochem Pharmacol 18: 2135, 1969.

Brosen K: Recent developments in hepatic drug oxidation: implications for clinical pharmacokinetics. Clin Pharmacokinet 18: 220–239, 1990.

Brosen K et al.: Inhibition by paroxetine of desipramine metabolism in extensive but not in poor metabolizers of sparteine. Eur J Clin Pharmacol 44: 349–355, 1993.

Cholerton S et al.: The role of individual human cytochromes P450 in drug metabolism and clinical response. Trends Pharmacol Sci 13: 434–439, 1992.

Ciraulo DJ, Shader RI: Fluoxetine drug-drug interactions. J Clin Psychopharmacol 10: 48–50, 123–117, 1990.

Greenblatt DJ, Shader RI: *Pharmacokinetics in Clinical Practice*. Philadelphia, WB Saunders, 1985.

Greenblatt DJ et al.: Absorption rate, blood concentration, and early response to oral chlordiazepoxide. Am J Psychiatry 134: 559–562, 1977.

Hunter KR et al.: Use of levodopa with other drugs. Lancet 2: 1283, 1970.

Klotz V et al.: The effects of age and liver disease on the disposition and elimination of diazepam in adult man. J Clin Invest 55: 347, 1975.

MacLeod SM et al.: Interaction of disulfiram with benzodiazepines. Clin Pharmacol Ther 24: 583, 1978.

Murray M: P450 enzymes: inhibition mechanisms, genetic regulation and effects of liver disease. Clin Pharmacokinet 23: 132–146, 1992.

Nelson DR et al: The P450 superfamily: update on new sequences, gene mapping, accession numbers, early trivial names of enzymes, and nomenclature. DNA Cell Biol 121: 1–51, 1993.

Otten SV et al.: Inhibition by fluoxetine of cytochrome P450-2D6 activity. Clin Pharmacol Ther 53: 401–509, 1993.

Rowland M, Tozer TN: *Clinical Pharmacokinetics*, Philadelphia, Lea & Febiger, 1980.

Sellers EM, Koch-Weser J: Potentiation of warfarin-induced hypoprothrombinemia by chloral hydrate. New Engl J Med 283: 827, 1970.

Sellers EM et al.: Differential effects of benzodiazepine disposition by disulfiram and ethanol. Arzneimittelforschung 37: 2, 1980.

Shader RI, Greenblatt DJ: Clinical indications for plasma level monitoring of psychotropic drug. Am J Psychiatry 136: 1590–1591, 1979.

Wagner JG: *Fundamentals of Clinical Pharmacokinetics*, Hamilton, IL, Drug Intelligence Publications, 1975.

2

Antidepressants

Overview

With the introduction of several new antidepressants over the past decade, no classification system has proven satisfactory. Formerly classified into two groups, tricyclic antidepressants and monoamine oxidase inhibitors, the advent of new drugs challenged our system of categorization. Terminology became strained and awkward—as these agents were referred to as tetracyclics, heterocyclics, and atypical antidepressants.

For the purposes of discussing drug-drug interactions we have divided the antidepressants into three categories: (1) cyclic antidepressants (which include tricyclic, heterocyclic, and atypical agents); (2) selective serotonin reuptake inhibitors (SSRIs); and (3) monoamine oxidase inhibitors (MAOIs). This grouping does not necessarily imply distinct pharmacologic boundaries or mechanisms of antidepressant action, but rather it suggests that members of each group share similar characteristics that predispose to common mechanisms of drug-drug interactions.

SECTION 2.1 CYCLIC ANTIDEPRESSANTS

DOMENIC A. CIRAULO, WAYNE L. CREELMAN, RICHARD I. SHADER, RICHARD L. O'SULLIVAN

ACETAZOLAMIDE (DIAMOX®)

Evidence of Interaction

Acetazolamide is a carbonic anhydrase inhibitor useful in the treatment of glaucoma, seizure disorders, and abnormal fluid retention (such as that seen with cardiac edema). It alkalizes urinary pH, thus potentially increasing the amount of an antidepressant that is un-ionized, which promotes reabsorption of the drug by the kidney and increases serum levels.

Mechanism
Pharmacokinetic alteration of renal reabsorption.

Clinical Implications
Described in detail in Chapter 1, this type of interaction is important only when drugs are eliminated primarily through the kidney. Antidepressants are primarily eliminated by hepatic metabolism; thus it is unlikely that this interaction is of clinical importance (Gram et al. 1971, Sjoqvist 1969).

AMANTADINE

Evidence of Interaction
After a cumulative dose of 450 mg bupropion over 72 hours, a 75-year-old man taking amantadine 300 mg daily for Parkinson's disease, haloperidol 2 mg daily, and benztropine 2 mg daily, became agitated and delirious, with visual and auditory hallucinations (Liberzon et al. 1990). After discontinuation of the bupropion, his symptoms cleared in 4 days.

Mechanism
An interaction has not been established.

Clinical Implications
This single case report does not establish an interaction between amantadine and bupropion, since the symptoms may have been produced by bupropion alone.

AMMONIUM CHLORIDE

Summary
Ammonium chloride acidifies the urine and could potentially reduce serum concentrations of antidepressants (Gram et al. 1971, Sjoqvist 1969). Since hepatic metabolism is responsible for elimination of cyclic antidepressants, this is not a clinically relevant effect.

ANALGESICS, OPIOID (*See also* METHADONE, *this chapter*)

Evidence of Interaction

Clomipramine, pargyline, and nialamide potentiate the analgesic effect of morphine and pentazocine in rodents (Lee et al. 1980). Morphine analgesia in rats was potentiated by amitriptyline, desipramine, and sertraline (Taiwo et al. 1985). This effect was blocked by prior administration of parachlorophenylalanine, which reduces brain serotonin to about 32% of normal levels (it also may reduce brain norepinephrine and dopamine to about 69% of normal levels (Koe et al. 1966, Miller et al. 1970). The effect of parachlorophenylalanine was not reversed by serotonin, which suggests that other neurotransmitters may also be involved. The morphine-potentiating effects of the antidepressants were blocked by methysergide (a serotonin antagonist), yohimbine, and phentolamine (α-adrenergic antagonists), but not by propranolol (a β-adrenergic antagonist). Another study found that morphine analgesia in rats was potentiated by desipramine or clomipramine, but that by 8–15 days of treatment this effect was no longer present and there was a reduction from baseline morphine analgesic activity (Kellstein et al. 1984). Other studies have also demonstrated that desipramine potentiates morphine analgesia (Ossipov et al. 1982).

Nefazodone alone had an analgesic effect in one animal model of pain, and potentiated the analgesic action of morphine 4-fold without affecting lethality in this mouse model (Pick et al. 1992). Naloxone did not block the analgesic effect of nefazodone alone, suggesting that the analgesic action of nefazodone is not mediated via the opiate system.

Propoxyphene may inhibit the metabolism of doxepin and perhaps other cyclic antidepressants (Abernethy et al. 1982). Elevated serum levels of doxepin developed in an 89-year-old man taking doxepin 150 mg daily after propoxyphene 65 mg every 6 hours was administered. The patient became lethargic and his symptoms did not clear completely until 5 days after propoxyphene was stopped.

Mechanism

Potentiation of the serotonergic system appears to be responsible for enhanced analgesic effects. This is supported by evidence that fluoxetine (a specific serotonin uptake inhibitor) and 5-methoxy-*N,N*-dimethyltryptamine (a specific serotonin agonist) potentiate the action of morphine while serotonergic antagonists or depleting agents antagonize its action. Desipramine inhibits metabolism of methadone and morphine and may increase plasma levels of these opioids (Goldstein et al. 1982, Liu et al. 1975, 1985). Methadone also inhibits the metabolism of desipramine (Maany et al. 1989). Propoxyphene inhibits oxidative metabolism, as evidenced by impaired antipyrine clearance in healthy volunteers who had taken 8 doses of propoxyphene 65 mg every 4 hours (Abernethy et al. 1982).

Clinical Implications

Several anecdotal reports suggest that cyclic antidepressants relieve pain, and they are useful alone in the treatment of headache. Combinations of agents may allow lower doses of opioids to be used, although there is some evidence that tolerance occurs with prolonged treatment. Further clinical studies are required (*see also* section on Selective Serotonin Reuptake Inhibitors).

ANESTHETICS (GENERAL) (*See also* SYMPATHOMIMETICS, *this chapter*)

Evidence of Interaction

After the administration of halothane and pancuronium, tachyarrhythmias developed in two patients without cardiovascular disease who were receiving long-term imipramine treatment (Edwards et al. 1979). This same drug combination in dogs increased the risk of premature ventricular contractions, ventricular tachycardia, ventricular fibrillation, and cardiac arrest.

Mechanism

Both imipramine and pancuronium have anticholinergic and adrenergic actions. When combined with halothane, which is known to predispose the myocardium to arrhythmias following administration of atropine or epinephrine, the likelihood of cardiac arrhythmias increases.

Clinical Implications

All strongly anticholinergic antidepressants (all tricyclic antidepressants and maprotiline) should be avoided when a patient receives the combination of halothane and pancuronium (or gallamine). It may be safer to use a muscle-blocking agent without vagolytic and sympathomimetic effects (e.g. *d*-tubocurarine). Enflurane may be a safer general anesthetic agent for patients receiving anticholinergic antidepressants.

ANTICHOLINERGIC AGENTS

Evidence of Interaction

Tricyclic antidepressants and maprotiline have significant anticholinergic effects. When given with antiparkinsonian agents (benztropine, trihexyphenidyl, etc.), significant additive atropinic effects may occur in some antipsychotics (especially thioridazine, chlorpromazine), antihistamines, glutethimide, meperidine, and others. Central nervous system symptoms of the anticholinergic syndrome include anxiety, agitation, disorientation, dysarthria, impairment of memory, hallucinations, myoclonus, and seizures. Systemic signs include tachycardia, arrhythmias, mydriasis, elevated body temperature, hot dry flushed skin, decreased bowel motility, and urinary retention.

Mechanism

Receptor site interaction.

Clinical Implications

Anticholinergic toxicity is an important syndrome, especially in geriatric patients. Cyclic antidepressants with strong anticholinergic effects include all tricyclics (amitriptyline, clomipramine, imipramine, protriptyline, trimipramine, nortriptyline, doxepin, desipramine). Antidepressants with little or no anticholinergic effects include selective serotonin reuptake inhibitors, trazodone, nefazodone, bupropion, and venlafaxine (Richelson et al. 1984). Treatment for the anticholinergic syndrome includes discontinuation of offending agents and slow intravenous or intramuscular administration of 1 to 2 mg of physostigmine, repeated as needed every 15 to 30 minutes. Peripheral anticholinergic symptoms can be treated with neostigmine but this agent does not cross the blood-brain barrier.

ANTICOAGULANTS

Evidence of Interaction

A single case report describes a 40-year-old woman whose hypoprothrombinemic response to warfarin was reduced when trazodone was administered (Hardy et al. 1986). While receiving warfarin after mitral valve replacement, trazodone 300 mg/day was administered to treat depression. A 30% reduction in prothrombin times was observed after 5 weeks of trazodone therapy, which returned to pretreatment levels when the antidepressant was discontinued.

In a controlled study by Vesell (1970), a single dose of dicumarol 4 mg/kg orally was given prior to administration of nortriptyline 4 mg/kg orally. Following 8 days of nortriptyline administration, serum half-life of dicumarol was significantly longer (105.7 ± 54.2 hours) than pretreatment half-life (35.3 ± 5.3 hours).

In a placebo-controlled study, Pond et al. (1975) found that warfarin elimination was not affected by concurrent nortriptyline or amitriptyline administration. The half-life of warfarin 25 mg taken with a single dose of synthetic vitamin K 10 mg was measured prior to initiation of nortriptyline 40 mg/day orally/divided dose or amitriptyline 75 mg/day orally/divided dose and during the last 4 days of the 13-day course of nortriptyline or amitriptyline. There was no consistent effect on warfarin elimination. A similar protocol was followed with dicumarol, 200 mg and 300 mg doses. There were inconsistent effects on dicumarol metabolism, with a suggestion that dicumarol absorption was increased in the presence of these highly anticholinergic antidepressants. An increase in elimination half-life of dicumarol was found in only 2 of 12 subjects.

In one report, it was suggested that concurrent treatment with amitriptyline contributed to hemorrhagic reactions in patients taking warfarin, although a causal relationship was not established (Koch-Weser 1973).

Mechanism

There is no consistent evidence supporting an interaction between warfarin or dicumarol and amitriptyline or nortriptyline. Some evidence suggests that nortriptyline may prolong dicumarol half-life, although a carefully controlled study found no interaction (Pond et al. 1975). These tricyclic antidepressants may increase dicumarol bioavailability by decreasing intestinal (gut) motility, thereby increasing absorption (Pond et al. 1975). Further complicating the matter is an animal study indicating that amitriptyline- and nortriptyline-impaired warfarin metabolism in the rat (Loomis et al. 1980). Antidepressant-induced displacement from protein binding sites and increases in unbound warfarin are possible when highly bound drugs are added to the anticoagulant.

Clinical Implications

Data on this interaction are limited. Due to genetic factors, dose, and route of administration, warfarin kinetics are complex and variable. If an interaction does occur it is probably uncommon. Patients receiving this combination should be monitored for increases in pro-thrombin time, which would indicate that a reduction in the warfarin dose is necessary. Anticoagulant response to warfarin, dicumarol, and related anticoagulants should be monitored closely when trazodone, nortriptyline, or other antidepressants (e.g. *see* section on Selective Serotonin Reuptake Inhibitors) are started or discontinued.

ANTICONVULSANTS (*See also* CHAPTER 6)

Phenytoin

There is contradictory evidence concerning the possibility of interaction between tricyclic antidepressants and phenytoin. In one study 3 subjects were given amitriptyline 25 mg twice daily with and without phenytoin (Pond et al. 1975). Phenytoin elimination half-lives were not different during concurrent treatment. Another report, however, suggested that phenytoin levels increased in 2 patients after imipramine was discontinued (Perucca et al. 1977). These patients had been receiving imipramine 75 mg daily over a 3-month period with increasing serum levels of phenytoin (1 patient increased from 30 to 60 mmol/liter, 7.6 to 15.1 mg/L). When imipramine was discontinued, levels fell. This case was complicated by coadministration of nitrazepam and clonazepam in one patient, and sodium valproate and carbamazepine in the other. Another study showed that nortriptyline 75 mg daily produced a small increase in phenytoin levels (Houghton et al. 1975). A case report described elevation of phenytoin levels from therapeutic levels (10–20 µg/ml) to 46 µg/ml after 4 months of trazodone 500 mg/day. The patient complained of dizziness and weakness, which abated when trazodone was reduced to 400 mg/day and phenytoin to from 300 mg to 200 mg/day (Dorn 1986).

Valproate

Conflicting data exist on the possible interaction of cyclic antidepressants and valproate. One study reported a rise in desipramine serum concentrations from 246 ng/ml to 324 ng/ml after valproate therapy was discontinued (Joseph et al. 1993). On the other hand, another report described increased levels of amitriptyline and nortriptyline when amitriptyline was prescribed with valproic acid (Vandel et al. 1988). Other studies have also reported increases in amitriptyline/nortriptyline levels in the presence of valproate (Bertschy et al. 1990).

Carbamazepine

In a study 36 children with attention deficit disorder were treated either with imipramine alone or imipramine with carbamazepine (Brown et al. 1992). Despite receiving higher doses of desipramine, children in the combined treatment group had lower serum antidepressant levels, suggesting that carbamazepine induced drug metabolism. Carbamazepine cotreatment also lowered levels of desipramine in another study (Baldessarini et al. 1988). In a 10-year study of almost 3,000 patients, comparisons were made between the concentration-to-dose ratio of patients taking only an antidepressant and those taking an antidepressant plus carbamazepine (Jerling et al. 1994). The mean ratio of amitriptyline and nortriptyline was 50% lower in patients taking both carbamazepine and an antidepressant compared with those taking the antidepressant alone, suggesting significant enzyme induction by carbamazepine.

Mechanism

The mechanism of interaction with phenytoin is unknown. Valproate may impair metabolism of some cyclic antidepressants, but additional data are needed. Carbamazepine is a well-known enzyme inducer and lowers serum levels of many drugs that undergo oxidative hepatic metabolism.

Clinical Implications

The interaction with phenytoin is not well established, but clinicians should be aware that there is the possibility that phenytoin levels may increase with antidepressant coadministration. More frequent monitoring of phenytoin levels may be necessary. Frequent monitoring of antidepressant levels during concurrent therapy with valproate or carbamazepine is warranted.

ANTIHYPERTENSIVES (*See also* RESERPINE, *this section*)

Evidence of Interaction

The interaction between the tricyclic antidepressants and guanethidine is well established. Imipramine 75 mg/day antagonized the antihypertensive effects of guanethidine in 3 hypertensive patients (Leishman et al. 1963). In that study a clinically effective dose of guanethidine (or bethanidine, debrisoquin, or methyldopa) was determined clinically and given throughout the study period. After 5 days of antihypertensive treatment, desipramine (70 mg [*N*

= 9], 125 mg [N = 1], 50 mg [N = 3], 150 mg [N = 1]), or protriptyline (20 mg daily [N = 1]) was added to the treatment regimen. Altogether, there were 7 patients taking guanethidine, 3 taking bethanidine, 2 taking debrisoquin, and 3 taking methyldopa (2 patients were studied twice). Desipramine and protriptyline reversed the antihypertensive effects of guanethidine in every patient. The reversal of the effect of guanethidine required 1 to 2 days for maximum antagonism, whereas reversal of bethanidine or debrisoquin occurred within a few hours. No patients had a rise in pressure greater than their prestudy level. After discontinuation of the antidepressant, 5 to 7 days were required for the antihypertensive action to reappear (for the 2 patients receiving 125 and 150 mg, 10 days were necessary for return of effect). The action of methyldopa was not antagonized by desipramine (see below).

Probably all cyclic antidepressants that inhibit the reuptake of norepinephrine block the antihypertensive effect of guanethidine. Amitriptyline 75 mg/day was administered to a patient receiving guanethidine 75 mg/day, methyldopa 750 mg/day, and trichlormethiazide 8 mg/day. Five days after the initiation of amitriptyline treatment, a reversal of antihypertensive effect was seen, requiring an increase in the guanethidine dose (to 300 mg/day). Amitriptyline was discontinued and 18 days were required to overcome the antagonism (Meyer et al. 1970). Differences between onset of, and recovery from, antagonism between amitriptyline and desipramine may be related to the relative abilities of the drugs and their metabolites to influence noradrenergic function. Desipramine is highly noradrenergic while amitriptyline is less so (its demethylated metabolite, nortriptyline, has substantial noradrenergic effects).

Studies that have not found an antidepressant-induced reversal of the antihypertensive effects of guanethidine, are misleading because they observed patients for too short a period (8 and 12 hours), whereas the antagonism develops after 1 or 2 days (Gulati et al. 1966, Ober et al. 1973).

A single case report described cardiac standstill in a 37-year-old man taking both guanethidine 125 mg/day (after failure to control hypertension with methyldopa and intramuscular hydralazine) and imipramine 75 mg daily in divided doses. It is not possible to definitively attribute these cardiac complications to a drug-drug interaction.

Other antihypertensives have also been investigated with respect to a possible interaction with antidepressants. Although animal data suggest that the hypotensive effect of methyldopa may be antagonized by antidepressants, human studies do not support an interaction. After intravertebral artery infusion of tricyclic antidepressants to anesthetized cats, methyldopa 20 mg/kg was administered via the same route. The usual hypotensive effect of methyldopa was blocked by both imipramine and desipramine 300 μg/kg (Van Zwieten 1975). Similar findings have been reported after intraventricular injection in rats (Finch 1975). Studies of humans, on the other hand, have not confirmed the animal findings. Five male volunteers (one "mildly hypertensive") were given either desipramine 25 mg 3 times daily or placebo in a double-blind crossover design 2 weeks apart. After 4 days of antidepressant or placebo, methyldopa 750 mg was administered. Desipramine did not reduce the hypotensive effect. This study confirmed the findings of Mitchell and associates (1970), who found no interaction in 3 patients receiving that combination.

The hypotensive effect of clonidine may be antagonized during concurrent antidepressant therapy. Briant and colleagues (1973) studied 5 hypertensive patients maintained on clonidine plus a diuretic for 2 to 3 years. Desipramine 75 mg/day or placebo was added to the drug regimen and the antidepressant caused a rise in blood pressure in 4 of 5 patients, averaging 22/15 mm Hg supine, 12/11 mm Hg standing. In 1 patient the blood pressure increased within 24 hours of taking the active drug. Another report described a woman whose blood pressure was controlled with clonidine 0.4 mg daily until she was given 50 mg per day of imipramine for 2 days, after which her blood pressure rose to 230/130 mm Hg (Hui 1983). Trazodone also antagonized clonidine (Hansten 1984).

Animal data support these findings. Van Zwieten (1975) found that the hypotensive effect of intravenously administered clonidine 1 μg/kg was antagonized in anesthetized cats pretreated with desipramine, imipramine, amitriptyline, protriptyline, and mianserin. Another study found that single doses of desipramine and amitriptyline attenuated clonidine-induced electroencephalogram synchronization in rats while mianserin potentiated it (Kostowski et al. 1984). Chronic antidepressant administration (14 days) either completely (desipramine, amitriptyline) or partially (mianserin) reduced the effect of clonidine. Other evidence suggested that mianserin did not reverse the antihypertensive effects of clonidine or methyldopa (Elliot et al. 1981, 1983). Although maprotiline reversed the antihypertensive effect of bethanidine, guanethidine, and debrisoquin, it did not alter the antihypertensive response to clonidine (Gundert-Remy 1983).

Lower doses of cyclic antidepressants may be required when diltiazem or verapamil are prescribed concurrently. Twelve healthy male volunteers received a 7-day course of verapamil 120 mg every 8 hours, diltiazem 90 mg every 8 hours, labetalol 200 mg every 12 hours, or placebo (Hermann et al. 1992). On the 4th day of the study period, imipramine (a single 100-mg oral dose) was administered. Verapamil, diltiazem, and labetalol increased the imipramine plasma versus time area-under-the-curve by 15%, 30%, and 53%, respectively. No consistent changes were found in the levels of the primary metabolites—desipramine, 2-hydroxyimipramine, or 2-hydroxydesipramine. Nifedipine has been implicated in the reversal of antidepressant response (Fadden 1992, Hullet et al. 1988), but the effect of nifedipine in animal models of depression is not entirely consistent with the case reports (Kostowski et al. 1990).

Mechanism

1. Guanethidine and related antihypertensives (bethanidine, debrisoquin) are taken up into noradrenergic neurons by the same pump that is responsible for the reuptake of norepinephrine. Tricyclic antidepressants block this pump, preventing guanethidine from reaching its site of action.
2. Clonidine is known to activate the presynaptic α-adrenoreceptors, which provide a negative feedback system in the peripheral and central nervous system. *In vitro* preparations of rat cerebral cortex slices were used to demonstrate that desipramine antagonized the inhibitory effect of clonidine on central adrenergic neurotransmission, perhaps by altering the sensitivity of the presynaptic receptor (Dubocovich et al. 1979). One study found no interaction between nortriptyline, imipramine, and desmethyldoxepin on platelet α_2-adrenoreceptors (Barnes et al. 1982).
3. Verapamil and diltiazem inhibit metabolism of drugs oxidized by the cytochrome P450-3A4 isoenzyme.

Clinical Implications

Guanethidine (and the related antihypertensives bethanidine, debrisoquin) should not be used with antidepressants that block the neuronal noradrenergic reuptake pump. Doses of doxepin less than 100 mg probably do not antagonize the hypotensive effect, but this may not produce an adequate antidepressant effect. Clonidine (and the related antihypertensives guanabenz and guanfacine) should also be avoided. The withdrawal syndrome associated with clonidine, characterized by rebound hypertension and tachycardia, may be exacerbated by amitriptyline and possibly other antidepressants (Stiff et al. 1983).

Methyldopa and thiazide diuretics are safe to use, but caution must be observed to avoid hypotension, especially in the elderly. Potassium must be monitored when the thiazides are used, since hypokalemia may increase cardiac irritability and the chance of arrhythmia. Some evidence suggests that mianserin does not reverse the antihypertensive effects of clonidine or methyldopa (Elliot et al. 1981, 1983). Although maprotiline reverses the antihypertensive effect of bethanidine, guanethidine, and debrisoquin, it does not alter the antihypertensive response to clonidine (Gundert-Remy 1983).

Verapamil and diltiazem may impair metabolism of imipramine and other psychotropic medications metabolized by the cytochrome P450-3A4 isoenzyme. Dosage reductions of the antidepressant may be required. (See also Reserpine, this section, and Antihypertensives, under section on Selective Serotonin Reuptake Inhibitors, and section on Monoamine Oxidase Inhibitors).

ANTIPSYCHOTICS (See CHAPTER 3)

ANTIMICROBIALS

Evidence of Interaction

A patient treated with a combination of rifampin, isoniazid, pyrazinamide, and pyridoxine was given nortriptyline 175 mg daily, to achieve antidepressant serum levels of 193 mmol/liter (Bebchuck et al. 1991). Following discontinuation of rifampin and isoniazid, nortriptyline serum levels rose to 671 mmol/liter, accompanied by adverse effects. Reduction of nortriptyline to 75 mg daily resulted in a return to therapeutic levels of the antidepressant.

In another case report (Gannon et al. 1992), a 65-year-old woman was taking nortriptyline 75 mg daily for 1 year prior to taking fluconazole (Diflucan®). Twelve days after the addition of the antifungal agent, the serum nortriptyline level rose to 252 ng/ml from a baseline of 149 ng/ml.

Mechanism

Rifampin is a potent inducer of oxidative metabolism, whereas fluconazole and related antifungals (ketoconazole, itraconazole) inhibit the metabolism of some drugs (especially those metabolized by cytochrome P450-3A4).

Clinical Implications

When rifampin is discontinued after concurrent therapy with nortriptyline or related antidepressants, the dosage of the antidepressant must be lowered. When fluconazole, ketoconazole, or itraconazole are prescribed concurrently with antidepressants, serum levels of the antidepressant should be monitored and clinicians should observe patients for signs and symptoms of toxicity.

BARBITURATES

Evidence of Interaction

Several reports suggest that barbiturates decrease plasma levels of antidepressants. One patient who had been receiving 100 mg of phenobarbital for 14 days had a 50% decrease in desipramine levels (Hammer et al. 1967). In a study of nortriptyline pharmacokinetics in identical twins, concurrent barbiturate treatment resulted in a 30% reduction in nortriptyline levels (Alexanderson et al. 1969). That study also found lower steady-state nortriptyline plasma levels in subjects treated with antidepressant plus barbiturate than with antidepressant alone. In another single case, amobarbital 200 mg at bedtime for 5 days reduced nortriptyline plasma levels (Burrows et al. 1971). In a report of 3 patients taking nortriptyline who had amobarbital added, statistically significant decreases in serum nortriptyline levels were seen only after 10 days of concurrent drug therapy (Silverman 1972). Protriptyline levels may also be decreased with coadministration of barbiturates (Moody et al. 1977).

Mechanism

Barbiturates induce hepatic enzymes and enhance antidepressant metabolism.

Clinical Implications

The role of barbiturates in clinical psychopharmacology is limited. Given their high abuse potential, lethality in overdoses, and enzyme induction, they are of limited usefulness in depressed patients. Benzodiazepine anxiolytics and hypnotics are safer and easier to use. Should barbiturates be used, however, plasma levels of antidepressants should be monitored.

CHOLESTYRAMINE

Summary

An *in vitro* study found that cholestyramine (Questran®) bound amitriptyline, desipramine, doxepin, imipramine, and nortriptyline (Bailey et al. 1992). Patients should take their antidepressant dose 2 hours before or 4 hours after cholestyramine.

DIGOXIN

Evidence of Interaction

There are two reports of digoxin toxicity occurring after the addition of trazodone (Dec et al. 1984, Rauch et al. 1984). In one patient the serum digoxin concentration rose from 0.8 to 2.8 ng/ml after 11 days of trazodone therapy. In a canine model, however, no elevation of serum digoxin level was found during combined digoxin/trazodone therapy.

Mechanism

Not established.

Clinical Implications

There is insufficient evidence to establish this as an important interaction. Clinicians may wish to closely monitor digoxin levels if trazodone is administered concurrently.

DISULFIRAM (*See* CHAPTER 8)

ESTROGENS

Evidence of Interaction

Some studies suggest that an interaction occurs between estradiol or conjugated estrogens and imipramine.

In one study, 30 women with a diagnosis of primary depression were given either placebo, imipramine plus placebo, or ethinyl estradiol in doses either 25 or 50 μg/day orally (Khurana 1972). Side effects occurred more commonly with the imipramine-estradiol combination and included tremor, hypotension, and drowsiness. Serum levels of antidepressants were not measured.

Another study examining oral contraceptives and clomipramine was unable to find evidence of increased toxicity (Beaumont 1973). The lower estrogen doses administered in that study probably account for the absence of untoward effects.

A study of 10 women on long-term, low-dose estrogen oral contraceptive steroids found that after a single oral dose of imipramine 50 mg absolute systemic bioavailability increased, resulting in decreased apparent oral clearance without a change in oral elimination half-life compared with controls (Abernethy et al. 1984a). After intravenous imipramine 12.5 mg, elimination half-life was prolonged in the contraceptive users but clearance and volume of distribution were similar to those of control subjects. These findings suggest that lower doses of imipramine should be used when patients are taking oral contraceptives.

Mechanism

Estrogenic compounds may impair N-oxidation and demethylation of imipramine. Ethinyl estradiol inhibits the metabolism of ethylmorphine and hexobarbital in rats (Tephly et al. 1968). Furthermore, other steroids such as norethindrone (a progestogen) inhibit the metabolism of antipyrine in women (Field et al. 1979) and imipramine in mice (Bellward 1974).

Clinical Implications

There are several clinical situations in which estrogens are used, including oral contraception, menopause, atrophic vaginitis, dysmenorrhea, dysfunctional bleeding (although the cyclic use of progestin is usually preferred), acne, hirsutism, osteoporosis, breast cancer, and suppression of postpartum lactation. Many of these clinical problems are also associated with depression, so that the combination of an estrogen and antidepressant is not uncommon. Although the potential for increased toxicity should be kept in mind, if side effects are carefully monitored and the imipramine dosage increased slowly, this drug combination is safe to use.

ETHANOL (*See also section on* SELECTIVE SEROTONIN REUPTAKE INHIBITORS AND ETHANOL)

Evidence of Interaction

Cyclic antidepressants may interact with alcohol to produce (1) enhanced sedation and impairment of psychomotor skills, (2) enhanced metabolism of the antidepressant, and/or (3) delayed absorption of alcohol from the gut.

Impairment of psychomotor skills has been evaluated with amitriptyline, nortriptyline, doxepin, clomipramine, trazodone, zimelidine, and bupropion. In one study amitriptyline 0.8 mg/kg orally was administered the night before and the morning of alcohol consumption (to produce a blood alcohol level of 80 mg/100 ml), the morning of the test only, or not at all (placebo on the two occasions). Both amitriptyline-treated groups showed impairment of driving skills (Landauer et al. 1969). Another study investigated the effect of 5 days of treatment with amitriptyline (100 mg daily in 2 divided doses) or placebo. Despite the production of blood alcohol levels similar to those in the previous study, no differences in driving performance were found between the amitriptyline and the placebo groups (Patman 1969).

A study of nortriptyline-alcohol interactions showed that nortriptyline (40–100 mg during 24 hours prior to ethanol) tended to improve scores on an audiofeedback test given when the subject had a blood alcohol level of 50 mg/100 ml. The short time period of drug administration limits the clinical significance of this finding (Hughes et al. 1963). Doxepin has been studied in two experiments. In the first, 22 subjects received doxepin (12–25 mg/m^2) plus alcohol to the point of intoxication (producing an average blood alcohol level of 73.6 mg/100 ml). This group had better scores on a driving test than a group of 12 control subjects who received alcohol alone (Milner et al. 1978). The second study compared doxepin to amitriptyline, nortriptyline (all were given 30 and 60 mg/day for 7 days), and clomipramine (30 and 75 mg/day for 7 days each). These agents were probably not equipotent so the comparison once again suffers. Despite this shortcoming, the important observation was made that the impairment effect diminishes with time. Impairment of psychomotor skills was seen after 7 days of treatment with amitriptyline or doxepin (when blood alcohol levels were 0.47%) but not after an additional 7 days (at twice the dose) (Seppala et al. 1975). Dorian and colleagues (1983) found that acute ethanol ingestion decreased apparent oral clearance of amitriptyline, impaired memory, and increased body sway.

Single doses of trazodone 100 mg, amitriptyline 50 mg, or placebo were administered alone or with ethanol 0.5 ml/kg to 6 healthy volunteers in a double-blind crossover study (Warrington et al. 1986). Both trazodone and amitriptyline impaired performance on critical flicker fusion frequency, choice reaction time, and manual dexterity. The antidepressants also increased drowsiness and reduced "clear-headedness," aggression, and inhibition. Ethanol alone, at mean blood concentrations that did not exceed 30 mg/100 ml, had similar pharmacodynamic effects. Ethanol, in combination with either antidepressant, caused a greater impairment in manual dexterity than was seen with the antidepressant alone. Blood alcohol levels were not altered by trazodone or amitriptyline. The time to reach maximum trazodone concentration was prolonged by ethanol coadministration, but all other pharmacokinetic parameters for trazodone and amitriptyline were not significantly affected by ethanol.

In another study, zimelidine 200 mg/24 hours was administered for 10 days to 12 healthy men, and ethanol 0.5 and 1.0 g/kg or placebo drinks were administered with either placebo capsules or zimelidine in the last 3 treatment days (Linnoila et al. 1985). Although the higher dose of ethanol increased plasma zimelidine and norzimelidine concentrations, no significant interactions were noted on a battery of tests measuring skilled performance.

Another study examined the interaction of ethanol with bupropion (Hamilton et al. 1984). In 12 healthy volunteers, bupropion (100 mg) reversed alcoholic-induced sedation, impairment of auditory vigilance, and some of the drug's effects on the electroencephalogram. The subjective sense of inebriation was not reversed by bupropion.

Amitriptyline may enhance alcohol-induced euphoria (Hyatt et al. 1987). Three men with alcohol abuse/dependence used amitriptyline in doses of 200 to 500 mg in combination with ethanol to "stay high cheaply." They reported that when taking amitriptyline they required smaller amounts of ethanol to become intoxicated.

The second type of alcohol antidepressant interaction is enhanced metabolism of the tricyclic antidepressant. In a study of recently detoxified inpatient alcoholics ($N = 11$) and depressed nonalcoholic controls ($N = 12$) treated with imipramine (50 mg three times a day orally), the former group had lower plasma levels of imipramine, and 2-hydroxyimipramine as well as a lower total (imipramine, desipramine, and their two hydroxy metabolites) than did control subjects. Alcoholics were noted to have persistent depressions, whereas the control group had significant improvement in depression (as measured by the Beck Depression Inventory) (Ciraulo et al. 1982). A follow-up study by the same investigators (Ciraulo et al. 1988a) found that alcoholics had a 3-fold greater intrinsic clearance of unbound imipramine than nonalcoholic controls and an approximately 2-fold decrease in elimination half-life. Desipramine clearance was affected to a greater extent than imipramine, although intravenous clearance was significantly greater in alcoholics. 2-Hydroxyimipramine, a metabolite of imipramine, also was cleared more rapidly in alcoholics (Ciraulo et al. 1990a).

In a study of amitriptyline in 10 alcoholic and 11 nonalcoholic depressed patients, alcoholics had lower steady-state nortriptyline levels (a metabolite of amitriptyline, Sandoz et al. 1983). Plasma levels of amitriptyline, hydroxyamitriptyline, and hydroxynortriptyline were not different between groups. These findings are puzzling because most studies indicate that demethylation is induced by chronic ethanol consumption. The large intersubject differences in a small sample may account for a failure to find differences in amitriptyline levels. Furthermore alcoholics received a mean dose 25 mg greater than nonalcoholics.

The final type of interaction is a delay in ethanol absorption when desipramine is given concurrently (Hall et al. 1976).

Mechanism

The mechanisms for the pharmacokinetic (metabolic) interaction are easiest to identify. Chronic administration of ethanol to humans causes proliferation of the smooth endoplasmic reticulum, increases microsomal protein and cytochrome P450, and often results in the augmentation of the drug-metabolizing capability of the liver. Although alcoholics are often cigarette smokers, the antidepressant studies (Ciraulo et al. 1982, 1988a) controlled for this factor.

The delayed absorption of alcohol in the presence of desipramine is most likely due to impaired gastric emptying secondary to the anticholinergic effect of desipramine.

Impairment of psychomotor skills and enhanced high, when certain tricyclic antidepressants and alcohol are given concomitantly, are most likely results of receptor site interactions, although specifics are not known.

Clinical Implications

Studies of psychomotor alterations during combined antidepressant treatment and alcohol consumption present conflicting data, which are difficult to interpret in light of an obvious clinical interaction. It is our impression that most, if not all, tricyclic antidepressants enhance the sedative effects and psychomotor impairment induced by ethanol. Perhaps the less sedating agents (e.g. nortriptyline) interact to a lesser degree. Certainly bupropion and selective serotonin reuptake inhibitors (SSRIs) show little interaction with ethanol.

With tricyclic antidepressants and ethanol, patients often say they feel intoxicated after fewer drinks. We advise patients to reduce or discontinue consumption of alcoholic beverages during antidepressant treatment. For those who continue to drink, tolerance to the interaction often develops.

With regard to the finding of lower plasma levels of imipramine and desipramine in chronic alcoholics as compared with depressed control subjects, higher doses of tricyclic antidepressants may be needed to achieve the therapeutic plasma levels early in abstinence. Depression, anxiety, and phobias are prominent symptoms among alcoholics and may require treatment with antidepressants. Some studies indicate a possible role for desipramine (Mason et al. 1991) and imipramine (Nunes et al. 1993) in depressed alcoholics.

HISTAMINE$_2$-BLOCKING AGENTS

Evidence of Interaction

Several reports have established that cimetidine may impair metabolism of tricyclic antidepressants, leading to elevated plasma levels and toxicity.

Anticholinergic toxicity developed in one patient who was taking cimetidine 1,200 mg/day upon initiation of moderate doses of imipramine 125 mg/day. Steady-state concentrations of imipramine increased from 187 to 341 ng/ml and elimination half-life from 22.8 to 43.7 hours (Miller et al. 1983a). Another patient taking both cimetidine and nortriptyline had an average 42% higher nortriptyline serum concentration on the drug combination (Miller et al. 1983b).

In a study of 6 subjects given imipramine 12.5 mg intravenously or 50 mg orally, alone and with cimetidine, imipramine clearance was reduced 41% while bioavailability was increased (from 40 to 75%) with concurrent cimetidine. Such an interaction could lead to important increases in imipramine plasma levels with chronic treatment (Abernethy et al. 1983).

Another clinical study examined the interaction of cimetidine with either imipramine or nortriptyline (Henauer et al. 1984). Cimetidine decreased clearance of imipramine and increased bioavailability. Cimetidine did not increase the bioavailability of nortriptyline, although peak levels and the area under the plasma level versus time curve was increased for 10-hydroxynortriptyline, its active metabolite.

Cimetidine 600 mg twice daily but not ranitidine 150 mg twice daily increased serum doxepin levels in a study in healthy volunteers (Sutherland et al. 1987). Cimetidine also impaired the metabolism of nefazodone.

Mechanism

Cimetidine impairs hepatic metabolism of antidepressants. Although cimetidine-induced alterations of hepatic blood flow are also a possible mechanism of interaction, this is a less likely explanation.

Clinical Implications

Considerable evidence suggests that some antidepressants such as imipramine have a minimal plasma level required for optimal response and that other antidepressants such as nortriptyline have an optimal therapeutic range ("therapeutic window"). If cimetidine therapy were to be discontinued during chronic imipramine therapy, it is possible that levels of the antidepressant would drop below the minimal therapeutic concentration. On the other hand, if a patient had been stabilized on imipramine, and cimetidine was then added, toxicity could result. Symptoms of tricyclic antidepressant toxicity include tachycardia, large pupils, injected sclera, elevated temperature with dry skin, urinary retention, decreased gut motility, and central nervous system symptoms such as anxiety, agitation, psychosis, disorientation, memory impairment, myoclonus, and seizures. Clinical implications of altered metabolite levels are not known.

The most reasonable clinical course would be to substitute ranitidine, famotidine, or nizatidine for cimetidine. Ranitidine will not impair oxidative metabolism (Abernethy et al. 1984b). Alternatively, plasma levels of antidepressants and their active metabolites should be monitored during concurrent administration of cimetidine and antidepressants.

LEVODOPA

Evidence of Interaction

An absorption interaction between imipramine and levodopa has been reported in both animals and humans. Imipramine-treated rats retained approximately 30% of single dose of 14C-levodopa in their stomachs for 2 hours, compared with retention in rats that had not received imipramine (Morgan et al. 1975).

A similar interaction was found in humans (Morgan et al. 1975). The absorption of a single dose of 14C-levodopa 500 mg was studied in 4 male subjects after 3 days of administration of imipramine 25 mg 4 times a day and placebo. On the morning of sampling, subjects took one 25-mg tablet of imipramine 2 hours prior to receiving radioactively labeled levodopa through a nasogastric tube (which was also used to obtain samples of gastric juice). Polyethylene glycol was also administered as a marker compound to assess the degree of gastric emptying; it demonstrated that gastric emptying was impaired during imipramine treatment. In addition, total gastric juice radioactivity (from labeled levodopa) was 11% of the initial dose at 6 hours during imipramine treatment, while it was less than 0.1% on placebo. Plasma concentrations of radioactivity were significantly lower at 45 and 105 minutes in the levodopa-imipramine group. While this study showed impaired rate of absorption of levodopa, it did not establish a difference in completeness of absorption between groups (24 hours cumulative urinary excretion of radioactivity was not significantly different between groups).

Mechanism

The anticholinergic activity of imipramine impairs gastric motility, thus reducing the rate of absorption of other drugs. There is some evidence that levodopa is metabolized in the stomach and the gastrointestinal tract, and there is the potential for a decrease in absolute amount of drug absorbed whenever transit time is slowed (Rivera-Calimlim et al. 1970).

Clinical Implications

The rate of absorption is not critical for drugs taken on a chronic basis. The combination of these agents may be commonplace in light of the frequent coexistence of depression and parkinsonism (Mindham 1970). There appears to be no evidence that the pharmacokinetic interaction is of clinical significance, and it is likely that effects on both cholinergic and catecholamine systems would be either synergistic or additive in the treatment of parkinsonism.

METHADONE

Evidence of Interaction

There is one study of 5 men in a methadone maintenance program who had higher desipramine serum levels while taking methadone than while taking the antidepressant alone (Maany et al. 1989). The combination of methadone 0.5 mg/kg daily and desipramine 2.5 mg/kg daily increased serum antidepressant levels from 72.6% to 168.9% compared with monotherapy.

Mechanism

Methadone probably impairs hydroxylation of desipramine.

Clinical Implications

Pharmacokinetic interactions of methadone with antidepressants are not well studied, although methadone probably impairs metabolism of several cyclic antidepressants. Clinicians should monitor patients taking methadone and cyclic antidepressants for adverse effects. Serum antidepressant levels may be helpful in guiding dosage in these patients.

METHYLPHENIDATE

Evidence for Interaction

Three clinical studies from the same group of investigators have suggested that methylphenidate increases plasma levels of imipramine and its metabolite desmethylimipramine (Perel et al. 1969, Wharton et al. 1971, Zeidenberg et al. 1971).

In their first report, they indicated that blood levels of parent drug and metabolite increased when methylphenidate was added to imipramine 150 mg every day. A follow-up study examined patients at both 450 mg of imipramine alone daily or 150 mg of imipramine plus 20 mg of methylphenidate. One patient received dextroamphetamine 5 mg twice a day in place of methylphenidate. Blood levels were found to be highly variable from patient to patient, as was the effect of methylphenidate. In 5 patients the ratios of imipramine concentrations at steady-state after 450 mg daily compared with imipramine 150 mg plus methylphenidate were 1.2, 1.2, 4.1, 2.7, and 1.6, indicating that methylphenidate increased plasma levels of imipramine, but the extent of the effect was highly variable.

The third study by the same group of investigators studied 7 patients with "recurrent refractory psychotic depression." Six patients were treated with imipramine in varying doses (from 75 to 225 mg daily) and one with nortriptyline 25 mg three times daily for 3 weeks and then methylphenidate 10 mg twice daily for 10 to 21 days followed by the original dose of tricyclic antidepressant given alone. Of the 7 patients treated with the combination, 5 had "prompt, striking, complete clinical remission." Plasma levels of imipramine and desmethylimipramine rose following addition of methylphenidate. Imipramine binding was not affected.

Mechanism

Methylphenidate inhibits the metabolism of imipramine, leading to elevated plasma levels and increased therapeutic effect. Methylphenidate may possess some antidepressant activity in its own right, which may account for the dramatic improvement in cases of refractory depression.

Clinical Implications

Combined treatment with imipramine and methylphenidate may offer little advantage over merely increasing the imipramine dosage to obtain higher plasma levels. For those patients who require an immediate mood response, some clinicians administer methylphenidate when tricyclic antidepressant therapy is initiated. Due to unpredictable alterations in tricyclic drug plasma levels, we advise against this practice. In some cases of refractory depression, the addition of a stimulant to an antidepressant may be helpful (Feighner et al. 1985). A study in children indicated that the combination of methylphenidate and desipramine led to more complaints of nausea, dry mouth, tremor, and higher ventricular rates as compared to monotherapy (Pataki et al. 1993).

MONOAMINE OXIDASE INHIBITORS (MAOIs)

Evidence of Interaction

Schuckit and associates (1971) reviewed the English language literature and found 25 case reports of morbidity in patients managed on combined therapy. After eliminating those cases in which a suicide attempt was made (6), other centrally acting drugs were taken (8), or the drugs were given parenterally (4), 6 of 7 cases were reviewed in depth (1 was omitted because of inadequate clinical details). The patients were all women between the ages of 37 and 66. All received imipramine; the monoamine oxidase inhibitors (MAOIs) included iproniazid (1 case), tranylcypromine (2 cases), isocarboxazid (2 cases), and pargyline (1 case). In 4 of the 6 cases the MAOI was used first, and in all 6, adverse effects were noted within 36 hours of the patient's beginning the combination. Symptoms included flushing, sweating, dizziness, tremor, fever, restlessness, confusion, hypotension, dyspnea, hallucinations, convulsions, and coma. All 6 patients recovered. It was the conclusion of Schuckit and co-workers that these symptoms could not clearly be attributed to the drug combination rather than to an idiosyncratic drug reaction. They also pointed out that there was a similarity between the reported symptoms and those seen with tricyclic antidepressant overdose alone.

Other clinical data are available from the British literature. In a study of 149 outpatients, ages 19 to 70, receiving various tricyclic antidepressant-MAOI combinations, there were 7 patients in whom uncomfortable side effects developed, but no serious reactions were noted (Gander 1965). Several other British investigators have reported similar findings (Randell 1965, Sargent 1965, 1971). Schuckit and co-workers (1971) reviewed the medical records of 50 patients receiving a tricyclic antidepressant (usually 75–100 mg of imipramine) in combination with an MAOI (an average dose of 30 mg of isocarboxazid "or its equivalent"). In 4 cases, side effects developed that may or may not have been attributed to the combination and that cleared spontaneously despite continued therapy. In a prospective group of 10 patients receiving a combination of amitriptyline 150 mg daily and tranylcypromine 30 to 40 mg daily, no significant side effects were noted.

Later studies appear to confirm the safety of the drug combination. Davidson and colleagues (1982, 1984) studied 19 treatment-resistant depressed patients and randomly assigned them to either electroconvulsive therapy (ECT) or combined amitriptyline (average dose of 71 mg/day) and phenelzine (average dose of 34 mg/day) for 3 to 5 weeks. No serious toxicity was noted in patients on the drug combination, although dosage was limited in 4 patients because of side effects. The issue of efficacy was raised by this study, which found ECT superior to drug treatment.

In a larger outpatient study ($N = 135$), trimipramine alone proved to be more efficacious than combinations of that drug with phenelzine or isocarboxazid or isocarboxazid alone. Side effects were minor, with trimipramine alone causing more tremor, and MAOI either alone or in combination causing more insomnia (Young et al. 1979).

In a study, 30 newly hospitalized patients with research diagnostic criteria of major or minor depressive disorder were randomly assigned to open treatment with amitriptyline alone (average daily dose of 165 mg), tranylcypromine (average daily dose of 30 mg) or the combination (80 and 13 mg, respectively, average daily dose) (White et al. 1980). Using the Hamilton and Zung depression scales, the study found that all 3 groups showed improvement (over 82% of all patients) with no one treatment group showing superior results; it also found no significant differences in side effects among the three groups.

On the other hand, there is one report of 3 deaths in patients receiving the combination of clomipramine and MAOI, reportedly in "therapeutic" doses (although at least 1 patient received clomipramine intravenously) (Beaumont 1973). Another report described fatal disseminated intravascular coagulation in a 34-year-old man when clomipramine (10 mg twice daily) was added to tranylcypromine (Tackley et al. 1987).

Mechanism

The mechanism for the interaction (whether it is sympathetic overstimulation or increased efficacy in depressed patients) appears to be the result of increased availability of norepinephrine, serotonin, and other neurotransmitters. MAOIs prevent intraneuronal degradation of norepinephrine, increasing the amount of neurotransmitter available for release. Tricyclic antidepressants inhibit reuptake of norepinephrine and serotonin into the presynaptic neuron. The combined effects may lead to enhanced clinical effect or toxicity depending upon which drug combinations are used and the route of administration (*see below*).

Clinical Implications

It is apparent from available data that the dangers of combined therapy have been exaggerated. The question of efficacy remains unanswered. There are several uncontrolled trials of the combination in refractory depression. Sethna studied 12 patients who had been refractory to treatment with MAOIs, tricyclic antidepressants, and ECT (9 patients) who were "practically free of depression or anxiety" (Sethna 1974). Winston et al. (1971) and Gander (1965) reported similar findings. These studies may be criticized on the basis of being open studies with mixed types of depressions, probably including some form of chronic anxiety or atypical depression. Controlled studies supporting the advantage of the combination over the use of each drug alone are not available.

Nevertheless there may be some patients refractory to conventional treatments who could benefit from combined treatment (Ananth et al. 1977), and the following guidelines are suggested:

1. It is preferable to use amitriptyline, trimipramine, or nortriptyline, because clinical experience and controlled studies have established their safety. Imipramine, desipramine, clomipramine, and SSRI should be avoided (*see also* section on SSRI). Experience with trazodone is limited, but there is one case of safe combination with phenelzine (Zetin 1984). There are no published studies with nefazodone but it is pharmacologically similar to trazodone. Nor are there any published studies of bupropion combined with MAOIs, but the manufacturer indicates that animal studies have indicated a possible toxicity with the combination and warns against concurrent use. Carbamazepine, which has a tricyclic structure, has been used suc-

cessfully with tranylcypromine but not isoniazid (Joffe et al. 1985, Wright et al. 1982).

2. Although some clinicians avoid tranylcypromine in favor of phenelzine, controlled studies support the safety of both drugs.
3. The route of administration should be oral.
4. Both drugs should be started simultaneously. Tricyclics should *never* be added to an MAOI regimen.
5. Doses should be lower than the usual therapeutic dose for either drug.

Moclobemide, a member of a new class of reversible inhibitors of MAO (RIMA), may pose less risk of drug interactions. This remains controversial, however, because even though one report suggested no interaction between moclobemide and fluoxetine or fluvoxamine (Dingemanse 1993a,b), another report described an interaction between clomipramine and moclobemide in a 76-year-old woman in whom confusion, fever, somnolence, muscle stiffness, myoclonus, and convulsions developed after she was switched from clomipramine 50 mg/day to moclobemide 300 mg/day (Spigset et al. 1993). Postmarketing surveillance of patients receiving concomitant or sequential treatment with SSRI and moclobemide, and a prospective analysis of combined treatment or medication switches without a drug-free washout period showed no adverse consequences (Delini-Stula et al. in press), although these data must be considered preliminary. At the present time moclobemide is not available in the United States, but is marketed in Canada and the United Kingdom.

PROPAFENONE (RYTHMOL®)

Evidence of Interaction
In a 68-year-old man toxic levels of desipramine developed at doses he had tolerated well previously when the antiarrhythmic propafenone was given in doses of 150 mg twice daily and 300 mg at bedtime (Katz 1991).

Mechanism
Propafenone inhibits cytochrome P450-2D6.

Clinical Implications
Clinicians should use lower doses of those antidepressants that are metabolized through the 2D6 isoenzyme when propafenone is given concurrently. Antidepressant plasma levels should be monitored.

S-ADENOSYLMETHIONINE

Evidence of Interaction

A 71-year-old woman taking S-adenosylmethionine 100 mg intramuscularly had her clomipramine dose increased from 25 mg daily to 75 mg daily and within 48 to 72 hours became anxious, agitated, and confused (Iruela et al. 1993). She became stuporous, with tachycardia, tachypnea, diarrhea, myoclonus, rigidity, tremors, hyperreflexia, shivering, diaphoresis, and hyperthermia. Intravenous dantrolene reduced rigidity, but did alter her level of consciousness. The symptoms gradually diminished over 4 days.

Mechanism

S-Adenosylmethionine increases central serotonin and norepinephrine. Combination with clomipramine resulted in a serotonin syndrome.

Clinical Implications

S-Adenosylmethionine is a donor of methyl groups in transmethylation reactions in the body. It is widely used in Europe as an antidepressant, although it is only available in parenteral form. The combination of S-adenosylmethionine with serotonergic antidepressants may predispose to the serotonin syndrome.

PHENYLBUTAZONE

Evidence of Interaction

Consolo and associates (1970) have reported that absorption of phenylbutazone was delayed in patients taking desipramine. Four patients received 400 mg of phenylbutazone 30 minutes after 50 mg of oral desipramine. Combined treatment delayed absorption so that peak plasma levels of phenylbutazone were not attained even 10 hours following the dose (without desipramine, peaks were attained at 4–6 hours). Urine excretion of oxyphenylbutazone (the major metabolite of phenylbutazone) did not differ between groups, indicating that even though the rate of absorption was delayed and peak decreased, total drug absorbed was not different between groups. These same investigators examined chronic treatment in 8 female patients. These patients received a single oral dose of 400 mg of phenylbutazone and, following 10 days of blood sampling, received desipramine (25 mg, 3 times per day) for 7 days. When the 2 drugs were given 30 minutes apart, a delay in absorption was apparent.

When 14 hours separated administration of the 2 drugs, a delay in absorption was not apparent, but plasma levels were lower in the combined group.

Mechanism

Desipramine possesses significant anticholinergic activity, which inhibits gastric emptying. Any agent that delays transit time will impair rate of absorption. This effect requires that the drugs be administered within a short time of each other. The observation that lower levels were achieved on combined drugs compared with the phenylbutazone group may indicate that some drug metabolism occurs in the gut.

Clinical Implications

A minimal therapeutic level of 100 μg/ml is required for the therapeutic activity of phenylbutazone. It is conceivable that coadministration of desipramine could interfere with achieving adequate plasma levels. Appropriate dose adjustments should be made. All antidepressants with anticholinergic activity interact similarly. Rat data indicate a similar interaction may occur with oxyphenylbutazone, cortisol, and, to a slight extent, salicylic acid (Consolo et al. 1969).

QUINIDINE AND QUININE

Evidence of Interaction

Both quinidine and quinine may impair desipramine 2-hydroxylation (Steiner et al. 1988). Ten subjects were administered 800 mg of quinidine for 2 days and a single 25-mg oral dose of desipramine was then given. Urinary levels of 2-hydroxydesipramine decreased by 96% in rapid hydroxylators (previously determined by debrisoquin hydroxylation) and 68% in slow hydroxylators. After treatment with 750 mg of quinine for 2 days, urinary levels of 2-hydroxydesipramine in rapid hydroxylators were 54% lower than during the control period, while in slow hydroxylators no difference was observed. 2-Hydroxylation of imipramine is also inhibited by quinidine, although desmethylation may not be affected (Brosen et al. 1989, Skjelbo et al. 1992).

Mechanism

Quinidine and quinine inhibit hepatic hydroxylation of desipramine, probably by affecting CYP2D6.

Clinical Implications

The addition of quinidine or quinine to desipramine may impair metabolism of the antidepressant, leading to toxicity. Plasma levels of desipramine should be monitored and appropriate dosage adjustments made. Many other antidepressants and other psychotropics undergo hydroxylation and may be affected similarly.

RESERPINE

Evidence of Interaction

When high doses of reserpine 7 to 10 mg/day were added to imipramine or desipramine (75 mg/day average dose), an initial period of manic excitement was noted, followed by dramatic improvement in depression in previously treatment-resistant cases (Poldinger 1963).

Another study using considerably higher doses of imipramine 300 mg/day in 15 nonresponders found that the addition of 7.5 to 10 mg of reserpine resulted in all but one patient showing initial improvement lasting 2 to 12 days. Return of depressive symptoms occurred in 8 patients, while in 6 the improvement lasted throughout a 6-month follow-up. All patients experienced a "conspicuous vasodilation" as well as an increase of intestinal peristalsis, which was accompanied by profuse diarrhea in one patient (Haskovec et al. 1967).

In another open study of 10 patients unresponsive to imipramine treatment (225 mg/day), 10 mg of reserpine was added for 2 days and depression-rating scales were used to assess clinical change (Carney et al. 1969). A significant decrease in Hamilton Depression Scale scores (18.3 before treatment, 10.2 after treatment) was noted; however, on a global clinical assessment only 2 patients became symptom free, and 6 of the 10 showed slight or no improvement. Since this was an open trial, which involved admitting outpatients to the hospital, the positive effects of the hospital milieu may have influenced the Hamilton scores. On the other hand, in one patient a manic episode did develop, which suggests (in light of other manic episodes with this drug combination) that the interaction is important for some patients.

Mechanism

Reserpine rapidly depletes catecholamine and serotonin from intraneuronal storage sites. Most of the catecholamine is deaminated intraneuronally by monoamine oxidase (unless this enzyme has been inhibited). Although the action of imipramine and other tricyclic antidepressants on the noradrenergic synapse is complex, it is generally thought that they increase availability of norepinephrine in the synaptic cleft. In reserpine-treated test animal brains, there is an increase in deaminated metabolites (the intraneuronal action of MAO) and a decrease in O-methylated metabolites (from the action of catechol-O-methyltransferase (COMT) in the synapse). When reserpine is combined with desipramine, the opposite occurs. The combination appears to produce a shift in norepinephrine metabolism from deamination to O-methylation in animals, and there is some evidence to suggest that this may occur in humans (Haskovec et al. 1967). This would indicate that norepinephrine is being released into the synapse (the site of action of COMT), thus causing a potentiation of the action of the antidepressant. This action would expectedly be rapid, short-lived, and probably corresponds to the brief manic phase seen in some patients.

Clinical Implications

Reserpine is an antihypertensive agent that is administered alone or with other drugs in many combination products. It has also been used to treat psychosis and tardive dyskinesia. It is not possible to determine from available data whether the combination of high dose reserpine and a tricyclic antidepressant is effective in treating refractory depressions. We would not recommend such a combination, as evidence supporting its efficacy is scant. Side effects range from uncomfortable (e.g. diarrhea, cutaneous vasodilation) to dangerous (e.g. mania).

Alseroxylon, deserpidine, rescinnamine, and syrosingopine are related to reserpine and may also interact with antidepressants although this is unstudied. All available tricyclic antidepressants and several newer antidepressants probably have the potential for interaction with reserpine, but clinical studies are lacking.

SULFONYLUREAS

Evidence of Interaction

Two women with type II diabetes mellitus had hypoglycemic reactions when a tricyclic antidepressant was added to a medication regimen containing a sulfonylurea (True et al. 1987). Eleven days after starting doxepin (from 25–75 mg daily dose) a 71-year-old woman taking tolazamide 1 g/day had a fall in blood sugar from 300 to 400 to 75 mg/dl. She presented to the emergency department in an unresponsive state and was admitted; however, her blood glucose fell to 35 mg/dl 12 hours following admission. She responded to fluid, electrolyte, and dextrose and was discharged taking doxepin 75 mg/day and tolazamide 100 mg/day (blood sugar 163 mg/dl).

The other woman was given nortriptyline 125 mg/day while taking chlorpropamide 250 mg/day (as well as hydrochlorothiazide and potassium chloride for hypertension). A week after starting nortriptyline her blood glucose fell from between 180 and 218 to 50 mg/dl, requiring glucagon treatment. Chlorpropamide was discontinued and the patient's blood glucose stabilized at 90 to 120 mg/dl.

Another report described a patient with type I diabetes in whom hypoglycemia developed when amitriptyline 25 mg was given (Sherman et al. 1988).

Mechanism
Unknown.

Clinical Implications
Hypoglycemia has been reported with nortriptyline and imipramine, although not with maprotiline (Grof et al. 1984, Shrivastava et al. 1983). Clinicians should be aware that the prescription of some antidepressants may lead to hypoglycemia, especially for patients on sulfonylureas. Decreases in dosage of the hypoglycemic medication and blood glucose monitoring may be necessary.

SYMPATHOMIMETIC AMINES

Evidence of Interaction
Intravenous administration of direct-acting sympathomimetic amines to subjects taking tricyclic antidepressants has produced conflicting data. Intravenous injections of adrenaline and noradrenaline to 6 human subjects taking protriptyline 20 mg 3 times a day for 4 days showed a 9-fold potentiation of the pressor effects of noradrenaline and 3-fold potentiation of adrenaline (Svedmyr 1968). Boakes and associates (1973) have found a similar response in subjects treated with imipramine. Subjects given imipramine 25 mg 3 times a day for 5 days showed 2- to 3-fold potentiation of the pressor effects of phenylephrine (200 mg/min, systolic pressure increased from 143 to 173 mm Hg, diastolic increased from 89 to 108 mm Hg), a 4- to 8-fold increase with noradrenaline (9 mg/min, systolic pressure increased from 131 to 174 mm Hg, diastolic increased from 84 to 99 mm Hg), and a 2- to 4-fold increase with adrenaline (18 mg/

min, systolic pressure increased from 123 to 153 mm Hg, diastolic increased from 60 to 72 mm Hg). No significant increases were seen with isoprenaline (used as an inhalant to treat bronchial asthma).

Another study compared blood pressure responses to norepinephrine in subjects receiving trazodone and imipramine (Larochelle et al. 1979). Trazodone did not potentiate pressor response to norepinephrine, whereas imipramine did. Desipramine and amitriptyline also increased pressor responses to norepinephrine (Mitchell et al. 1970).

Mechanism

Cyclic antidepressants may exert their effect by inhibiting reuptake of norepinephrine from the synaptic cleft or by affecting presynaptic receptor sensitivity, thereby decreasing or blocking feedback inhibition resulting in increased noradrenergic activity. Exogenous administration of either noradrenaline or direct acting sympathomimetic amines results in increased sympathetic tone.

Clinical Implications

Sympathomimetic amines given orally for such problems as cold symptoms may have the potential to increase sympathetic response; however, oral routes of administration have not been used in drug interaction studies. It is our clinical impression that for most healthy patients the oral combination poses no risk. Similarly, there is no evidence of increased toxicity in asthmatics who inhale sympathomimetics while taking tricyclic antidepressants. Intravenous administration of levarterenol increases sympathetic response, and a rise in blood pressure and heart rate should be expected. There is some question as to whether local anesthetics containing noradrenaline might produce similar problems, although we expect that this is quite uncommon. Some dentists feel that the use of local anesthetics with norepinephrine or levonordefrin is dangerous for patients taking cyclic antidepressants (Goulet et al. 1992). Yagiela et al. (1985) recommended that the maximum amount of norepinephrine that patients on cyclic antidepressants receive is 0.05 mg per session (5.4 ml of local anesthetic with epinephrine 1:100,000). Care must be taken to avoid injection into a blood vessel.

TRIIODOTHYRONINE (T3)

Evidence of Interaction

The observation that imipramine toxicity was enhanced in the presence of hyperthyroidism led Prange and associates to question whether small amounts of thyroid hormone might enhance the therapeutic effect of antidepressant treatment (Prange et al. 1969). Later animal findings showed that T3 enhanced the activity of imipramine in the pargyline-DOPA mouse activation test (a screening test for antidepressant activity of drugs) (Prange et al. 1976). In the first study, 20 euthyroid patients (16 women, 4 men) with retarded depression were studied to determine the effect of combined imipramine-T3 treatment. All patients had retarded depression (most were unipolar). Treatment consisted of 150 mg of imipramine plus 25 μg of T3 or placebo starting on the 5th day of drug treatment. Several patients receiving T3 appeared improved 8 hours after the initial dose, and as a group the T3 patients improved more quickly than the placebo group (Hamilton Depression Scale scores 8 at 17.4 days for the T3 group and at 24.8 days for the placebo group). Subsequent studies by the same investigators demonstrated that women with nonretarded depressions responded to T3 augmentation but that T3 added no advantage to imipramine treatment of men (Prange et al. 1976). Coppen et al. (1972) found that 14 days of 25 μg of T3 given with imipramine was superior to imipramine alone but the number of subjects was so small that the study results are difficult to interpret. In fact, the response was dramatic—mean Hamilton scores for depressed female patients receiving the T3-imipramine combination fell from 22 to 0.

Another study by Feighner and associates (Feighner et al. 1972) evaluated the response of primary depressive subjects to imipramine 200 mg plus placebo ($N = 12$; 4 female and 8 male subjects) or imipramine 200 mg plus T3 ($N = 9$; 2 male and 7 female subjects) and found no enhancement of antidepressant activity. The reason for the difference from previous studies is unclear, but the following points have been raised as possible explanations: (1) a relatively small N with a large number of males; (2) failure to delay the start of the study to eliminate positive responders to hospitalization alone; (3) the use of a higher dose of imipramine (200 vs. 150 mg) than previous studies; and (4) a heterogeneous population of depressed patients (the criteria for primary depression were used).

Positive results with an amitriptyline-T3 combination have been reported by Wheatley (1972) in a double-blind study of 52 depressed outpatients. He found that patients who received 40 μg of T3 with amitriptyline 100 mg improved faster than those who received the antidepressant with either placebo or a lower dose of T3 (20 μg). Women did better than men, and patients with high thyroid indices did better than those with low indices. An open study with clomipramine found similar results (Tsutsui et al. 1979).

Prange et al. (1976) suggested that T3 corrects refractoriness in approximately 50% of patients. Preliminary studies seem to support this impression. Earle (1970) found that 14 of 23 patients unresponsive to tricyclic antidepressants (12 taking imipramine 150 mg daily) showed rapid improvement in depressive symptoms when T3 (25 μg/day) was added. It is uncertain whether these patients would have improved if the dose of antidepressant was increased without the addition of T3 since we now know that 150 mg may be an inadequate dose of imipramine. Ogura et al. (1974), in a study of 44 depressed (unipolar and bipolar) outpatients, found that the addition of T3 to an antidepressant regimen resulted in improvement in depression in 66% of patients. A double-blind study of Goodwin and associates (1982) investigated the response of 12 treatment-resistant depressed patients (6 male, 6 female patients; unipolar, $N = 4$; bipolar II, $N = 4$; bipolar I, $N = 4$) to a combination of T3 with either imipramine ($N = 8$) or amitriptyline ($N = 4$). Significant differences were found when scores on the 15-point modified Bunney-Hamburg Scale on tricyclic antidepressants alone were compared with scores after 4 weeks of the combination. Nine of the 12 patients had a decrease in depression ratings that was significant at least at the $P < 0.02$ level. Eight patients achieved ratings below 5 while taking the combination. Both male and female subjects, as well as imipramine or amitriptyline patients, showed a potentiation of antidepressant response with the addition of T3.

In a randomized, double-blind, placebo-controlled study, Joffe and colleagues found that both liothyronine 37.5 μg and lithium (mean level 0.68 nmol/liter in responders) improved antidepressant response when added to drug treatment of 50 patients who previously failed to respond to an adequate trial of either desipramine ($n = 46$) or imipramine ($N = 5$), at a minimum tricyclic dose of 2.5 mg/kg for 5 weeks (Joffe et al. 1993a). Of the 50 completers, 10 of 17 responded to the addition of liothyronine and 9 of 17 responded to lithium, while only 3 of 16 responded to placebo. One possible complicating factor in this study was the greater number of women in the liothyronine group than the lithium group (although this difference did not reach statistical significance), because some authorities believe that women are better responders to thyroid augmentation than are men.

In a crossover study comparing triiodothyronine to placebo Gitlin and associates (1987) found no significant differences, although their study has been criticized on the basis of small sample size and the crossover design that ignores the possibility that the addition of thyroid could produce a long-lasting effect that would carry over into the placebo period.

Another negative study was reported by Thase and colleagues (1989) who administered triiodothyronine 25 μg to 20 patients who had previously failed to respond to imipramine. Although 25% responded to adjunctive therapy, the same number of historical control subjects responded to continued imipramine treatment. A study by Targurn and colleagues (1984) found that thyroid augmentation was useful only for those patients with an increased thyroid-stimulating hormone response to thyroid-releasing hormone, which suggests that subtle thyroid abnormalities may be present in at least some patients who do not respond to antidepressants.

An initial report describing 3 cases of triiodothyronine augmentation of fluoxetine suggested that nonresponse to the SSRI antidepressants may be reversed by thyroid supplementation (Joffe et al. 1992).

Mechanism

The mechanism by which T3 either accelerates or potentiates clinical response to antidepressants is unknown but several interesting hypotheses have been proposed (see Goodwin 1982, Prange et al. 1969). A generalized thyroid defect has never clearly been associated with mood disorders; however, some evidence suggests a link. Whybrow and associates (1972) showed that in depressed patients not selected for thyroid dysfunction, response to imipramine was positively correlated with pretreatment chemical indices of thyroid function. In addition to these data, Prange and colleagues (1969) found that as a group the 20 depressed patients they studied had slow normal ankle reflex time (an index of thyroid function), which increased after T3-antidepressant treatment. Perhaps small doses of T3 in some way lead to a change in thyroid activity, which is necessary for recovery from a depressive episode. Joffe et al. (1990) suggested that T3 augmentation suppresses endogenous T4 production, and that an increase in the T3 to T4 ratio is an important factor in antidepressant augmentation.

Thyroid hormones increase β-adrenergic receptors in the heart (Williams et al. 1977) and it is possible that they do so in brain as well (Goodwin et al. 1982). Further evidence of a receptor site interaction is found in the data of Frazer and associates, who demonstrated that the addition of T3 to imipramine-treated rats altered the effect of tricyclic antidepressants on the postsynaptic generation of cyclic adenosine monophosphate (cAMP) (Frazer et al. 1974).

Clinical Implications

The addition of triiodothyronine to patients who have not responded to an adequate trial of antidepressant therapy is a reasonable therapeutic strategy, although one study of psychiatrists in the northeastern United States found that it was rarely used as a first step in nonresponsive patients (Nierenberg 1991). Thyroid is usually added as liothyronine (Cytomel), in doses of 25 to 75 μg. One report suggested that triiodothyronine was superior to thyroxine in augmentation of antidepressants (Joffe et al. 1990). Response to the addition of thyroid usually occurs within 3 weeks. There are no long-term studies addressing the issue of optimal length of triiodothyronine supplementation. Possible adverse consequences of thyroid augmentation include cardiovascular effects (tachycardia, atrial irritability, altered ventricular function, high output failure), anxiety, insomnia, and increased sweating.

SECTION 2.2 SSRI DRUG-DRUG INTERACTIONS

DOMENIC A. CIRAULO, RICHARD I. SHADER, and DAVID J. GREENBLATT

OVERVIEW OF THE PHARMACOLOGY OF SSRIs (*See* TABLE 2.1)

SSRIs are a chemically diverse group of antidepressants that are more specific in their inhibition of serotonin reuptake than the older antidepressants. Their most important characteristic relevant to the study of pharmacokinetic drug-drug interactions is their inhibition of cytochromes P450-2D6, P450-3A4, and for fluvoxamine the added inhibition of P450-1A2 (*for a review, see* Harvey et al. 1995). Through its actions on the parent drug and/or metabolites, cytochrome P450-2D6 is responsible for the metabolism of many psychotropic drugs, including amitriptyline, clomipramine, imipramine, desipramine, nortriptyline, perphenazine, and thioridazine. Hydroxylation of the secondary and tertiary amine antidepressants is a function of 2D6 (e.g. desipramine to 2-OH-desipramine), whereas conversion of tertiary to secondary amines is mediated by 1A2 and 3A3/4 (e.g. imipramine to desipramine). 2D6 is also involved in the metabolism of other drugs such as β-adrenergic blocking agents (metoprolol, timolol), antiarrhythmic drugs (encainide, mexiletine), and codeine. Cytochrome P450-3A4 metabolizes triazolam, alprazolam, and midazolam, as well as the initial demethylation step of tricyclic antidepressants. Cytochrome P450-1A2 also contributes to the metabolism of imipramine and theophylline, among other drugs. Some evidence

Table 2.1.
Pharmacology of SSRI

	Fluoxetine (Prozac®)	Fluvoxamine (Luvox®)	Paroxetine (Paxil®)	Sertraline (Zoloft®)	Citalopram (not marketed in United States)
Time to peak plasma level after oral dose	6–8 hr	5 hr	5 hr	4.5–8.4 hr postdose	2–4 hr
Protein binding	94.5%	77%	93–95%	98%	50%
Elimination half-life	Parent 1–3 days acute 4–6 days chronic Metabolite 4–16 days (acute or chronic)	15 hr	21 hr	26 hr (parent) 62–104 hr (metabolite)	33 hr
Active metabolite	Norfluoxetine	No	No clinically important metabolites	Desmethyl-sertraline	Desmethyl-citalopram

Table 2.2.
Probable Cytochrome P450 Isoenzymes Involved in Tricyclic Antidepressant Metabolism

Antidepressant	Phase I Metabolism	P450 Isoenzyme
Desipramine	Hyroxylation	2D6
Imipramine	Demethylation	1A2, 3A3/4
	Hydroxylation	2D6
Nortriptyline	Hydroxylation	2D6
Amitriptyline	Demethylation	1A2 and others?
	Hydroxylation	2D62

suggests that sertraline may be less potent than other SSRIs in its ability to inhibit CYP2D6 (von Moltke et al. 1994) (*see* Tables 2.2 and 2.3).

Pharmacodynamic interactions may occur with the SSRIs because of their potent serotonergic actions. When given with other pro-serotonergic drugs such as tryptophan or lithium, they may lead to a serotonin syndrome characterized by diarrhea, nausea, headache, hyperthermia, myoclonus, tremor, hyperreflexia, ataxia, seizures, agitation, confusion, excitability, and delirium (Nierenberg et al.

Table 2.3.
Cytochrome P450 Inhibition

	3A4	2D6	1A2
Fluoxetine	+	+++	+
Norfluoxetine	++ to +++	+++	+
Sertraline	++	+	+
Desmethylsertraline	++	+	+
Paroxetine	+	+++	+
Fluvoxamine	++	+	+++
Nefazodone	+++	+	−
Venlafaxine		+	

+ = mild; ++ = moderate; +++ = strong; − = no significant effect; blank space indicates data not available.

1993, Sternbach 1991a). The serotonin syndrome has long been recognized as a possible consequence of the combination MAOI antidepressants and other drugs such as tryptophan, meperidine, or lithium. More recently, however, there have been reports of a serotonergic syndrome occurring with the combination of SSRI with lithium, tryptophan, or MAOI. There are even reports of serotonergic syndromes occurring when strongly serotonergic tricyclic drugs such as clomipramine are given alone (Lejoyeux et al. 1992, 1993).

Another interesting pharmacodynamic interaction with the SSRI is enhanced downregulation of β-adrenergic receptors that occurs when they are coadministered with some tricyclic antidepressants (TCA). This interaction may result in potentiation of therapeutic response.

ANTICONVULSANTS

Evidence of Interaction

Fluoxetine.   There are several cases reported of toxic phenytoin levels developing shortly after the addition of fluoxetine 20 mg daily (Jalil 1992, Woods et al. 1994) or 40 mg daily (Darley 1994). In a study of the interaction of fluoxetine and carbamazepine, 6 healthy volunteers were administered carbamazepine 400 mg daily for 3 weeks, followed by 7 days of combined therapy with fluoxetine 20 mg daily (Grimsley et al. 1991, 1992). As a result, the plasma versus time area-under-the-curve (AUC) for carbamazepine and its major metabolite carbamazepine-10,11-epoxide increased by 27% and 31%, respectively. Other studies produced contradictory findings. Spina and colleagues (1993b) administered fluoxetine 20 mg daily ($N = 8$) or fluvoxamine 100 mg daily ($N = 7$) to epileptic patients on chronic carbamazepine therapy. They found no change in steady-state carbamazepine levels. Another study examined the effect of fluoxetine and norfluoxetine on carbamazepine-10,11-epoxide formation in perfused rat liver, in vitro human liver microsomes, and 14 patients (Gidal et al 1993). There was no effect on carbamazepine clearance in perfused rat liver, and inhibition of carbamazepine-10,11-epoxide formation occurred only at concentrations 20 times those found clinically. Patients receiving carbamazepine monotherapy and those receiving carbamazepine with fluoxetine had similar ratios of carbamazepine to the epoxide metabolite. Despite the contradictory findings in clinical studies, several case reports have described toxicity when carbamazepine and fluoxetine were combined (Dursun et al. 1993, Pearson 1990). In one of these patients, symptoms were consistent with a serotonin syndrome (agitation, diaphoresis, hyperreflexia, shivering, incoordination), but other patients had symptoms consistent with carbamazepine toxicity (slurred speech, vertigo, tinnitus, blurred vision, diplopia, tremor). Case reports indicated increased carbamazepine plasma levels as high as 63% above baseline, although the changes in plasma levels have been highly variable.

A case report described a possible interaction between valproate and fluoxetine (Sovner et al. 1991). A 57-year-old woman with atypical bipolar disorder and severe mental retardation was taking divalproex sodium (Depakote®) in daily doses of up to 3,500 mg/day with levels of 100 to 120 mg/liter. Prior to initiation of fluoxetine 20 mg daily she was taking 3,000 mg of divalproex sodium with a level of 93.5 mg/liter. Two weeks after the addition of fluoxetine her valproic acid level was 152 mg/liter, although clinical toxicity did not develop.

Fluvoxamine. High doses of fluvoxamine (100–300 daily) may impair carbamazepine metabolism (Bonnet et al. 1992, Fritze et al. 1991), but lower doses may not (Spina et al. 1993b).

Paroxetine. Paroxetine did not affect metabolism of phenytoin, carbamazepine, or valproate in 20 patients with epilepsy who were well controlled on monotherapy (Anderson et al. 1991).

Sertraline. Sertraline in doses of 200 mg daily for 17 days led to a slight, but nonsignificant, increase in plasma versus time area-under-the-curve for phenytoin and a 14% decrease for carbamazepine (Harvey et al. 1995).

Mechanism

Inhibition of metabolism can be explained at least partially, based on the known effects of SSRI on the cytochrome P450 system. Multiple pathways are involved in the metabolism of carbamazepine and phenytoin, but 3A3/4 is important for the former, and 2C9 for the latter anticonvulsant.

Clinical Implications

Several reports document impaired metabolism of phenytoin, carbamazepine, and perhaps valproate when administered with fluoxetine and perhaps with other SSRIs. The data are far from consistent however, with some studies indicating no interaction. Until more information is available, careful monitoring of anticonvulsant serum levels and frequent evaluation of clinical signs and symptoms of drug toxicity are warranted when these medication combinations are used.

ANTIDEPRESSANTS (See also MONOAMINE OXIDASE INHIBITORS)

Evidence of Interaction

SSRIs interact with other antidepressants in two ways (Ciraulo et al. 1990b). First, they impair oxidative metabolism, resulting in higher plasma levels of antidepressants metabolized via this route. As discussed above, CYP2D6, CYP3A4, and CYP1A2 may be affected (see Table 2.3). Various SSRIs may differ in their effects on different subfamilies, although further studies are needed to identify differences among the class and other isoenzymes that could be affected.

The second type of interaction derives from preliminary evidence in animals suggesting that fluoxetine, when given in combination with desipramine, may lead to a more rapid downregulation of β-adrenoreceptors. Downregulation of these receptors is thought by some to be an important mechanism of antidepressant action.

With respect to the pharmacokinetic interactions of SSRIs with other antidepressants, several anecdotal reports suggest that fluoxetine inhibits oxidative metabolism. Vaughan described a 31-year-old woman who was being treated with nortriptyline. At doses of 125 mg/day and 175 mg/day, her plasma levels of nortriptyline were 77 and 88 ng/ml, respectively. The nortriptyline dose was reduced to 100 mg daily and fluoxetine 20 mg daily was started. After 2 weeks of combined therapy the patient reported decreased energy, sedation, and psychomotor retardation. A plasma nortriptyline level done 10 days after the onset of symptoms was 162 ng/ml, a level generally considered above the therapeutic range. Nortriptyline was discontinued and symptoms resolved in 3 weeks. Another woman received fluoxetine 20 mg, lithium 1200 mg, and desipramine 150 mg daily for 3 days until the fluoxetine was discontinued when a skin rash developed. Decreased energy, drowsiness, and psychomotor retardation also developed in the patient, and desipramine was increased to 350 mg/day but symptoms persisted. A plasma desipramine level was 632 ng/ml. A previous level on the same does of desipramine prior to fluoxetine was 133 ng/ml (Vaughan 1988).

In another report, a 33-year-old man had been taking fluoxetine 40 mg daily and desipramine 150 mg daily for 5 weeks (Goodnick 1989). Although his depression improved, the patient reported dry mouth, tinnitus, memory impairment, and decreased alertness. Fluoxetine was discontinued and plasma desipramine levels were followed. The levels were 938.0 ng/ml 595.9 ng/ml, and 47.8 ng/ml at 2, 9, and 49 days after discontinuation, respectively.

A third report described a 75-year-old woman who was being treated with desipramine 300 mg daily, L-tryptophan 2 g at bedtime, and multivitamins when fluoxetine 20 mg daily was added to the regimen (Bell et al. 1988). Desipramine levels prior to the fluoxetine had been 150 ng/ml, 109 ng/ml, and 131 ng/ml. Five days after fluoxetine was started, her desipramine level was 212 ng/ml. Four days after fluoxetine was increased to 40 mg daily, her desipramine level was 419 ng/ml. Increased levels were associated with clinical deterioration. After the desipramine dose was reduced to 200 mg and the fluoxetine discontinued, desipramine levels declined and symptoms improved.

Since those initial clinical case reports appeared, others have been published (Aranow 1989, Preskorn 1990). One study attempted to quantify the alterations in metabolism (Bergstrom et al. 1992). In that study, 6 subjects were given desipramine 50 mg and 6 subjects were given imipramine 50 mg, on 3 separate occasions—alone, 3 hours after a single 60-mg oral dose of fluoxetine, and 3 hours after the eighth dose of fluoxetine given 60 mg daily. With daily fluoxetine dosing, desipramine concentrations were approximately 10 times higher and clearance was 10-fold lower. Imipramine concentrations were about 3 times higher and clearance 4 times lower with daily fluoxetine. Even after a single 60-mg dose there was about a 50% decline in clearance of the two tricyclic antidepressants. Amitriptyline elimination half-life may also be impaired by fluoxetine (Muller et al. 1991).

A possible interaction between fluoxetine and bupropion has also been reported (van Putten et al. 1990). In that case, a 42-year-old man was started on bupropion 1 day after stopping fluoxetine 60 mg daily. Over the next 2 weeks he had myoclonus, agitation, psychosis, and delirium. Since norfluoxetine has a long half-life and is a potent enzyme inhibitor, it may have elevated bupropion levels to cause toxicity. There is also another report of catatonia developing when bupropion was given following fluoxetine therapy (Preskorn 1991).

Fluvoxamine increased plasma levels of imipramine and desipramine in 4 patients in whom adverse effects developed (Spina et al. 1992). Another report described a 40% increase in plasma imipramine level (Maskall et al. 1993). Subsequent studies have found that the effect of fluvoxamine on imipramine metabolism is greater than the effect on desipramine metabolism (Spina et al. 1993a,c). Fluvoxamine also impaired the metabolism of trimipramine (Seifritz et al. 1994) and clomipramine (Bertschy et al. 1991).

Sertraline (50 mg/day) when added to desipramine (200 mg/day) led to an increase in desipramine plasma level from 44 ng/ml to 108 ng/ml, resulting in dysphoria and tremors in a 50-year-old woman (Barros et al. 1993). Another patient had an increase in desipramine level from 152 ng/ml to 240 ng/ml 1 month after sertraline (50 mg/day) was added to desipramine (Lydiard et al. 1993). Sertraline and its metabolite desmethylsertraline may be less potent inhibitors of desipramine metabolism than fluoxetine and norfluoxetine (von Moltke et al. 1994). In a study of 18 healthy volunteers who were extensive metabolizers of dextromethorphan (a 2D6 probe drug) (Preskorn et al. 1994), the average maximum desipramine concentration increased from 51.2 ng/ml to 193.3 ng/ml after 21 days of treatment with fluoxetine (20 mg daily) compared with an increase from 24.5 ng/ml to 32.8 ng/ml after sertraline 50 mg daily. Furthermore, 3 weeks after discontinuation, the inhibition of desipramine hydroxylation was still apparent (due to persistent levels of norfluoxetine), whereas the effects of sertraline abated within 1 week. The dosages of the antidepressants used in this study may not have been therapeutically equivalent.

Paroxetine and its M2 metabolite are inhibitors of 2D6, and significantly reduced desipramine clearance in one study (Brosen et al. 1993) and increased desipramine plasma levels 5-fold in another (Harvey et al. 1995). Sertraline metabolism was not affected by desipramine (Harvey et al. 1995).

Citalopram had no effect on amitriptyline, nortriptyline, or maprotiline plasma levels when coadministered (Baettig et al. 1993).

In addition to a pharmacokinetic interaction, a potentially significant receptor site interaction has also been reported. The combination of fluoxetine and desipramine may lead to a more rapid and greater downregulation of β-adrenergic receptors than seen with desipramine alone (Nelson et al. 1991, Rothschild 1994). If such an effect is important in the antidepressant action of drugs, as some investigators believe, the combination may provide a more rapid and/or more effective treatment of some depressions. Male Sprague-Dawley rats were given intraperitoneal injections of desipramine (5 mg/kg once a day), fluoxetine (10 mg/kg once or twice a day), or a combination for either 4 or 14 days (Baron et al. 1988). After 4 days there was a 27% decline in cerebral cortical β-adrenergic receptor density with the combination treatment, whereas there was no change with either drug alone. After 14 days of treatment, desipramine resulted in a 14% decrease. While both drugs alone resulted in a decrease in isoproterenol-stimulated cAMP accumulation, the combination produced greater decrements. To the extent that β-adrenergic receptor downregulation is related to antidepressant response, the combination may, theoretically at least, provide a more rapid antidepressant response.

Mechanism

The evidence suggests that several SSRIs impair oxidative metabolism, through varying effects on the cytochrome P450 system. Differences in the subtypes of cytochrome P450 that are affected by the various SSRIs are incompletely studied. Tables 2.2 and 2.3 can be used as a general guide to allow clinicians to anticipate and therefore avoid drug interactions; however, caution should be exercised whenever adding or discontinuing SSRIs in a patient taking other medications, because our knowledge of the P450 subfamilies is still incomplete. It appears that 2D6 is responsible for hydroxylation of secondary and tertiary amines, whereas demethylation may be mediated by 1A2 and 3A3/4.

With respect to β-adrenergic downregulation, it is hypothesized that the serotonergic system plays a role in the regulation of beta adrenergic receptors. For example, lesions of serotonergic terminals or inhibition of serotonin synthesis prevents or reverses the β-adrenergic downregulation secondary to desipramine (Baron et al. 1988). It is also possible, however, that the combination treatment merely resulted in higher desipramine brain levels.

Clinical Implications

Coadministration of SSRI with cyclic antidepressants that are hydroxylated through cytochrome P450-2D6 may lead to higher plasma levels of the latter. In some cases initial demethylation may also be affected, but data are limited. Unless appropriate dosage reductions are made, toxicity may result. Because fluoxetine and its major metabolite norfluoxetine have long elimination half-lives (2–3 and 7–9 days, respectively), switching from fluoxetine to another antidepressant may require smaller than usual initial doses of the new medication. Recovery from enzyme inhibition will take several weeks after fluoxetine therapy, but will require shorter times for paroxetine and sertraline.

The enhanced β-adrenergic receptor downregulation observed with the combination of fluoxetine and desipramine is of theoretical importance. Potentially, the combination may provide more rapid or more effective treatment of some types of depression. The clinical importance of the interaction awaits additional study. The mechanism is not fully understood, because a pharmacokinetic interaction cannot be ruled out. It is possible that the combination treatment merely led to high central nervous system (CNS) desipramine levels.

BARBITURATES

Evidence of an Interaction

In mice, fluoxetine (0.3–10 mg/kg) caused a dose-dependent increase in sleep time and hexobarbital brain levels (Fuller et al. 1976). Hexobarbital half-life was increased from 18 minutes in control mice to 95 minutes in the fluoxetine-treated group.

Phenobarbital may reduce serum levels of paroxetine (Greb et al. 1989a,b)

Mechanism

Fluoxetine and other SSRIs may inhibit barbiturate metabolism. Data on SSRIs as object drugs are limited, but one study suggests that phenobarbital may enhance metabolism of paroxetine.

Clinical Implications

Fluoxetine and other SSRIs will probably inhibit the metabolism of other barbiturates in addition to hexobarbital. Furthermore the barbiturates may reduce serum levels of SSRIs, although few data are available. Clinicians should monitor serum levels of barbiturates during combined treatment and observe patients for barbiturate toxicity or decreased antidepressant response.

BENZODIAZEPINES (*See* CHAPTER 4)

BENZTROPINE

Evidence of Interaction

In 5 patients taking either fluoxetine or paroxetine, in combination with an antipsychotic and benztropine, delirium developed (Roth et al. 1994). In 2 patients delirium was evident 2 days after benztropine (0.5 mg twice daily in 1 case, 3 times daily in the other) was started. The other patients had been stabilized on an antipsychotic and benztropine, but delirium developed shortly after either fluoxetine or paroxetine was added.

Mechanism

The mechanism is unknown.

Clinical Implications

Although data are limited to one series of cases, clinicians should monitor for altered mental status when using benztropine with SSRIs. Symptoms appear to develop rapidly within a few days of adding benztropine. In the reported cases, benztropine doses were moderate (1–3 mg daily).

β-ADRENERGIC BLOCKING AGENTS

Evidence of Interaction

A 54-year-old man was treated with metoprolol (Lopressor®) 100 mg daily for 1 month prior to the addition of fluoxetine 20 mg daily. Within 2 days of starting fluoxetine bradycardia (pulse rate fell from 64 to 36 beats/min) and lethargy developed. These adverse effects abated upon discontinuation of the medication and did not reappear when fluoxetine was given with sotalol (Betapace®) (Walley et al. 1993).

An interaction of fluoxetine with propranolol has also been reported (Drake et al. 1994). In a 53-year-old man who had been taking propranolol 80 mg daily and lorazepam 4 mg daily for 2 years without cardiac symptoms, complete heart block and loss of consciousness developed 2 weeks after fluoxetine 20 mg daily was added to his medication regimen.

Mechanism

Fluoxetine is a potent inhibitor of hepatic metabolism. Although the cytochrome P450-mediated metabolism of propranolol and metoprolol is complex, there is evidence that cytochrome P450-2D6 is involved to some extent and this is inhibited by fluoxetine (Marathe et al. 1994). Sotalol is not metabolized by the liver and undergoes renal excretion, which explains why it did not interact with fluoxetine, whereas metoprolol did.

Clinical Implications

β-Adrenergic blocking agents that are extensively metabolized by the liver will be likely to interact with SSRIs. There are no data available on whether β-blockers interfere with the metabolism of SSRIs. If it is clinically appropriate, sotalol or other β-blockers that do not undergo hepatic metabolism could be substituted for propranolol and metoprolol in patients taking SSRIs. Alternatively, lower doses of propranolol or metoprolol should be used.

BUSPIRONE

Evidence of an Interaction

A case report described a 35-year-old man who had depression, generalized anxiety, and panic attacks who had been unsuccessfully treated with a number of medications (Bodkin et al. 1989). He was started on buspirone 60 mg daily, and after 2 weeks had decreased symptoms of anxiety but worsening depression. Trazodone 200 mg/day was added without benefit. Fluoxetine 20 mg/day was then started, and within 48 hours symptoms of anxiety returned. Buspirone was increased to 80 mg/day for 1 week, but still the anxiety symptoms persisted. A satisfactory antidepressant and antipanic effect was obtained with fluoxetine 20 mg and trazodone 250 mg, but the patient remained anxious.

In contrast to that case report, is a preliminary study of buspirone augmentation of fluoxetine or fluvoxamine in 25 treatment-refractory depressed patients (Joffe et al. 1993b). Of 25 patients, 17 improved on the combination with "minimal" side effects. Buspirone augmentation of drug response to SSRI in obsessive compulsive disorder has been tried with mixed results, with success reported in open trials, and no effect in a controlled study (Grady et al. 1992, Jenike et al. 1991, Markovitz et al. 1990). Paradoxical worsening of obsessive symptoms was noted in a 31-year-old woman 3 days after buspirone 10 mg three times daily was started (Tanquary et al. 1990). In addition, a seizure has been reported in 1 patient taking the combination (Grady et al. 1992). A 31-year-old woman taking fluoxetine 80 mg/day for obsessive compulsive disorder had a grand mal seizure 3 weeks after buspirone 30 mg daily was added.

Mechanism

The mechanisms of the interactions are not known.

Clinical Implications

The efficacy of buspirone augmentation of antidepressant and antiobsessive effects of SSRI is not established. A definite drug-drug interaction has not been established either, but clinicians should be aware of the possibility of rare adverse effects from the combination, including worsening of psychiatric symptoms and seizures.

CALCIUM CHANNEL BLOCKERS

Evidence of Interaction

Sternbach (1991b) reported 3 cases of calcium channel blocker interaction with fluoxetine. In a 79-year-old woman taking sustained release verapamil 240 mg daily, chlorpropamide 250 mg three times daily, bumetanide 1 mg daily, and aspirin, edema (at first pedal, then pretibial with neck vein distension) developed 6 weeks after fluoxetine 20 mg every other day was started. The edema subsided within 2 to 3 weeks after the verapamil dose was lowered to 120 mg daily. In a 45-year-old man, dull, throbbing headaches developed after he began taking fluoxetine 40 mg daily and sustained release verapamil 240 mg daily, which subsided when he discontinued verapamil (although his migraine headaches, which were the reason for verapamil therapy, returned). A third patient, a 76-year-old woman, became nauseated and flushed on the combination of fluoxetine 20 mg every other day and nifedipine 60 mg daily. When nifedipine dosage was reduced to 30 mg daily her symptoms resolved over 2 to 3 weeks.

Mechanism

The mechanism for this interaction is not established but may involve impaired metabolism of calcium channel blockers by fluoxetine. All calcium channel blockers marketed in the United States undergo hepatic metabolism, making them susceptible to pharmacokinetic interactions.

Verapamil and diltiazem inhibit oxidative metabolism, but the effects of calcium channel blockers on SSRIs are not known. Nifedipine does not inhibit oxidative metabolism but does increase hepatic blood flow.

Clinical Implications

The combination of fluoxetine with calcium channel blockers may increase the adverse effects of the latter, such as edema, headache, nausea, and flushing. This appears to be adequately controlled by dosage reduction of the calcium channel blocker.

CYPROHEPTADINE (PERIACTIN®)

Evidence of Interaction

It is a common clinical practice to use cyproheptadine, a histamine$_1$ and serotonin antagonist, to counteract the frequent sexual dysfunction in patients taking SSRIs, although the efficacy of the drug for this purpose is not well established. Some clinicians instruct patients to take cyproheptadine on a regular basis, whereas others recommend a single dose 2 hours prior to sexual intercourse. Although a wide dosage range is used, the total daily dose should not exceed 0.5 mg/kg. Fluoxetine-induced anorgasmia was reversed in one patient by a single 8-mg dose of cyproheptadine and in another by daily doses of 16 mg daily (McCormick et al. 1990).

As might be anticipated, the reversal of sexual dysfunction has been associated with antagonism of antidepressant and antibulimic effects of fluoxetine. A 24-year-old woman with a 7-year history of bulimia nervosa was treated with fluoxetine 60 mg daily with a positive response after 2 weeks of therapy (Goldbloom et al. 1991). One month later, anorgasmia developed, which was treated with cyproheptadine, 2 mg daily and then 4 mg daily. A few days following the increase to 4 mg, the patient reported increased depression, an urge to binge, and chocolate cravings. In the same report a 32-year-old woman with an 11-year history of bulimia nervosa was treated successfully with fluoxetine 40 mg daily, and after 4 months anorgasmia developed, which responded to cyproheptadine 4 to 8 mg daily. After the addition of the cyproheptadine she had a recurrence of binge eating and weight gain.

Reversal of antidepressant effect was reported in 3 men treated with fluoxetine for depression in whom ejaculatory disturbances developed and who received cyproheptadine 2 to 6 mg daily (Feder 1991). Reversal of effect occurred rapidly, from several hours after the cyproheptadine to 2 days later.

Mechanism

Reversal of antidepressant effect is most likely a consequence of the serotonin antagonist activity of cyproheptadine. Reversal of the antibulimic effect is probably due to a combination of antihistaminic and antiserotonin actions.

Clinical Implications

The use of cyproheptadine to reverse sexual dysfunction resulting from SSRI therapy is often an effective treatment. Since reversal of antidepressant response is possible, it is preferable to begin with low doses of cyproheptadine and instruct patients to take it 2 hours prior to intercourse. Chronic treatment may be tolerated by some patients if intermittent use is not effective. Patients with bulimia nervosa may be at high risk for relapse because of the antihistaminic effects on appetite and weight gain, as well as the antiserotonergic effects of cyproheptadine. Alternative antidepressant therapy with agents less likely to produce sexual dysfunction, such as bupropion or nefazadone should be considered for patients with major depression who are unable to tolerate SSRIs.

DIGOXIN

Summary

SSRIs do not alter digoxin pharmacokinetics (Bannister et al. 1989, Forster et al. 1991, Kaye et al. 1989, Ochs et al. 1989).

ETHANOL

Evidence of an Interaction

Fluoxetine does not affect psychomotor performance or subjective effects of ethanol, nor does it affect ethanol metabolism (Lemberger et al. 1985). Six healthy men were given fluoxetine capsules (30 or 60 mg) or placebo with ethanol (45 ml absolute ethanol per 70 kg body weight, equivalent to 4 ounces of whiskey) or ethanol-placebo. Effects were tested after a single fluoxetine dose and after 9 days of fluoxetine administration. Stability of stance, manual coordination, motor performance, and subjective responses were assessed. Subjects achieved peak blood concentrations of ethanol of 50 to 70 mg/dl at 60 to 90 minutes. No differences in ethanol kinetics were seen between groups. Ethanol did not affect kinetics of fluoxetine or norfluoxetine. Pretreatment with fluoxetine did not affect psychomotor activity following ethanol administration.

In another study, 12 healthy volunteers were given amitriptyline, fluoxetine, and placebo for 7 days with 28 days intervening drug treatments (Allen et al. 1988). On the 8th day ethanol was given (mean blood alcohol levels via breathalyzer were 78 mg/dl, 77 mg/dl, and 81 mg/dl in the 3 groups, respectively). Mean plasma levels of the study drugs were as follows: amitriptyline 26.1 ng/ml, nortriptyline 25.6 ng/ml, fluoxetine 115.4 ng/ml, norfluoxetine 102.6 ng/ml. The ethanol-fluoxetine combination had few clinically significant interactions. For example, reaction time and digit symbol substitution did not differ among the groups after ethanol administration. Body sway measured with eyes open, on the other hand, was less in the fluoxetine group 1 hour after ethanol compared with the amitriptyline or placebo group. Three hours post–ethanol dose, however, only the placebo group showed less sway. The data available with other SSRIs also suggest that SSRI do not potentiate the psychomotor impairment and CNS depression produced by ethanol alone (Allen et al. 1988, 1989, Hindmarch et al. 1989, 1990, Linnoila et al. 1993, van Harten et al. 1992).

Another type of ethanol-antidepressant interaction is the ability of serotonergic agents to reduce ethanol consumption. Fluoxetine, fluvoxamine, sertraline, zimelidine, norzimelidine, fenfluramine, citalopram, tianeptine, and alaproclate decreased ethanol consumption by rats, while amitriptyline, desipramine and doxepin had no effect (Amit et al. 1984, Daoust et al. 1992, Haraguchi et al. 1990, Hyttel et al. 1985, Lu et al. 1992, 1993, Lyness et al. 1992, McBride et al. 1988, Meert 1993, Murphy et al. 1988, Zabik et al. 1985). In a study that may be significant in light of the efficacy of naltrexone in alcoholism treatment, fluoxetine decreased ethanol consumption in rats, but was not as potent in that effect as the opioid antagonist, nalmefene (Hubbell et al. 1991). In 2 studies, desipramine also decreased ethanol consumption in animal models (Gatto et al. 1990, Murphy et al. 1985).

In a clinical study, zimelidine reduced ethanol consumption in problem drinkers (Naranjo et al. 1984a). In that study 13 healthy male drinkers (ages 22–51 years), who drank an average 6.2 "standard drinks per day" at baseline, were given zimelidine (200 mg daily) or placebo in 5, 2-week periods in a double-blind, randomized crossover experiment. Zimelidine decreased the number of drinks consumed and increased the percentage of days abstinent. As a group there were no significant differences between the number of drinks consumed on drinking days during zimelidine and placebo (7.23 vs. 6.63). There were, however, interindividual variations, with some subjects drinking less per episode, others having fewer drinking days but consuming the usual quantity, while still others reduced both frequency and quantity. The onset of effect is apparently rapid, as opposed to the 2- to 3-week delay in antidepressant effects. The mechanism for zimelidine's ability to reduce ethanol consumption may be blocking of the positive, reinforcing characteristics of ethanol or accentuation of aversive effects of ethanol. The neurobiologic basis of this may lie in the serotonergic system. The reduction of ethanol consumption in this study was modest, less than a one-drink reduction per episode, and chemical hepatitis developed in 3 subjects, which reversed upon discontinuation of zimelidine. Amit et al. (1985) studied the effects of zimelidine on the ethanol consumption of social drinkers. Healthy male volunteers who were social drinkers (defined as "consuming moderate amounts of alcohol one to three times per week but not having any admitted history of alcoholism") participated in 3 experimental sessions. One group ($N = 12$) received ethanol (in four equal doses of 0.25 g/kg of body weight at 10-minute intervals) plus zimelidine (200 mg or 300 mg), or placebo at weekly intervals. The other group ($N = 12$) received mixers without alcohol and the same drugs. Subjective self-rating scales and independent observers found no drug effect on alcohol-induced intoxication or euphoria. An open-ended self-report, however, found that 14.5 and 20% more subjects on zimelidine, 200 and 300 mg, respectively, had alcohol-induced euphoria attenuated as compared with placebo. Furthermore, after only one session of ethanol and zimelidine, subjects expressed a decreased desire to drink and a reduction in the actual amount of alcohol consumed the week following the experimental session. Administration of 200 mg of zimelidine plus ethanol resulted in a 35% reduction in alcohol consumption compared with baseline, while 300 mg of zimelidine led to a 21.3% reduction. These findings suggest that zimelidine reduced the positive reinforcement of ethanol.

In another study of problem drinkers, fluoxetine 60 mg daily (but not 40 mg daily or placebo) decreased mean daily alcohol drinks from 8.3 to 6.9 (Naranjo et al. 1990). In a study of male alcoholics treated with up to 80 mg of fluoxetine daily or placebo, the active treatment group had a 14% lower alcohol intake during the first week only, with no differences in intake, desire for alcohol, or rating scale scores of psychiatric symptoms during the rest of the 28-day study (Gorelick et al. 1992). Similarly, Kranzler et al. (1995) found that fluoxetine did not reduce relapse frequency or severity in alcohol-dependent patients.

Mechanism

Ethanol consumption may be reduced through serotonergic mediated appetite/consumption mechanisms (Gill et al. 1989, Gorelick

1989, Naranjo et al. 1984b, 1989). Some have proposed a role for the renin-angiotensin system (Grupp et al. 1988).

Clinical Implications

Depression and alcoholism frequently coexist. Since SSRIs do not appear to interact with ethanol in a clinically important way, they may provide a margin of safety in depressed patients who use ethanol. It should be noted however that fatal overdoses have occurred with fluoxetine alone or when it was combined with alcohol (Kincaid et al. 1990, Rohrig et al. 1989).

Animal studies have demonstrated that the SSRIs reduce ethanol consumption. Zimelidine, citalopram, and fluoxetine have produced modest reductions of alcohol intake in problem drinkers. Studies in alcoholics have not demonstrated a lasting or clinically significant effect. We recommend the use of SSRI in alcoholics with primary depression, because it provides a margin of safety not offered with alternative antidepressants. As noted above however, overdose of SSRI with ethanol may lead to fatalities or other medical complications (Lazarus 1990). Liver disease may also influence dosage, since impaired metabolism is likely in patients with cirrhosis (Schenker et al. 1988).

HALLUCINOGENS

Evidence of Interaction

A 16-year-old boy who had been taking fluoxetine 20 mg daily for 1 year took 2 doses of blotter acid and developed stupor and a grand mal seizure (Picker et al. 1992). Thirty previous experiences with lysergic acid diethylamide (LSD) at lower doses had not produced a seizure in this patient even while he was taking fluoxetine.

Two cases of worsening of the LSD flashback syndrome by SSRI have been reported (Markel et al. 1994). The first patient was an 18-year-old girl who had stopped using LSD 10 months prior to her treatment for depression and panic attacks. During that period of drug abstinence she had 4 LSD flashbacks. Two days after starting sertraline 50 mg daily, she had the worst flashback she had ever experienced, which lasted over 15 hours. She was then given paroxetine, which also led to a severe flashback lasting the entire day. After SSRIs were stopped the patient did not experience any flashbacks during a 6-month follow-up. A second patient in the same report was a 17-year-old boy with prior LSD use in whom severe flashbacks developed 2 weeks after paroxetine was administered.

Mechanism

The mechanism of the hallucinogenic effect of LSD is not known, although it probably involves sensitization of one or more subtypes of the serotonin receptor. The way in which SSRI may increase the flashback phenomenon is unknown.

Clinical Implications

We have had the opportunity to prescribe SSRIs to many adults and adolescents who have a history of LSD use. Our experience has been that patients who have had dysphoric experiences and/or flashbacks from LSD often have recurrence of these effects when SSRIs are started. The onset of these unpleasant effects are rapid, appearing most often after the first dose or after the first several doses of the SSRIs. We have not seen seizures with the combination, but our experience of patients who use LSD while taking SSRIs is very limited.

HISTAMINE$_2$ BLOCKING AGENTS (CIMETIDINE)

Summary

Limited evidence suggests that cimetidine impairs paroxetine metabolism (Greb et al. 1989a,b). Other SSRIs may also be affected but no data are available.

LITHIUM (See CHAPTER 4)

L-TRYPTOPHAN

Evidence of an Interaction

Steiner and Fontaine reported 5 cases of toxicity with the combination of L-tryptophan and fluoxetine (Steiner et al. 1986). Three men and two women with obsessive-compulsive disorder were treated with fluoxetine in doses of 50 to 100 mg daily for periods ranging from 3 to 9 months. L-Tryptophan was added in doses of 2 to 4 g/day for 7 to 22 days. A toxic syndrome of varying intensity developed in all patients. Symptoms included agitation, restlessness, poor concentration, insomnia, aggressive behavior, chills, headaches, palpitations, worsening obsessive-compulsive symptoms, nausea, abdominal cramps, and diarrhea. Two of the patients had previously been treated with L-tryptophan at twice the dosage without ill effect, and 2 of the patients had previously taken L-tryptophan with clomipramine without problems.

A second type of interaction has been reported in animal studies. Both fluoxetine and L-tryptophan lower blood pressure in hypertensive rats (Fuller et al. 1979). The combination produces an additive decrement in blood pressure (Sved et al. 1982). Implications for humans with hypertension are unknown.

Mechanism

Fluoxetine is a selective inhibitor of serotonin reuptake into presynaptic nerve terminals and L-tryptophan is a serotonin precursor. The combination results in enhanced serotonergic activity.

Clinical Implications

The case reports cited above were all patients with obsessive-compulsive disorder, an illness that typically requires treatment with higher fluoxetine doses than those used for depression. We have seen patients who have tolerated L-tryptophan while taking 20-mg doses of fluoxetine; nevertheless, clinicians should be aware of possible toxicity with the combination.

The reduction of blood pressure in hypertensive rats treated with fluoxetine and L-tryptophan is an interesting observation, but its significance in humans has not been studied.

MONOAMINE OXIDASE INHIBITORS (MAOIs)

Evidence of an Interaction

In 1988, the manufacturer of fluoxetine reported that 3 fatalities occurred when tranylcypromine was prescribed subsequent to fluoxetine. Consequently, they recommended a 5-week washout period between fluoxetine discontinuation and institution of MAOI therapy. Prior to the dissemination of that warning, a 31-year-old woman who had been taking fluoxetine 20 mg daily for 14 days was switched to tranylcypromine 10 mg daily 2 days after stopping fluoxetine (Sternbach 1988). She increased the dose of tranylcypromine to 20 mg daily 6 days after the fluoxetine was discontinued. Two to three hours after she took the increased dose, she experienced "uncontrollable shivering, double vision, nausea, confusion . . . anxiety . . . and audible chattering of her teeth." Her blood pressure was 110/80 mm Hg and temperature 37.2°C. Her symptoms cleared 24 hours after tranylcypromine was discontinued. Six weeks later a fluoxetine challenge in the absence of tranylcypromine was negative. Except for the absence of hyperthermia, the clinical presentation was consistent with a serotonergic syndrome.

Since those reports appeared, additional information on fluoxetine MAOI interactions has been made available. In a report, Beasley and colleagues (1993) described 8 severe reactions to the drug combination involving 7 deaths that were known to the manufacturer of fluoxetine. Five patients died when tranylcypromine was added within a few days after stopping fluoxetine; 1 died after phenelzine was started shortly after discontinuing fluoxetine. The 7th patient died after tranylcypromine was added to fluoxetine. The clinical presentation of these cases was characteristic of the serotonin syndrome, with hyperthermia, headache, agitation, myoclonus, disorientation, hypertension, delirium, seizures, and ventricular tachycardia. One patient in whom severe symptoms developed but who survived began treatment with tranylcypromine 7 days after stopping fluoxetine. Two days later toxicity began to develop—slurred speech, nystagmus, confusion, ataxia. She was treated successfully with discontinuation of tranylcypromine and administration of cyproheptadine.

There is also a case report of sertraline (at first 50 mg daily, which was then reduced to 25 mg daily) added to tranylcypromine 10 mg daily plus clonazepam 1.5 mg daily, after which adverse effects developed—anergy, decreased libido, chills, restlessness, unsteadiness, constipation, and urinary hesitancy (Bhatara et al. 1993).

Although there is one report of safely combining selegiline (Eldepryl®) with sertraline or paroxetine in depressed patients with Parkinson's disease (Toyama et al. 1994), the manufacturer of Eldepryl® in a warning letter to physicians in November 1994 reported instances of muscular rigidity, autonomic instability, severe agitation, and delirium when SSRIs were combined with selegiline. There are several published reports of an adverse interaction between selegiline and fluoxetine (Dingemanse et al. 1990, Jermain et al. 1992, Montastruc et al. 1993, Suchowersky et al. 1990).

The reversible inhibitor of monoamine oxidase A, moclobemide, has been linked to a serotonergic syndrome when combined with citalopram and clomipramine, but one group of investigators has used it safely in combination with sertraline or fluvoxamine in treatment resistant depressions (Dingemanse et al. 1993a.b) (for a more complete discussion of moclobemide, *see* section below on Monoamine Oxidase Inhibitors [MAOIs]).

Mechanism

The serotonergic syndrome is well described. It is believed to be the same mechanism underlying the well-recognized meperidine-

MAOI interaction. Symptoms include excitement, diaphoresis, rigidity, hyperthermia, hyperreflexia, tachycardia, hypotension, coma, and death. Animal studies confirm that rats pretreated with tranylcypromine develop a hyperthermic syndrome after fluoxetine (Marley et al. 1984). Pretreatment with parachlorophenylalanine blocks the toxic effects, suggesting that serotonin is responsible for the syndrome. Graham et al. (1988) and Marley et al. (1984) propose that it is the balance between an antidepressant's serotonin and dopamine reuptake blocking potencies that determines the risk of the syndrome. In this model, antidepressants, which have marked effects on serotonin reuptake but little effect on dopamine (e.g. fluoxetine, clomipramine) would be a high risk for interactions with MAOI. Drugs with intermediate ratios (e.g. amitriptyline, imipramine) would be at lower risk, and mianserin, which affects neither dopamine or serotonin, would be at least risk.

Clinical Implications

With the advent of more selective serotonergic agents, overstimulation of the serotonergic system has become a more common clinical problem. A minimum of 5 weeks should separate fluoxetine discontinuation from administration of MAOI. This will permit elimination of both fluoxetine and norfluoxetine. If especially high doses of fluoxetine have been administered, an even longer drug-free period may be necessary (Coplan et al. 1993). With those SSRIs for which the parent drug and metabolite having shorter elimination half-lives than fluoxetine (e.g., sertraline) or no clinically important metabolites (e.g., fluvoxamine), a 2-week drug-free period is recommended. It is important for clinicians to remember that the half-lives of a drug are variable from one patient to another, and the mean values provided by the manufacturer should only serve as a guide to prescribing. Serum SSRI levels may be helpful in assessing adequate washout periods between SSRIs and MAOIs.

NEUROLEPTICS/ANTIPSYCHOTICS (*See* CHAPTER 3)

OPIOIDS

Evidence of an Interaction

Fluoxetine, like many other antidepressants, can potentiate the analgesic effects of some opioids. Pretreatment with fluoxetine increased and prolonged catalepsy induced by morphine, codeine, and fentanyl. Antinoceptive action was potentiated for morphine and fentanyl, but not codeine or pentazocine (Larson et al. 1977). A case report described an interaction between pentazocine and fluoxetine (Hansen et al. 1990). A 39-year-old man taking fluoxetine 40 mg daily was given an oral analgesic containing pentazocine 100 mg and naloxone 0.5 mg (Talwin Nx®). Within 30 minutes, lightheadedness, anxiety, nausea, paresthesia, tremor, ataxia, and elevated blood pressure developed. He was treated with diphenhydramine 50 mg intramuscularly, and symptoms lasted for about 4 hours.

There have been two case reports of SSRI interactions with cough and cold products containing dextromethorphan. In one case a 51-year-old man taking paroxetine took a combination product containing dextromethorphan, doxylamine, pseudoephedrine, and acetaminophen (Nyquil®)(Skop et al 1994). After 2 days of treatment with the combination, nausea, tremor, diaphoresis, confusion, headache, shortness of breath, vomiting, muscular rigidity, frontal release signs, and elevated blood pressure developed. There was a good response to drug discontinuation and intravenous lorazepam. The other case report described a 32-year-old woman taking fluoxetine 20 mg daily who, on the 17th day of treatment, started a cough syrup containing dextromethorphan (Achamallah 1992). A day later, 2 hours after taking 2 teaspoons of the syrup, she had hallucinations of vivid colors and she perceived distortions in the shape and dimensions of her surroundings. Her symptoms persisted for 6 to 8 hours and she described them as similar to her prior experience with LSD 12 years earlier. Interpretation of this case is complicated by reports of flashbacks in former LSD users taking only SSRI (*see* Hallucinogens, this section).

Mechanism

The combination of SSRI with pentazocine, dextromethorphan, or other opioids affecting serotonin may lead to serotonergic overstimulation. A pharmacokinetic interaction between SSRI and dextromethorphan is also possible.

With respect to analgesic effects, several studies have indicated that serotonergic activity is important in the analgesic effects of morphine. Depletion of serotonin by drugs such as *p*-chlorophenylalanine or 5,6-hydroxytryptamine diminishes morphine analgesia. Lesions in the midbrain or medullary serotonin system also block morphine's analgesic effects. Enhanced serotonergic activity by administration of agonists, uptake inhibitors, or precursors potentiates morphine analgesia.

Clinical Implications

SSRI in combination with opioid drugs that affect serotonin, such as dextromethorphan, meperidine, and perhaps pentazocine, may cause a serotonergic syndrome similar to that seen with the MAOI and these opioids. This reaction has not been clearly established for SSRIs, and issues related to dose and pharmacokinetic interactions remain unstudied. Nevertheless, until more information is available, clinicians may wish to avoid the combination and warn patients about over-the-counter medications that contain dextromethorphan.

Fluoxetine potentiates the analgesic effects of morphine and fentanyl in rats (Kellstein et al. 1988). Clinical studies are lacking, but it should be noted that tolerance occurs to antidepressant potentiation of opioid analgesia (Malec et al. 1980).

STIMULANTS

Summary

Pemoline (Metz et al. 1991), amphetamine (Linet 1989), and methylphenidate (Bussing et al. 1993, Gammon et al. 1993) have been used to potentiate SSRI response in depression and attention deficit disorder. Minimal adverse effects have been reported, usually related to stimulant effects (e.g., anxiety, insomnia).

TERFENADINE (SELDANE®)

Evidence of Interaction

There is a single case report purportedly linking fluoxetine and terfenadine to symptoms of shortness of breath, sinus tachycardia, and atrial premature contractions (Swims 1993). The patient described was taking multiple medications, including a sympathomimetic (isometheptene contained in Midrin®), ibuprofen, misoprostol (Cytotec®), and ranitidine (Zantac®). Symptoms of shortness of breath and irregular heartbeat developed about 1 month after fluoxetine 20 mg daily was added to terfenadine 60 mg twice daily in addition to the aforementioned medications.

Mechanism

Terfenadine has been linked to drug interactions when given with drugs that inhibit cytochrome P450-3A4 (e.g. ketoconazole). Although some have dismissed the interaction because fluoxetine itself does not substantially affect 3A4, they have overlooked the fact that norfluoxetine, its major metabolite does inhibit 3A4, the isoenzyme responsible for terfenadine metabolism. Other SSRIs and nefazodone also inhibit 3A4.

Clinical Implications

Even though there is only one case report of the interaction, it is potentially serious because terfenadine can impair cardiac conduction and cause arrhythmias. We would recommend avoiding the combination of terfenadine with any SSRI, nefazadone, or other drug that inhibits cytochrome P450-3A4 (see Table 2.3). Astemizole (Hismanal®) is also contraindicated in patients taking drugs that inhibit 3A4.

TETRAHYDROCANNABINOL

Evidence of an Interaction

δ-9-Tetrahydrocannabinol-induced aggressive behavior in rats previously deprived of rapid eye movement (REM) sleep was potentiated by fluoxetine and tryptophan, but blocked by parachlorophenylalanine, cyproheptadine, and cinanserin (Carlini et al. 1982).

Mechanism

Increased serotonergic activity potentiates the aggressive behavior, and drugs that decrease serotonergic activity block the aggression. It is believed that both dopamine and serotonin play a role in this animal model of aggression (Carlini et al. 1982).

Clinical Implications

Human studies of this interaction are lacking.

THEOPHYLLINE

Evidence of Interaction

There are several case reports documenting theophylline toxicity when the drug was given in combination with fluvoxamine (Diot 1991). In a 78-year-old woman taking sustained release theophylline 400 mg twice daily, theophylline toxicity developed 2 days after fluvoxamine 50 mg was started (Van den Brekel et al. 1994). Anorexia, nausea, supraventricular tachycardia, a grand mal seizure, and coma developed, as her theophylline level increased from 74 mmol/L to 197 mmol/L. She recovered and theophylline was restarted at the previous dose without fluvoxamine, and therapeutic levels were maintained. In another case, theophylline toxicity, with ventricular tachycardia, developed in a 70-year-old man when his fluvoxamine dose was increased from 50 to 100 mg daily (Thomson et al. 1992). A third report (Sperber 1991) described an 11-year-old boy taking sustained release theophylline 300 mg twice daily whose serum theophylline levels doubled when he was given fluvoxamine (25 mg twice daily, then lowered to 25 mg once daily).

Mechanism

Fluvoxamine is a potent inhibitor of cytochrome P450-1A2, which metabolizes theophylline.

Clinical Implications

Fluvoxamine should be avoided when patients are taking theophylline. Alternative SSRIs that do not inhibit 1A2, such as sertraline, fluoxetine, or paroxetine, may be used. Theophylline toxicity is a serious, sometimes fatal, medical condition. Early signs are nausea (which may be confused with SSRI effects), diarrhea, dizziness, headache, hyperreflexia, and tachycardia. In severe cases myoclonic jerks, grand mal seizures, and ventricular tachycardia may develop.

WARFARIN

Evidence of Interaction

Data on interactions of SSRIs with warfarin are contradictory. With respect to fluoxetine, studies in rats and humans have yielded conflicting results (Rowe et al. 1978). Rats were pretreated with fluoxetine (10 mg/kg) or saline 15 minutes prior to the oral administration of warfarin. Plasma half-life of warfarin in the fluoxetine group was 22.8 hours compared with 8 hours in the saline group. In the same report, the warfarin half-life in 3 healthy male volunteers did not change with pretreatment of a single oral dose of fluoxetine 30 mg 3 hours prior to warfarin, fluoxetine 30 mg daily for 1 week, or when warfarin was given alone (36 hours, 33 hours, and 33 hours, respectively). Warfarin-induced prolongation of prothrombin time was not affected by fluoxetine.

On the other hand, case reports continue to appear suggesting an interaction between fluoxetine and warfarin. In one case, bruising developed in a woman taking fluoxetine after warfarin was added (Claire et al. 1991). In another case, a 47-year-old man who had been stabilized on warfarin had an increase in International Normalized Ratio (INR, a measure of anticoagulant activity) 10 days after fluoxetine 20 mg daily was added (Woolfrey et al. 1993). That same report identified another patient, a 72-year-old woman, whose INR became elevated 10 days after starting fluoxetine 20 mg daily.

The plasma versus time area-under-the-curve for warfarin was increased by multiple doses of sertraline and prothrombin time was increased 8.9% in one study (van Harten 1993, Wilner et al. 1991).

In a separate study, paroxetine did not increase plasma warfarin concentrations but the combination was associated with bleeding (van Harten 1993).

Two weeks of therapy with fluvoxamine increased warfarin concentrations by 65% and resulted in increased prothrombin times (van Harten 1993).

Mechanism

There are three potential mechanisms for SSRI interactions with warfarin. The first is the possibility that highly protein-bound SSRI (e.g. fluoxetine, sertraline, paroxetine) could displace warfarin from binding sites transiently increasing its effects.

The second type of interactions are those involving drug metabolism. As described by Harvey et al. (1995), the metabolism of warfarin is complex. Warfarin is a racemic mixture, with the (S)-enantiomer providing most of the anticoagulant action. The cytochrome responsible for metabolism of (S)-warfarin is 2C9. The inactive (R)-warfarin is hydroxylated through the 1A2 and 3A4 isoenzymes, and (R)-warfarin inhibits 2C9, even though that enzyme is not involved in its metabolism. The effects of SSRI on 2C9 are not well studied, making it impossible at this time to predict the effects of different SSRI on metabolism of the (S)-enantiomer. The interaction with fluvoxamine, however, may be understood on the basis of its inhibition of 1A2, which results in increased levels of the inactive (R)-enantiomer. This enantiomer, in turn, inhibits metabolism of the active (S)-enantiomer by influencing 2C9 activity.

A third possibility is that fluoxetine itself has anticoagulant effects in some patients (Aranth et al. 1992, Yaryura-Tobias 1991).

Clinical Implications

In a small human sample given clinically relevant doses of fluoxetine, no alterations were seen in warfarin half-life or prothrombin time. Animal studies, however, using very large fluoxetine doses, showed impaired clearance of warfarin. Fluoxetine, sertraline, and paroxetine are highly protein bound, and there is a potential for a protein-binding interaction with warfarin. Isolated case reports continue to appear suggesting the possibility of increased anticoagulant effect in some patients on fluoxetine and warfarin. The possibility of bleeding as an adverse effect of fluoxetine alone has also been raised by case reports (Aranth et al. 1992, Yaryura-Tobias 1991). A metabolic drug interaction may be most likely with fluvoxamine. Until additional information on the effects of specific SSRI on warfarin metabolism is available, clinicians should be aware of a potential interaction. A protein-binding interaction would be of most concern when adding a highly protein bound SSRI to warfarin, since this could transiently increase free warfarin and enhance the anticoagulant effect. It should be emphasized that this is a transient effect. Interactions involving impaired metabolism usually take longer to develop, as steady-state levels of the SSRI are reached. The frequency of these types of interactions between SSRI and warfarin is not known.

SECTION 2.3 MONOAMINE OXIDASE INHIBITORS (MAOIS)

WAYNE L. CREELMAN and DOMENIC A. CIRAULO

INTRODUCTION

Monoamine oxidase is an enzyme that is located principally on the outer mitochondrial membrane. This enzyme acts via a pathway of oxidative deamination to inactivate over 15 different monoamines formed in the human body, some of which serve very important roles as neurotransmitters, neuromodulators, or hormones (Murphy et al. 1984). Several substrate selective MAOIs were developed in the late 1960s, which provided the first evidence for two forms of the enzyme. MAO-A selectively deaminates serotonin and norepinephrine, whereas MAO-B selectively degrades benzylamine and phenylethylamine. Dopamine is metabolized by both MAO-A and MAO-B, but is considered by some authorities to be the preferred substrate for MAO-B in humans. Specificity of a substrate for the enzyme is dependent on concentration, so that specificity is relative rather than absolute.

The purpose of this chapter is to discuss the interactions of several prescribed and over-the-counter medications, with MAOI antidepressant drugs—phenelzine (Nardil®), tranylcypromine (Parnate®), and isocarboxazid (formerly marketed as Marplan®, but no longer available in the United States). There are other MAOIs that are not used to treat depression, such as pargyline (formerly marketed in the United States as an antihypertensive, Eutonyl®), procarbazine (marketed as Matulane®, an antineoplastic agent), isoniazid (an antituberculosis agent), and furazolidone (marketed as Furoxone®, a synthetic antimicrobial), which are all nonselective inhibitors of MAO-A and MAO-B. These nonselective MAOIs irreversibly inactivate the monoamine oxidase A and B enzymes. Irreversible inhibition is sometimes referred to as "suicide enzyme inhibition," because irreversible covalent bonds are formed at the active site of the enzyme. This action has clinical importance because it accounts for the long duration of pharmacodynamic effect of these drugs even though many of them, such as phenelzine and tranylcypromine, have short elimination half-lives.

Intestinal MAO is primarily type A, whereas MAO in brain is mainly (70–75%) type B; however, little is known about regional brain differences of these two MAO subtypes in humans.

There are surprisingly few studies of the pharmacokinetics of phenelzine or tranylcypromine, the two most widely prescribed MAOI antidepressants in this country. Phenelzine was once thought to undergo acetylation as its primary metabolic step, but more recent studies have challenged that assertion and they suggest that oxidative metabolism to phenylacetic acid and its ring-hydroxylated metabolite may be the major pathway of degradation. Tranylcypromine is rapidly absorbed with peak plasma levels occurring within 1 to 2 hours, and it has an elimination half-life of less than 2 hours. A single 10-mg dose can produce MAO inhibition lasting 1 week. After 4 weeks of treatment, tyramine sensitivity lasts for several days, but the occasional patient may maintain sensitivity for several weeks.

Phenelzine and tranylcypromine are thought to act at different sites on the MAO enzyme, with phenelzine inactivating the flavin group, whereas tranylcypromine acts at the sulfhydryl group. Return of MAO activity is more rapid after tranylcypromine is discontinued than after phenelzine is stopped, which may reflect slow reversibility, rather than complete irreversibility, of its action on the enzyme.

Selegiline (Eldepryl®, often referred to in the research literature as l-deprenyl) is an MAOI marketed for the treatment of Parkinson's disease. At low doses it is an irreversible selective inhibitor of MAO-B, but it loses its selectivity as dosage is increased, and in some cases, especially with chronic dosing, may be nonselective even at a 10-mg dose. For all practical purposes, clinicians in the United States do not have at the present time a truly selective MAOI to treat depression.

Moclobemide is a reversible MAO-A inhibitor, which is available in Canada and the United Kingdom but not in the United States. It is rapidly absorbed after oral dose with maximum plasma concentrations occurring between 0.5 to 2 hours. It is not highly bound, so protein binding interactions do not occur. The reversibility of its MAO inhibition leads to a smaller increase in blood pressure in response to tyramine, especially in healthy volunteers, but in depressed patients the increase may produce clinical symptoms. Moclobemide is much less likely to produce hypertension in response to ingested tyramine than is tranylcypromine. The former drug produces a 2- to 4-fold enhancement of the pressor response to tyramine, whereas the latter causes a 30-fold increase. Some studies have indicated that moclobemide does not interact with SSRI or tricyclic antidepressants, although a serotonergic syndrome has been reported when it was given shortly after clomipramine was stopped, and fatalities have resulted when it was taken in overdose with clomipramine or citalopram. Moclobemide is oxidatively metabolized and it is a potent inhibitor of cytochrome P450-2D6, making it susceptible to pharmacokinetic interactions.

Despite the introduction of new MAOIs in other countries, clinicians in the United States are limited to the older agents. The two most important types of interactions with these MAOIs are the hypertensive crisis due to interactions with sympathomimetic drugs or tyramine and a serotonergic syndrome due to combination of MAOIs with SSRIs or those opioids that have serotonergic effects (Blackwell 1991). Some pharmacokinetic interactions also occur with the MAOI, but these are not well studied. Major interactions are summarized in Table 2.4.

AMANTADINE

Evidence of Interaction

A possible interaction between phenelzine and amantadine has been noted in the clinical literature (Jack et al. 1984). Amantadine hydrochloride is a dopaminergic agent frequently used as adjunctive therapy in the treatment of Parkinson's disease and as treatment of the neuroleptic-induced parkinsonian side effects of antipsychotic medication. A 49-year-old woman was administered haloperidol and amantadine hydrochloride in progressively increasing dosage, up to 15 and 300 mg/day, respectively. Haloperidol was discontinued and phenelzine was started because of treatment refractoriness, with the daily dose increased to 60 mg over 3 days. The patient's blood pressure increased from a baseline of approximately 140/90 mm Hg to 160/110 mm Hg. Prior to the administration of phenelzine and amantadine, the patient had never had elevated blood pressure.

Table 2.4.
MAOI Drug-Drug Interactions[a]

Drug	Interaction
Antiasthmatics	Oxtriphylline, a theophylline derivative, and albuterol when given to patients on phenelzine may lead to apprehension, tachycardia, and palpitations. One case report describes the onset of hypomania following the addition of isoetharine (an inhaled β-adrenergic agonist) to phenelzine.
Antibiotics	Sulfisoxazole, when added to phenelzine may result in ataxia, vertigo, tinnitus, muscle pain, paresthesias.
Anticholinergics	Atropine and scopolamine are potentiated by MAOI.
Antidepressants	Although the danger of this combination may have been exaggerated there are several reports indicating that combined therapy may lead to a potentially fatal interaction. Commonly described symptoms are diaphoresis, tremor, fever, confusion, agitation, dyspnea, hallucinations, hypotension, and convulsions. Coma and death may ensue. Recent studies suggest that the combination may be safe when certain guidelines are followed. Both drugs should be started simultaneously in lower than usual doses and only via the oral route. Amitriptyline, trimipramine, and nortriptyline appear to be the safest. Imipramine, desipramine, clomipramine, and selective serotonin reuptake inhibitors should be avoided.
Antihypertensives	Reserpine given with MAOI may result in autonomic excitation, delirious agitation, and hypertension. Clonidine administered with MAOI may lead to hypertensive reaction, but clinical experience is lacking. Some experts believe propranolol should not be used with MAOI to avoid hypertensive reactions, but that low doses have been safely used. MAOI potentiates the hypotensive action of thiazides. The antihypertensive effects of guanethidine are blocked by MAOI.
Atracurium	A case report described a 61-year-old woman with narcolepsy taking tranylcypromine (20 mg b.i.d.). She developed hypertension (systolic 350 mm Hg) 2 minutes after induction with etomidate (0.3 mg/kg) intravenous infusion followed by atracurium (0.8 mg/kg). Over 3 minutes, systolic pressure declined to 180 mm Hg and by 15 minutes was 150/80 mm Hg. Because etomidate has been used without incident in patients taking tranylcypromine, this report suggests that atracurium may be the agent responsible for the adverse reaction (Sides 1987).
Barbiturates	Tranylcypromine may prolong barbiturate-induced hypnosis.

Table 2.4.—continued

Drug	Interaction
Benzodiazepines	The combination is widely used without serious interactions. Two case reports exist describing generalized edema when chlordiazepoxide was given with phenelzine or tranylcypromine, but this could develop with an MAOI alone. One group reports a number of patients developing a disinhibited state when given this combination. Chorea has also been reported.
Buspirone	The manufacturer has reported four cases of elevated blood pressure with this drug combination. Many patients taking the combination, however, do not experience blood pressure alterations.
Ethanol	Alcoholic beverages with high tyramine content may produce a hypertensive reaction in patients on MAOI. Pargyline may produce a disulfiram-like reaction when ethanol is ingested.
Ginseng	May cause headache, tremulousness or hypomanic symptoms when taken by patients on phenelzine (Jones et al. 1987).
Hypoglycemic agents	Enhanced hypoglycemic response have been reported in some patients receiving MAOI with insulin or sulfonylurea hypoglycemics.
Lithium	The combination may be useful in treatment of refractory depressions
Narcotic analgesics	Hypo- and hypertension, excitment, diaphoresis, rigidity, hyperreflexia, hyperthermia, tachycardia, coma, and death have been reported with meperidine-MAOI combinations. Dextromethorphan may also cause a hypertensive, hypermetabolic reaction with MAOI (i.e. a serotonin syndrome). Morphine, codeine, and fentanyl are less likely to interact when used in reduced dosages.
Neuroleptics	The combination may lead to enhanced anticholinergic side effects, and extrapyramidal symptoms. Clinical use includes protection against MAOI-tyramine hypertensive crisis and treatment of anhedonic schizophrenics. A combination of tranylcypromine and trifluoperazine is marketed outside the United States and is considered by many to be safe.
Protein dietary supplement	There is a case report of a patient on MAOI (phenelzine) who, following ingestion of a powdered protein diet supplement, experienced a hypertensive crisis. This product and similar ones contain yeast, yeast spirulina, or yeast extract (Zetin et al. 1987).
Succinylcholine	Phenelzine may reduce cholinesterase levels and lead to prolonged apnea during electroconvulsive therapy or surgical procedures. Other MAOI do not appear to have this effect.

Table 2.4.—continued

Drug	Interaction
Sympathomimetics Indirect (amphetamine, methamphetamine, cyclopentamine, ephedrine, pseudoephedrine, guanethidine, L-dopa, α-methyldopa, dopamine, mephentermine, phentermine, metaraminol, methylphenidate, phenylpropanolamine, reserpine, tyramine) Direct (epinephrine, norepinephrine, phenylephrine, isoproterenol, methoxymine)	Both direct and indirect sympathomimetic amines may interact with MAOI although the latter are more dangerous. Concomitant use may lead to hypertension, agitation, fever, convulsion, and coma. On the other hand, recent case reports suggest that dextroamphetamine, methylphenidate, and phentermine may have a role when coprescribed with MAOI in treatment-resistant depressions.
Tryptophan	Occasionally used as a hypnotic in patients taking MAOI or to potentiate antidepressant effect. It may cause delirium, myoclonus, or hypomania.
Verapamil	Verapamil blocks phenelzine-induced hypomania (Dubovsky et al. 1985).

[a]Modified from Ciraulo et al.: Drug-drug interactions with monoamine oxidase inhibitors. In: Shader, RI (ed.): *MAOI Therapy.* Audio Visual Medical Marketing, New York, 1988b, p. 63. For references not listed, please see text.

Mechanism

It is well known that a hypertensive reaction can occur secondary to the combination of L-dopa or dopamine and phenelzine, and this case report may be the first documented reaction between another dopaminergic agent (amantadine) and phenelzine.

Clinical Implications

Although the evidence is limited to one case, it is possible that elevated blood pressure may result from an interaction between amantadine and phenelzine. This is probably an uncommon drug combination, but if these medications are used together, monitoring of blood pressure is indicated.

ANTIBIOTICS

Evidence of Interaction

A probable adverse interaction between the MAOI phenelzine and sulfisoxazole, a sulfonamide antimicrobial agent has been reported (Boyer and Lake 1983). A 37-year-old woman was being treated with phenelzine 15 mg 3 times daily for depression. Three weeks after beginning phenelzine therapy, the patient was prescribed a 10-day course of oral sulfisoxazole, 1 g every 6 hours for a urinary tract infection. Approximately 1 week after starting the antibiotic concurrently with phenelzine, the patient felt extremely weak walking up steps, fell, and was momentarily unable to stand. For the following 72 hours (during the remainder of her sulfisoxazole course), the patient also experienced ataxia, vertigo, tinnitus, muscle pain, and paresthesia. The symptoms started to resolve immediately after discontinuation of sulfisoxazole and were entirely absent 10 days after their first presentation.

Mechanism

Phenelzine interacts with several compounds by inhibiting the hepatic enzymes responsible for drug metabolism. The role of acetylation as the primary degradation pathway for both phenelzine has recently been challenged, although it is the major metabolic pathway for sulfisoxazole. Irrespective of this dispute, it is still likely that the combination of sulfisoxazole and phenelzine impaired this patient's acetylation capacity, resulting in higher than usual plasma levels and side effects of one or both medications (Boyer and Lake 1983).

Clinical Implications

Although the authors of the report underscore the fact that one case does not conclusively establish the existence of a predictable adverse reaction between sulfisoxazole and phenelzine, because sulfisoxazole is frequently prescribed, it is important for clinicians to be aware of the possibility of toxicity when these drugs are administered concurrently.

ANTICHOLINERGICS

Evidence of Interaction

Several authors emphasize the potential dangers of coprescribing MAOI medications with anticholinergic drugs, especially atropine and scopolamine, which are both potentiated by MAOI (Davidson et al. 1984, Walker et al. 1984).

Mechanism

Although MAOI possess little anticholinergic activity as measured by *in vitro* laboratory measures, patients often report symptoms such as dry mouth, constipation, and urinary hesitancy (especially with phenelzine), suggesting that these drugs may act indirectly to enhance anticholinergic activity.

Clinical Implications

Because the anticholinergic properties of atropine and scopolamine are potentiated by MAOI, it may be advisable to discontinue an MAOI prior to elective surgery. The dosages of antihistamines, antiparkinsonian agents, and other anticholinergic agents will often need to be reduced.

ANTICONVULSANTS (*See* CHAPTER 6)

ANTIHYPERTENSIVES (*See also* β-ADRENERGIC BLOCKERS)

Evidence of Interaction

Some serious complications have been reported with antihypertensive-MAOI combinations, including α-methyldopa, clonidine, reserpine, and guanethidine (Davidson et al. 1984, Davies 1960). Despite animal studies that suggest possible adverse interactions between pargyline and methyldopa, there exists only one case report in the human literature describing hallucinosis as a result of the combination. A hypertensive woman who was being treated with pargyline at a dosage of 25 mg given 4 times daily, developed hallucinations approximately 1 month after initiating concomitant treatment with methyldopa at a dosage of 250 to 500 mg daily. This is unusual in light of several other patients who received the combination with no unusual reactions or toxic effects (Paykel 1966).

Although reserpine is rarely been used in hypertensive patients requiring treatment for depression, there are case reports that document central excitation and hypertension as a consequence of combined therapy. This reaction, however, appears to be less likely if reserpine is administered prior to the monoamine oxidase inhibitor. One case report described a chronically depressed woman treated first with nialamide alone at a dosage of 100 mg given 3 times daily, followed by the addition of reserpine on the third day of treatment at a dosage 0.5 mg given 3 times daily. The woman became hypomanic approximately 24 hours after initiating the reserpine, which progressed to frank mania (Gradwell 1960). Other case reports have documented disturbance of affect and memory associated with autonomic excitation, delirious agitation, and disorientation. It has also been reported that antihypertensive effects of guanethidine can be antagonized by nialamide. Five hypertensive patients whose blood pressure had been controlled well with guanethidine in a dosage of 25 to 35 mg daily were then given single 50-mg doses of nialamide, which caused mean blood pressure readings to rise from about 140/85 to 165/100 mm Hg (Fann et al. 1971).

Mechanism

Methyldopa may cause the sudden release of accumulated catecholamines, which are presumed to be at higher levels in individuals being treated with MAOI. This sudden release of accumulated catecholamines could be responsible for a hypertensive crisis. Because reserpine depletes intracellular catecholamines by causing their release from bound stores, the acute administration of reserpine to a patient taking an MAOI can lead to a hypertensive crisis. The initial release of norepinephrine and serotonin can produce dangerous elevations of temperature as well as blood pressure. The mechanism of guanethidine and MAOI is not fully understood, but may involve antagonism of guanethidine-induced catecholamine depletion.

Clinical Implications

Although concurrent use of pargyline and methyldopa has been reported to be a safe combination in general, it may be prudent whenever possible to avoid giving methyldopa after pargyline to prevent any possible sudden release of accumulated stores of catecholamines. There appears to be little documentation about the use of methyldopa and other MAOIs. Reserpine has depressive effects and should be avoided in patients requiring treatment for depression. Guanethidine should be avoided in patients taking MAOI.

ASPARTAME

Evidence of Interaction

The acute ingestion of aspartame particularly when combined with carbohydrates can increase the level of tyrosine in the brain. A 22-year-old woman who used about 10 packets of an artificial sweetener that contained aspartame was given a trial of tranylcypromine 10 mg/day to treat her "tricyclic-resistant" depression (Ferguson 1985). After being on the regimen of 10 mg/day of tranylcypromine for approximately 2 weeks, the patient noticed severe throbbing headaches, and felt flushed and sweaty when consuming aspartame. On each of 5 separate occasions, the headaches stopped within a few hours after she stopped consuming the artificial sweetener. Unfortunately, the patient refused to have her blood pressure checked at these times. However, the patient's headaches were sufficiently unpleasant, and the correlation between the ingestion of the aspartame sweetener and the headaches were so closely linked that the patient changed her sweetener to saccharin, which did not produce headaches.

Mechanism

Elevated CNS level of tyrosine may occur in patients who consume carbohydrate loads and aspartame.

Clinical Implications

This is the only case report of an aspartame-MAOI adverse reaction, and given the wide use of aspartame it is probably not a common clinical problem.

BARBITURATES/SEDATIVE-HYPNOTICS

Evidence of Interaction

Several case reports and warnings exist in the clinical literature regarding the augmentation of barbiturate and sedative-hypnotic effects when combining these medications with MAOIs (Becker et al. 1974, Donlon 1982). Clinical experience suggests that considerable caution should be exercised when barbiturates are used with MAOI even though the MAOI are almost devoid of sedative effects. MAOIs prolong the hypnotic activity of barbiturates (Domino et al. 1962). A 20-year-old woman taking 10 mg of tranylcypromine 3 times daily became extremely agitated, necessitating seclusion and treatment with amobarbital sodium 250 mg intramuscularly for sedation. Approximately 3 hours after the barbiturate injection, the patient was found vomiting, semi-comatose, with widely dilated pupils and blood pressure of 82/64 mm Hg. The patient remained semi-comatose for approximately 36 hours and then gradually responded to supportive treatment.

Mechanism

Tranylcypromine may inhibit the metabolism of amobarbital. In animals premedication with tranylcypromine prolongs the duration of amobarbital hypnosis by at least 2½ times (Domino et al. 1962).

Clinical Implications

Clinicians should generally be aware of the potential toxicity resulting from the administration of MAOI and barbiturate sedative-hypnotic medications.

BENZODIAZEPINES

Evidence of Interaction

One review article reported that a number of patients have developed disinhibited states attributable to the combination of MAOI and benzodiazepines. As part of this syndrome these patients became irresponsible, socially indiscreet, and inappropriately happy (Davidson et al. 1984). There are 2 cases of generalized edema occurring when chlordiazepoxide was given with MAOI (Goonewardene et al. 1977, Pathak 1977) and 1 case of chorea (MacLeod 1964).

Mechanism

Unknown.

Clinical Implications

Although MAOIs and benzodiazepines can usually be safely combined, disinhibited states may sometimes occur. Benzodiazepines, themselves, can produce a disinhibition reaction. With respect to generalized edema, phenelzine, tranylcypromine, and possibly other MAOIs may produce this adverse reaction when administered alone.

B-ADRENERGIC BLOCKERS

Evidence of Interaction

The use of propranolol with MAOI has resulted in severe hypertensive crises (Risch 1982). Some clinicians assert that lower doses of propranolol can be well tolerated in combination with phenelzine (Davidson et al. 1984). Bradycardia developed in 2 patients taking nadolol (Corgard®) or metoprolol (Lopressor®) when phenelzine was added to their treatment (Reggev et al. 1989).

Mechanism

The hypertensive response apparently results from β-receptor blockade, in the presence of unopposed α-adrenergic activity. Phenelzine may impair metabolism of some β-blockers.

Clinical Implications

When β-blockers are used with MAOIs, doses should be reduced and blood pressure and pulse rate monitored.

BUSPIRONE

Summary

The manufacturer reported 6 cases of elevated blood pressure with the combination of MAOI and buspirone. Some patients, however, appear to tolerate the combination well (for a detailed discussion, see Ciraulo et al. 1990c).

DIETARY AMINES

One of the most worrisome adverse drug reactions involving MAOI is the tyramine-induced hypertensive crisis or the "cheese reaction." The interaction between MAOI and tyramine, an indirect-acting sympathomimetic amine, which is plentiful in the typical diet, can potentially produce a serious and sometimes fatal increase in blood pressure (hypertensive crisis). The knowledge that tyramine was responsible for the "cheese reaction" led to dietary precautions that have greatly improved the safety of MAOI usage. Tables 2.5–2.7 list the tyramine content of common foods and beverages (Shulman et al. 1989).

Foods with a high tyramine content must be avoided. These foodstuffs would include most unpasteurized cheeses containing strong, aromatic chemical structures including cheddar, camembert, and blue cheese (Folks 1983, Nies and Robinson 1982, Sullivan and Shulman 1983). Yeast extracts, pickled herring, aged and unpasteurized meats and sausages also must be avoided (Gelenberg 1982). Limited amounts of foodstuffs with moderate tyramine content are allowable, and these include avocados, meat extracts, certain ales and beers, as well as most white wines and champagne. There is one documented hypertensive crisis resulting from avocados (used in guacamole) and MAOI.

Some controversy exists regarding the consumption of alcohol with MAOI. Some clinicians recommend that red wines be avoided, but white wines, vodka, gin, rye, or scotch are allowable because they are low in tyramine content (Murphy et al. 1984). Shader (1986) reported that in his experience patients taking MAOI can safely drink up to 4 ounces of white wine or distilled spirits. One author (Jenike 1983) noted that there is no tyramine in most alcoholic beverages and suggested that patients can drink gin, vodka, and whiskey without danger of an interaction with an MAOI. He further stated that fermentation of most beers does not ordinarily involve the processes that produce tyramine, although he noted that some imported beers have caused hypertensive reactions in patients tak-

Table 2.5.
Tyramine Content of Miscellaneous Foods

Food	Tyramine Concentration μg/g	Tyramine Content per Serving, mg
Fish		
Pickled herring brine	15.1	—
Lump fish roe	4.4	0.2 mg/50 g
Sliced schmaltz herring in oil	4.0	0.2 mg/50 g
Pickled herring	Nil	Nil
Smoked carp	Nil	Nil
Smoked salmon	Nil	Nil
Smoked white fish	Nil	Nil
Meat and sausage (/30 g)		
Salami	188	5.6
Mortadella	184	5.5
Air-dried sausage	125	3.8
Chicken liver (day 5)	51	1.5
Bologna	33	1
Aged sausage	29	0.9
Smoked meat	18	0.5
Corned beef	11	0.3
Kielbasa sausage	6	0.2
Liverwurst	2	0.1
Smoked sausage	1	<0.1
Sweet Italian sausage	1	<0.1
Pepperoni sausage	Nil	Nil
Chicken liver	Nil	Nil
Pate (/30 g)		
Salmon mousse	22	0.7
Country style	3	0.1
Peppercorn	2	0.1
Fruit		
Banana peel	51.7	1.424 mg/peel
Avocado	Nil	Nil
Ripe avocado	Nil	Nil
Banana	Nil	Nil
Raisins (California seedless)	Nil	Nil
Figs (California Blue Ribbon)	Nil	Nil
Yeast Extracts		
Marmite concentrated yeast extract	645	6.45 mg/10 g
Brewer's yeast tablets (Drug Trade Co.)	—	191.27 μg/400 mg
Brewer's yeast tablets (Jamieson)	—	66.72 μg/400 mg
Brewer's yeast flakes (Vegetrates)	—	9.36 μg/15 g
Brewer's yeast debittered (Maximum Nutrition)	—	Nil
Other		
Sauerkraut (Krakus)	55.47	13.87
Beef bouillon mix (Bovril)	—	231.25 μg/package
Beef bouillon (Oetker)	—	102 μg/cube
Soy sauce	18.72	0.2 mg/10 mL
Beef gravy (Franco American)	0.85	<0.1 mg/30 mL
Chicken gravy (Franco American)	mL	<0.1 mg/30 mL
Chicken bouillon mix (Maggi)	0.46	Nil
Vegetable bouillon mix	Nil	Nil
Yogurt	Nil	Nil
Fava beans	Nil	Nil

Reprinted from Shulman KI, Walker SE, MacKenzie S, Knowels S: Dietary restriction, tyramine, use of monamine oxidate inhibitors. J Clin Psychopharmacol 9(6):397–402, copyright Williams & Wilkins, 1989.

Table 2.6.
Tyramine Content of Cheeses

Type	Tyramine Content, μg	Tryramine Content per Serving, mg[a]
English stilton	1156.91	17.3
Blue cheese	997.79	15.0
3-yr-old white	779.74	11.7
Extra-old	608.19	9.1
Old cheddar	497.90	7.5
Danish blue	369.47	5.5
Danish blue	294.67	4.4
Mozzarella	158.08	2.4
Cheese spread, Handisnack	133.81	2.0
Swiss gruyere	125.17	1.9
Muenster, Canadian	101.69	1.5
Old Coloured, Canadian	77.47	1.2
Feta	75.78	1.1
Parmesan, grated (Italian)	74.57	1.1
Gorgonzola (Italian)	55.94	0.8
Blue cheese dressing	39.20	0.6
Medium (Black Diamond)	37.64	0.6
Mild (Black Diamond)	34.75	0.5
Swiss Emmenthal	23.99	0.4
Berie (M-C) with rind	21.19	0.3
Cambozola blue vein (germ)	18.31	0.3
Parmesan, grated (Kraft)	15.01	0.2
Brie (d'OKA) without rind	14.65	0.2
Farmers, Canadian plain	11.05	0.2
Cream cheese (plain)	9.04	0.1
Cheeze Whiz (Kraft)	8.46	0.1
Brie (d'OKA) with rind	5.71	0.1
Brie (M-C) without rind	2.82	<0.1
Sour cream (Astro)	1.23	<0.1
Boursin	0.93	<0.1
Havarti, Canadian	Nil	Nil
Ricotta	Nil	Nil
Processed cheese slice	Nil	Nil
Bonbel	Nil	Nil
Cream cheese (Philadelphia)	Nil	Nil

[a]Based on a 15-g (single slice) serving.
Reprinted from Shulman KI, Walker SE, MacKenzie S, Knowles S: Dietary restriction, tyramine, and the use of monoamine oxidase inhibitors. J Clin Psychopharmacol 9:397–402, copyright Williams & Wilkins, 1989.

Table 2.7.
Tyramine Content of Beer, Wine, and Distilled Spirits

Tyramine Content of Beer			
		Tyramine Concentration, μg/mL	Tyramine Content per Serving, mg[a]
Amstel	Amstel	4.52	1.54
Export Draft	Molson	3.79	1.29
Blue Light	Labatts	3.42	1.16
Guinness Extra Stout	Labatts	3.37	1.15
Old Vienna	Carling	3.32	1.13
Canadian	Molson	3.01	1.03
Miller Light	Carling	2.91	0.99
Export	Molson	2.78	0.95
Heineken	Holland	1.81	0.62
Blue	Labatts	1.80	0.61
Coors Light	Molson	1.45	0.49
Carlsberg Light	Carling	1.15	0.39
Michelob	Anheuser Busch	0.98	0.33
Genesee Cream	Genesee	0.86	0.29
Stroh's	Stroh's	0.78	0.27

Tyramine Content of Wines					
Wine	Color	Type	Country	Tyramine Concentration, μg/mL	Tyramine Content per Serving, mg[b]
Rioja (Siglo)	Red	—	Spain	4.41	0.53
Ruffino	Red	Chianti	Italy	3.04	0.36
Blue Nun	White	—	Germany	2.70	0.32
Retsina	White	—	Greece	1.79	0.21
La Colombaia	Red	Chianti	Italy	0.63	0.08
Brolio	Red	Chianti	Italy	0.44	0.05
Beau-Rivage	White	Bordeaux	France	0.39	0.05
Beau-Rivage	Red	Bordeaux	France	0.35	0.04
Maria Christina	Red	—	Canada	0.20	0.02
Cinzano	Red	Vermouth	Italy	Nil	Nil
Le Piazze	Red	Chianti	Italy	Nil	Nil

Other		
Type	Tyramine Concentration, μg/mL	Tyramine Content per Serving, mg
Harvey's Bristol Cream	2.65	0.32 mg/4 oz.
Dubonnet	1.59	0.19 mg/4 oz.
London distilled dry gin (Beefeater)	Nil	Nil
Vodka	Nil	Nil
Rare blended scotch whiskies	Nil	Nil

[a]Based on a 341-mL serving (one bottle).
[b]Based on a 120-mL (4-ounce) serving.
Reprinted from Shulman KI, Walker SE, MacKenzie S, Knowles S: Dietary restriction, tyramine, and the use of monoamine oxidase inhibitors. J Clin Psychopharmacol 9:397–402, Copyright Williams & Wilkins, 1989.

ing MAOIs. Most, but not all, white wines are free of tyramine. There is substantial variability in the tyramine content of different brands of beer and wine (see Table 2.7). In addition to tyramine interaction with ethanol, pargyline may inhibit acetaldehyde metabolism, leading to disulfiram-like reaction (Collins et al. 1975).

Generally, foods that have low or no tyramine content are permissible in the MAOI diet; these include bananas, pasteurized cheeses, or any of the distilled spirits (in moderation). Most authorities believe that greater than 10 mg of tyramine must be ingested to produce a hypertensive reaction in a patient taking MAOIs. After the discontinuation of MAOI usage, many clinicians suggest that at least 2 weeks may be required for sufficient synthesis of new MAO enzyme so that restriction of tyramine-rich foods should last a minimum of 2 weeks after stopping MAOI. (DeCastro 1985, Rabkin et al. 1985, Smookler et al. 1982). Tyramine challenge produces smaller increases in blood pressure in patients taking the reversible MAOI moclobemide compared with irreversible MAOI. This may be because tyramine is able to displace moclobemide from its MAO binding site.

"ECSTASY" (3,4-METHYLENEDIOXYMETHAMPHETAMINE [MDMA])

Evidence of Interaction

There is a case report of an 18-year-old woman taking phenelzine 60 mg daily and lithium (serum level 0.7–0.9 mEq/L) who ingested juice that allegedly contained MDMA (Kaskey 1992). Within 15 minutes increased muscular tension and tremor developed and she became comatose with decorticate-like posturing. She had a temperature of 100.5°F and a blood pressure of 150/100 mm Hg. She recovered within 5 hours. Another case of an MAOI/MDMA interaction has also been reported (Smilkstein et al. 1987).

Mechanism

MDMA may increase central serotonergic effects.

Clinical Implications

Evaluation of interactions of therapeutic agents with illicit drugs is complex. Although patients may believe they are taking MDMA, it is often surreptitiously adulterated or substituted with other drugs, especially stimulants. There is certainly a theoretical basis for suspecting that MDMA would lead to a serotonin syndrome in patients taking MAOI, although one of us (DAC) has seen patients use MDMA while on MAOI without adverse effects. Caution would dictate that patients who continue to use illicit drugs or who are at high risk for relapse to drug use should not be treated with MAOI.

ETHANOL

Evidence of Interaction

The hypertensive crisis associated with the concurrent usage of some red wines or imported beers (those that have high tyramine contents) with MAOIs is now well known (Table 2.7). A fatal malignant hyperthermic reaction as a result of ingestion of tranylcypromine combined with white wine and cheese has also been described (Mirchandani et al. 1985). In a comprehensive review of psychotropic drugs and alcohol (Weller et al. 1984), the authors underscored the fact that alcohol increases central amine synthesis and release, which may account for the observed potentiation of the sedative effects of alcohol when used with MAOI. The authors also indicated that some MAOIs (e.g., pargyline) inhibit alcohol dehydrogenase, thus delaying clearance of alcohol from the body and potentially lengthening the individual's duration of intoxication.

Mechanism

Fermentation of wine does not usually produce tyramine, but contamination with other than the usual fermenting organisms has resulted in appreciable amounts of tyramine in chianti and could occur in any red wine (Jenike 1983). On a pharmacodynamic level, MAOI generally will cause an accentuation or prolongation of the usual actions of alcohol, such as sedation, associated with its usage (Blackwell et al. 1984).

Clinical Implications

Differing views exist with regard to the combination of MAOIs and "safe" alcoholic beverages. In view of the possibility of tyramine-mediated hypertensive crises, potentiation of alcohol sedative properties, and lengthening of intoxication periods, patients should be cautioned against the combined use of alcohol and MAOI (Weller et al. 1984). Some clinicians suggest that patients taking an MAOI should not drink fermented beverages (including beer and wine), and if they drink distilled spirits quantities should be limited because MAOIs potentiate the effects of alcohol (Domino and Selden 1984). Other clinicians suggest that it is incorrect to state that alcohol is contraindicated with MAOI, because there is virtually no tyramine (the agent responsible for the hypertensive events) in most alcoholic beverages, especially gin, vodka, whiskey, and most white wines. Instructions to avoid imported beer and red wine while permitting distilled spirits is consistent with this approach, which may increase medication compliance (Jenike 1983). Each clinician must decide which approach suits the specific circumstances of the individual patient.

HYPOGLYCEMIC DRUGS

Evidence of Interaction

Monoamine oxidase inhibitors potentiate hypoglycemic agents (Becker et al. 1974, Gelenberg, 1982, Nies and Robinson 1982). Dangerous hypoglycemia has been reported to occur in patients receiving both insulin and MAOI treatment (Davidson et al. 1984). Enhanced hypoglycemic responses have been documented in diabetics on tolbutamide when also treated with mebanazine (Adnitt et al. 1960, 1968, Cooper 1966).

Mechanism

Several mechanisms have been proposed to explain the potentiation of hypoglycemic agents by MAOIs. MAOIs lower blood glucose and interfere with the adrenergically mediated compensatory reaction to hypoglycemia. Another contributing factor may be that the insulin resistance said to occur during depression is reversed with adequate drug treatment.

Clinical Implications

Clinicians may wish to monitor blood glucose frequently in patients taking MAOIs and hypoglycemic agents. Cyclic antidepressants may also interact with hypoglycemic drugs (see section on Cyclic Antidepressants).

LITHIUM (See CHAPTER 4)

LOCAL ANESTHETICS WITH VASOCONSTRICTORS (DENTAL)

Evidence of Interaction

The clinical literature is replete with warnings regarding the combining of MAOIs and local anesthetics that contain vasoconstrictors (Davidson et al. 1984, Nies and Robinson 1982, Risch et al. 1982). Although direct-acting sympathomimetic compounds (norepinephrine, epinephrine, etc.) do not cause the serious hypertensive reactions that the indirect-acting sympathomimetic compounds cause, nevertheless several anecdotal case reports have indicated that when these compounds are used as vasoconstrictors in combination with dental anesthesia, they may interact with MAOIs to produce hypertension (Risch et al. 1982).

Mechanism

The mechanism may involve a postsynaptic "denervation hypersensitivity" caused by the chronic administration of MAOI.

Clinical Implications

When dental anesthesia is necessary, it may be preferable to use lidocaine or mepivocaine without epinephrine or any other sympathomimetic substances. Levonordefrin has less of a hypertensive effect than epinephrine, yet still provides the vasoconstrictor effect and may be a suitable alternative for patients taking MAOIs. The most recent reviews of dental anesthesia emphasize that there are greater risks when patients taking tricyclic agents are given sympathomimetic vasoconstrictors as compared with patients taking MAOIs (Goulet et al. 1992).

MONOAMINE OXIDASE INHIBITORS (MAOIs)

Evidence of Interaction

A potential problem may occur in switching from one MAOI to another. For many years clinicians believed that switching from tranylcypromine to phenelzine was not a major problem because MAO activity recovered more rapidly after tranylcypromine discontinuation (5 days) than after phenelzine discontinuation. Unfortunately, the time required for recovery of MAO activity is highly variable and unpredictable among patients. Regardless of the order of switch, hypertensive MAOI-MAOI reactions have been observed in several patients when inadequate washout periods have occurred.

Mechanism

The mechanism is unknown, but may involve the metabolism of tranylcypromine to compounds that are indirect-acting sympathomimetic amines.

Clinical Implications

Patients should not be directly switched from one MAOI to another (Davidson et al. 1984). The minimum recommended interval of time between two different MAOI would be 1 week, but more conservative clinicians recommend that the first MAOI be discontinued for 2 to 3 weeks before starting a second MAOI. Although the period of washout after moclobemide, a reversible MAOI, should be shorter, clinical experience is limited.

NARCOTIC ANALGESICS

Evidence of Interaction

Many anecdotal case reports described patients who had toxic reactions when placed on MAOI and a narcotic analgesic (Gelenberg 1981, Janowsky et al. 1981, Meyer et al. 1981, Vigran 1964). Hypertensive crises have also been reported when MAOIs and dextromethorphan were combined (Janowsky et al. 1985, Nierenberg et al. 1993). Although hypertension has been described in the MAOI/meperidine interactions, hypotension is a more common occurrence. Other signs and symptoms of this interaction include excitement, sweating, rigidity, neuromuscular irritability, and hyperreflexia. In the extreme case, signs and symptoms have included respiratory depression, agitation, hyperactivity, disorientation, cyanosis, coma, extensor plantar responses, hypertension, tachycardia, hyperthermia, and occasionally death (Meyer and Halfin 1981). This has been referred to as "the serotonin syndrome" (Sternbach 1991a). Selegiline, an MAOI that is selective for MAO-B at low doses, also reacts with meperidine (Zornberg et al. 1991).

Mechanism

The mechanism of the MAOI/meperidine and MAOI/dextromethorphan interactions probably involves the alteration of cerebral serotonin levels. In addition, opioid analgesics may be potentiated by MAOI via inhibition of hepatic metabolism (Janowsky et al. 1981), although a pharmacodynamic mechanism is also possible.

Clinical Implications

The use of meperidine or dextromethorphan in patients treated with MAOIs must be avoided. This prohibition also applies to the reversible MAOI such as moclobemide, and to the somewhat selective MAO-B inhibitor selegiline. This restriction does not apply to the larger issue of using non-meperidine narcotics in patients who are also on MAOI therapy. Should narcotics be necessary in a patient taking MAOI, authorities recommend beginning narcotic therapy from ⅕ to ½ the usual dosage and titrating the dosage very carefully on the basis of response. Patients should be carefully observed for 15 to 20 minutes after the dose for change in vital signs or level of consciousness. Meperidine should not be used; acceptable narcotic medications would include codeine, oxycodone (Gratz et al. 1993), fentanyl, alfentanil, or morphine, which have not caused this very serious reaction. They will, however, have their usual opiate effects potentiated.

NEUROLEPTICS/ANTIPSYCHOTICS

Evidence of Interaction

A number of clinical investigators have noted that MAOI treatment may inhibit phenothiazine metabolism, potentiate hypotensive or extrapyramidal reactions, and prolong the central anticholinergic side effects of phenothiazine medication (Donlon 1982, Tollefson 1983). One study found that the combination of MAOIs with neuroleptics was useful in the treatment of anhedonic schizophrenics (Hedberg et al. 1971).

Mechanism

MAOIs retard dealkylation, demethylation, and hydroxylation. MAOIs may also alter the action of other drugs by pharmacodynamic or receptor site interactions.

Clinical Implications

There may be additive hypotensive effects and enhanced anticholinergic reactions with the combined use of MAOI and phenothiazine medications. The clinician should be prepared to monitor for these effects and make appropriate dosage adjustments. The combination product of tranylcypromine and trifluoperazine is widely used outside of the United States.

STEROIDS

Evidence of Interaction

Fludrocortisone has offered effective relief from the problem of MAOI-induced orthostatic hypotension (Rabkin et al. 1984, 1985). Some studies indicate that up to 25% of patients taking phenelzine or tranylcypromine will experience orthostatic hypotension.

Mechanism

The mechanism by which steroids increase blood pressure is not completely understood. Hypotheses include (1) salt retention leading to edema within arteriole walls; (2) sensitization of blood vessels to the effects of catecholamines and angiotensin; (3) elevation of renin substrate; (4) antidiuretic hormone effects.

Clinical Implications

Although a variety of conservative measures may be taken such as decreasing dosage, increasing salt intake, wearing custom-fitted support hose, fludrocortisone can also counteract orthostatic hypotension induced by MAOI treatment.

Because orthostatic hypotension can often limit the use of MAOI therapy, doses of fludrocortisone between 0.3 and 0.6 mg/day may allow MAOI treatment to continue even when orthostatic symptoms develop. Often after 4 to 6 weeks, the patient will no longer need the fludrocortisone. It should be noted, however, that the prescription of fludrocortisone is not without risk, particularly with elderly patients or those individuals with limited cardiac or renal function because it can cause edema, hypervolemia, and even congestive heart failure.

SUCCINYLCHOLINE

Evidence of Interaction

Phenelzine may reduce cholinesterase levels and lead to prolonged apnea during electroconvulsive therapy or surgical procedures. Four patients undergoing treatment with phenelzine had low serum pseudocholinesterase levels, and apnea developed in 1 for more than 1 hour following a modified electroconvulsive treatment (Bodley et al. 1969). In the other 3 patients, serum pseudocholinesterase levels returned to normal after the withdrawal of phenelzine therapy.

Mechanism

Low serum pseudocholinesterase levels appeared to be responsible for increased levels of succinylcholine with resultant prolonged apnea. Some authorities believe that with appropriate dosage adjustments, succinylcholine may be used in patients taking MAOIs who require ECT or surgery. In actual practice, irreversible MAOIs are often discontinued 10 to 14 days prior to elective procedures requiring succinylcholine. Tranylcypromine does not inhibit pseudocholinesterase.

SYMPATHOMIMETIC AMINES

Evidence of Interaction

Both indirect-acting sympathomimetics (more dangerous) as well as direct-acting (less dangerous) sympathomimetics may cause a hypertensive crisis when administered with MAOI. The following indirect-acting vasopressors produce their pressor effects through the release of bound intraneuronal stores of norepinephrine and dopamine: amphetamine, methamphetamine cyclopentamine, ephedrine, pseudoephedrine, L-dopa, dopamine, mephentermine, phentermine, metaraminol, methylphenidate, phenylpropanolamine, and tyramine. The indirect-acting agents are generally believed to be more dangerous than direct-acting amines, with the indirect agents ephedrine, pseudoephedrine, and phenylpropanolamine being especially hazardous.

Several case reports described the coadministration of MAOIs and amphetamines (Feighner et al. 1985, Kline 1981, Krisko et al. 1969). Some have documented the occurrence of hypertensive crises, while others suggested that the combination may be used without problems. One report noted that phentermine was prescribed for a 35-year-old man for weight reduction. After a 2-week trial the patient was given tranylcypromine, and although instructed to discontinue phentermine and wait 7 days before starting tranylcypromine, the patient used both drugs concurrently (Raskin 1984). There were no documented blood pressure changes with the combined medication. Another example involved a 40-year-old man taking amphetamines for 3 years and who was instructed to discontinue the amphetamines and substitute tranylcypromine. The patient decided to continue taking the amphetamines with tranylcypromine, and no problems occurred with this combination (Raskin 1984).

Another paper reported a case series demonstrating the safety and efficacy of adding a stimulant to an MAOI in the treatment of intractable depression (Feighner et al. 1985). The indirect stimulants used in this case series were methylphenidate and dextroamphetamine with daily divided dosage ranging 5 to 20 mg/day for dextroamphetamine and 10 to 15 mg/day for methylphenidate. The most common MAOIs administered were tranylcypromine and phenelzine. There were no hypertensive crises in this series and the combination proved to be of benefit in treatment-resistant depression.

Earlier case reports, on the other hand, support the commonly held notion that MAOIs and stimulants in combination can cause serious toxicity. One report involved a 41-year-old woman who had progressive agitation, hyperkinesis, fever, coma, opisthotonos, and convulsions after ingesting 10 mg of tranylcypromine plus a combination product containing dextroamphetamine and amobarbital. The woman's temperature was above 109°F for over 30 minutes in a rare "drug fever" resulting from the simultaneous ingestion of tranylcypromine and dextroamphetamine (Krisko et al. 1969).

Another report describes a 49-year-old woman who suffered a subarachnoid hemorrhage following ephedrine and MAOI treatment (Hirsch et al. 1965). This woman was being treated for depression with the MAOI nialamide (100–150 mg/day). She experienced episodes of lightheadedness and postural dizziness; oral ephedrine was given to raise her blood pressure. Within 1 hour a severe vertex headache developed, associated with neck stiffness, diaphoresis, left-sided chest pain, nausea, vomiting and leg-muscle spasms. A systolic blood pressure taken shortly thereafter was 160 mm Hg. A lumbar puncture documented subarachnoid hemorrhage. The toxic syndrome eventually cleared with no apparent neurologic or psychiatric residual symptoms.

In another series of case reports, drug interactions between L-dopa, tranylcypromine, and carbidopa were studied in 4 patients with idiopathic parkinsonism (Teychenne et al. 1975). Pressor responses were induced by the combination of L-dopa and tranylcypromine. Because these hypertensive reactions were inhibited by carbidopa, they were probably mediated at a peripheral level.

Mechanism

Most indirect-acting vasopressors produce their pressor effects through the release of bound intraneuronal stores of norepinephrine and dopamine. Combining MAOI medication with indirect-acting vasopressors increases the pressor effect of neurotransmitters, resulting in hypertensive crises. Similarly, the combination of L-dopa with MAOI prolongs and potentiates the pressor effects of dopamine, although this can be blocked by carbidopa.

The direct-acting vasopressors are believed to be less dangerous than the indirect-acting sympathomimetic amines because they do not release intracellular stores of monoamines, but rather bind to postsynaptic receptors. They also do not depend on monoamine oxidase for metabolic inactivation and are primarily degraded by the extracellular enzyme catecholamine-O-methyl-transferase (Risch et al. 1982). However, in isolated incidences, they can cause a hypertensive effect with MAOI.

Clinical Implications

Since the recognition of the mechanism of action regarding hypertensive crises, careful patient instruction about foodstuffs, drug interactions of prescribed and over-the-counter drugs have made this worrisome side effect a rare problem (Shader et al. 1985). When patients do experience hypertensive reaction heralded by headache, diaphoresis, and elevation of blood pressure, the prompt intervention with α-blocking drugs such as phentolamine or the calcium channel blocker, nifedipine, will usually lower blood pressure. In general, the administration of a stimulant drug (indirect acting vasopressor) such as amphetamine to patients also receiving an MAOI is a potentially worrisome combination. When prescribing both MAOI and stimulant medication, the physician should start the MAOI first, with the addition of dextroamphetamine or methylphenidate in 2.5-mg increments to stabilize blood pressure and enhance clinical response (Feighner et al. 1985). For the most part these combinations should be used only in treatment-refractory depression that is unresponsive to either medication alone, and by clinicians experienced in their use. The indirect-acting vasopressors are far more dangerous than the direct-acting vasopressors with respect to hypertensive crisis reactions and should be avoided in patients taking MAOI.

THEOPHYLLINE

Evidence of Interaction

One case report described an adverse reaction between phenelzine and the theophylline derivative oxtriphylline (Shader et al. 1985). The patient was a 28-year-old woman who responded well to phenelzine at a daily dosage of 45 mg. When bronchitis developed, she was instructed to use a cough syrup before bedtime that had been previously used safely on other occasions. The patient awoke approximately 2 hours later with tachycardia, palpitations, and a sense of apprehension that remained at a distressing level for more than 4 hours. The patient's cough syrup was a combination of oxtriphylline and guaifenesin. Upon repeated challenge with the same cough syrup, the patient had a similar apprehensive state. Rechallenging the patient with guaifenesin alone did not produce adverse effects, whereas oxtriphylline tablets alone did.

Mechanism

Oxtriphylline, a choline salt of theophylline, is a xanthine-bronchodilating agent. β-Adrenergic effects may be enhanced when oxtriphylline is given with an MAOI.

Clinical Implications

The combination of MAOI and xanthine bronchodilating agents may lead to anxiety, palpitations, and tachycardia in some individuals. Albuterol may lead to similar symptoms. Another antiasthmatic drug, isoetharine (an inhaled β-adrenergic agonist) induced hypomania in a patient also taking phenelzine.

TRYPTOPHAN

Evidence of Interaction

The addition of tryptophan to an MAOI has been used successfully for treatment of refractory patients who did not respond to treatment with an MAOI alone (Glassman et al. 1969). Several authors have reported behavioral or neurologic toxicity with this combination, sometimes with acute behavioral and neurologic toxicity observed immediately after tryptophan administration in patients taking MAOIs. One case report involving a 21-year-old man (Thomas et al. 1984) documented marked behavioral changes consistent with a transient hypomanic episode while he was taking 90 mg/day of phenelzine in addition to 6 g of L-tryptophan. In another series of patients (Pope et al. 1985), the authors described 8 cases of delirium, agitation, and myoclonus apparently attributable to the combination of tranylcypromine and L-tryptophan. Similar cases have been reported by other investigators (Alvine et al. 1990, Levy et al. 1985). Goff (1985) described 2 cases of hypomania attributed to the combination. Fatalities have been reported with the combination of lithium, phenelzine, and L-tryptophan (Brennan et al. 1988, Staufenberg et al. 1989).

Mechanism

The cause of the behavioral toxicity with the combination of MAOI and L-tryptophan remains unclear, but is probably due to stimulation of the serotonergic system.

Clinical Implications

If patients taking MAOI also receive L-tryptophan, it would be safer to start at a low dose of L-tryptophan, such as 0.25 or 0.5 g and gradually titrate the dosage upward. Patients should be monitored for signs and symptoms of the serotonin syndrome and/or a switch to hypomania.

REFERENCES

Abernethy DR et al.: Impairment of hepatic drug metabolism by propoxyphene. Ann Intern Med 97: 223, 1982.

Abernethy DR et al.: Imipramine-cimetidine interaction: impairment of clearance and enhanced bioavailability. Clin Pharmacol Ther 33: 237, 1983.

Abernethy DR et al.: Imipramine disposition in users of oral contraceptive steroids. Clin Pharmacol Ther 35: 792, 1984a.

Abernethy DR et al.: Ranitidine does not impair oxidative or conjugative metabolism: non-interaction with antipyrine, diazepam, and lorazepam. Clin Pharmacol Ther 35: 188, 1984b.

Achamallah NS et al.: Visual hallucinations after combining fluoxetine and dextromethor-phan. Am J Psychiatry 149: 1406, 1992.

Adnitt PI et al.: Hypoglycemic action of monoamine oxidase inhibitors (MAOI). Diabetes 17: 628, 1960.

Adnitt PI et al.: The hypoglycemic action of monoamine oxidase inhibitors (MAOI). Diabeteologia 4: 349, 1968.

Alexanderson A et al.: Steady state plasma levels of nortriptyline in twins: influence of genetic factors and drug therapy. Br Med J 4: 764, 1969.

Allen D et al.: Interactions of alcohol with amitriptyline, fluoxetine and placebo in normal subjects. Int J Clin Pharmacol 4: 7, 1989.

Allen D et al.: A comparative study of the interaction of alcohol with amitriptyline, fluox-etine and placebo in normal subjects. Prog Neuropsychopharmacol Biol Psychiatry 12: 63, 1988.

Alvine G et al.: Case of delirium secondary to phenelzine/L-tryptophan combination. J Clin Psychiatry 51: 311, 1990.

Amit Z et al.: Zimelidine: a review of its effects on ethanol consumption. Neurosci Biobehav Rev 8: 35, 1984.

Amit Z et al.: Reduction in alcohol intake in humans as a function of treatment with zimel-idine: implications for treatment. In: *Research Advances in New Psychopharmacologi-cal Treatment for Alcoholism,* Amsterdam, Excerpta Medica, Elsevier, 1985, p. 189.

Ananth J et al.: A review of combined tricyclic and MAOI therapy. Compr Psychiatry 18: 221, 1977.

Anderson BB et al.: No influence of the antidepressant paraoxetine on carbamazepine, val-proate and phenytoin. Epilepsy Res 10: 201, 1991.

Aranow RB et al.: Elevated antidepressant plasma levels after addition of fluoxetine. Am J Psychiatry 146: 911, 1989.

Aranth J et al.: Bleeding, a side effect of fluoxetine (letter). Am J Psychiatry 149: 412, 1992.

Baettig D et al.: Tricyclic antidepressant plasma levels after augmentation with citalopram: a case study. Eur J Clin Pharmacol 44: 403, 1993.

Bailey DN et al.: Interaction of tricyclic antidepressants with cholestryamine in vitro. Ther Drug Monit 14: 339, 1992.

Baldessarini RJ et al.: Anticonvulsant cotreatment may increase toxic metabolites of anti-depressants and other psychotropic drugs. J Clin Psychopharmacol 8: 381, 1988.

Bannister SJ et al.: Evaluation of the potential for interactions of paroxetine with diazepam, cimetidine, warfarin, and digoxin. Acta Psychiatr Scan 80: 102, 1989.

Barnes JC et al.: Lack of interaction between tricyclic antidepressants and clonidine at the α_2-adrenoreceptor on human platelets. Clin Pharmacol Ther 32: 744, 1982.

Baron BM et al.: Rapid down regulation of beta-adrenoceptors by co-administration of desi-pramine and fluoxetine. Eur J Clin Pharmacol 154: 125, 1988.

Barros G et al.: An interaction of sertraline and desipramine (letter). Am J Psychiatry 150: 1751, 1993.

Beasley CMJ et al.: Possible monoamine oxidase inhibitor-serotonin uptake inhibitor inter-action: fluoxetine clinical data and preclinical findings. J Clin Psychopharmacol 13: 312, 1993.

Beaumont G: Drug interactions with clomipramine (Anafranil). J Int Med Res 1: 480, 1973.

Bebchuk JM et al.: Drug interactions between rifampin and nortriptyline: a case report. Int J Psychiatry Med 21: 183, 1991.

Becker CE et al.: A quick guide to common drug interactions. Patient Care : 1, 1974.

Bell IR et al.: Fluoxetine induces elevation of desipramine level and exacerbation of geriatric nonpsychotic depression. J Clin Psychopharmacol 8: 447, 1988.

Bellward GD et al.: The effects of pretreatment of mice with norethindrone on the metab-olism of [^{14}C]-imipramine by the liver microsomal drug-metabolizing enzymes. Can J Physiol Pharmacol 52: 28, 1974.

Bergstrom RF et al.: Quantification and mechanism of the fluoxetine and tricyclic antide-pressant interaction. Clin Pharmacol Ther 51: 239, 1992.

Bertschy G et al.: Fluvoxamine-tricyclic antidepressant interaction: an accidental finding. Eur J Clin Pharmacol 40: 119, 1991.

Bertschy G et al.: Valpromide-amitriptyline interaction. Increase in the bioavailability of amitriptyline and nortriptyline caused by valpromide. Encephale 16: 43, 1990.

Bhatara VS et al.: Possible interaction between sertraline and tranylcypromine. Clin Pharm 12: 222, 1993.

Blackwell B: Monoamine oxidase inhibitor interactions with other drugs. J Clin Psychopharmacol 11: 55, 1991.

Blackwell B et al.: Drug interactions in psychopharmacology. Psychiatr Clin North Am 7: 625, 1984.

Boakes AJ et al.: Interactions between sympathomimetic amines and antidepressants agents in man. Br Med J 1: 311, 1973.

Bodkin JA et al.: Fluoxetine may antagonize the anxiolytic action of buspirone. J Clin Psychopharmacol 9: 150, 1989.

Bodley PO et al.: Low serum pseudocholinesterase levels complicating treatment with phenelzine. Br Med J 3: 510, 1969.

Bonnet P et al.: Carbamazepine, fluvoxamine. Is there a pharmacokinetic interaction? (letter). Therapie 47: 165, 1992.

Boyer WF, Lake CR: Interaction of phenelzine and sulfisoxazole. Am J Psychiatry 140: 264, 1983.

Brennan D et al.: Neuroleptic malignant syndrome without neuroleptics. Br J Psychiatry 152: 578, 1988.

Briant RH et al.: Interaction between clonidine and desipramine in man. Br Med J 1: 522, 1973.

Brosen K et al.: Quinidine inhibits the 2-hydroxylation of imipramine and desipramine but not the demethylation of imipramine. Eur J Clin Pharmacol 37: 155, 1989.

Brosen K et al.: Inhibition by paroxetine of desipramine metabolism in extensive but not in poor metabolizers of sparteine. Eur J Clin Pharmacol 44: 349, 1993.

Brown CS et al.: Possible influence of carbamazepine on plasma imipramine concentrations in children with attention deficit hyperactivity disorder. J Clin Psychopharmacol 12: 67, 1992.

Burrows GD et al.: Antidepressants and barbiturates. Br Med J 4: 113, 1971.

Bussing R et al.: Methamphetamine and fluoxetine treatment of a child with attention deficit hyperactivity disorder and obsessive compulsive disorder. J Child Adol Psychopharmacol 3: 53, 1993.

Carlini EA et al.: Effect of serotonergic drugs on the aggressiveness induced by delta 9-tetrahydrocannabinol in REM-sleep-deprived rats. Braz J Med Biol Res 15: 281, 1982.

Carney MWP et al.: Effects of imipramine and reserpine in depression. Psychopharmacologica 14: 349, 1969.

Ciraulo DA et al.: Imipramine disposition in alcoholics. J Clin Psychopharmacol 2: 2, 1982.

Ciraulo DA et al.: Clinical pharmacokinetics of imipramine and desipramine in alcoholics and normal volunteers. Clin Pharmacol Ther 43: 509, 1988a.

Ciraulo DA et al.: Drug-drug interactions with monoamine oxidase inhibitors. In: Shader RI (ed.): MAOI Therapy, New York, Audio Visual Medical Marketing, 1988b, p. 63.

Ciraulo DA et al.: Intravenous pharmacokinetics of 2-hydroxyimipramine in alcoholics and normal controls. J Stud Alcohol 51: 366, 1990a.

Ciraulo DA et al.: Fluoxetine drug-drug interactions: I. Antidepressants and antipsychotics. J Clin Psychopharmacol 10: 48, 1990b.

Ciraulo DA et al.: Question the experts: buspirone and MAOI. J Clin Psychopharmacol 10: 306, 1990c.

Claire RJ et al.: Potential interaction between warfarin sodium and fluoxetine (letter). Am J Psychiatry 148: 1604, 1991.

Collins MA et al.: Tetrahydroisoquinolines in vivo, I: rat brain formation of salsolinol, a condensation product of dopamine and acetaldehyde under certain conditions during ethanol intoxication. Life Sci 16: 585, 1975.

Consolo S et al.: Effect of desimpramine on intestinal absorption of phenylbutazone and other drugs. Eur J Pharmacol 6: 322, 1969.

Consolo S et al.: Delayed absorption of phenylbutazone caused by desmethylimipramine in humans. Eur J Pharmacol 10: 239, 1970.

Cooper AJ et al.: Action of mebanazine, a monoamine oxidase inhibitor antidepressant drug in diabetes, II. Int J Neuropsychiatry 2: 343, 1966.

Coplan JD et al.: Detectable levels of fluoxetine metabolites after discontinuation: an unexpected serotonin syndrome (letter). Am J Psychiatry 150: 837, 1993.

Coppen A et al.: The comparative antidepressant value of L-tryptophan and imipramine with and without attempted potentiation by triiodothyronine. Arch Gen Psychiatry 26: 234, 1972.

Daoust M et al.: Tianeptine, a specific serotonin uptake enhancer, decreases ethanol intake in rats. Alcohol Alcohol 27: 15, 1992.

Darley J: Interaction between phenytoin and fluoxetine. Seizure 3: 151, 1994.

Davidson J: Adding a tricyclic antidepressant to a monoamine oxidase inhibitor. J Clin Psychopharmacol 2: 216, 1982.

Davidson J et al.: Practical aspects of MAO inhibitor therapy. J Clin Psychiatry 45: 81, 1984.

Davies TS: Monoamine oxidase inhibitors and rauwolfia compounds (letter). Br Med J : 739, 1960.

Dec GW: Trazodone-digoxin interaction in an animal model. J Clin Psychopharmacol 4: 153, 1984.

Decastro RM: MAOIs, the cheese reaction, and sleep apnea. J Clin Psychopharmacol 5: 59, 1985.

Delini-Stula A et al.: Pharmacological interactions of SSRI and RIMA—new selective antidepressants affecting the serotonin system and the phenomenon of the 5-HT-syndrome. J Clin Psychopharmacol (in press), 1995.

Dingemanse J et al.: Interaction of fluoxetine and selegiline (letter). Can J Psychiatry 35: 571, 1990.

Dingemanse J: An update of recent moclobemide interaction data. Int Clin Psychopharmacol 7: 167, 1993a.

Dingemanse J et al.: Pharmacodynamic and pharmacokinetic interactions between fluoxetine and moclobemide. Clin Pharmacol Ther 53: 178, 1993b.

Diot P et al.: Possible interaction entre theophylline et fluvoxamine. Therapie 46: 170, 1991.

Domino EF et al.: Barbiturate intoxication in a patient treated with a MAO inhibitor. Am J Psychiatry 118: 941, 1962.

Domino EF et al.: Red wine and reactions. J Clin Psychopharmacol 4: 173, 1984.

Donlon PT: Cardiac effects of antidepressants. Geriatrics 37: 53, 1982.

Dorian P et al.: Amitriptyline and ethanol: pharmacokinetic and pharmacodynamic interaction. Eur J Clin Pharmacol 25: 325, 1983.

Dorn JM: A case of phenytoin toxicity possibly precipitated by trazodone. J Clin Psychiatry 47: 89, 1986.

Drake W et al.: Heart block in a patient on propranolol and fluoxetine. Lancet 343: 425, 1994.

Dubocovich ML et al.: Cocaine and desipramine antagonize the clonidine-induced inhibition of [^{3}H]-noradrenaline release from the rat cerebral cortex [Proceedings]. Br J Pharmacol 67: 144, 1979.

Dubovsky SL et al.: Phenelzine-induced hypomania: effect of verapamil. Biol Psychiatry 20: 1009, 1985.

Dursun SM et al.: Toxic serotonin syndrome after fluoxetine plus carbamazepine (letter). Lancet 342: 442, 1993.

Earle BV: Thyroid hormone and tricyclic antidepressants in resistant depressions. Am J Psychiatry 126: 1667, 1970.

Edwards RP et al.: Cardia responses to imipramine and pancuronium during anesthesia with halothane or enflurane. Anesthesiology 50: 421, 1979.

Elliot HS et al.: Pharmacodynamic studies on mianserin and its interaction with clonidine. Eur J Clin Pharmacol 21: 97, 1981.

Elliot HS et al.: Assessment of the interaction between mianserin and centrally-acting and antihypertensive drugs. J Clin Pharmacol 15: 3235, 1983.

Fadden JS: Nifedipine and nonresponse to antidepressants (letter). J Clin Psychiatry 53: 416, 1992.

Fann WE et al.: Chlorpromazine reversal of the anti-hypertensive action of guanethidine. Lancet 2: 436, 1971.

Feder R: Reversal of antidepressant activity of fluoxetine by cyproheptadine in three patients. J Clin Psychiatry 52: 163, 1991.

Feighner JP et al.: Hormonal potentiation of imipramine and ECT in primary depression. Am J Psychiatry 128: 1230, 1972.

Feighner JP et al.: Combined MAOI, TCA, and direct stimulant therapy of treatment resistant depression. J Clin Psychiatry 46: 206, 1985.

Ferguson JM: Interaction of aspartame and carbohydrates in an eating-disordered patient. Am J Psychiatry 142: 271, 1985.

Field B et al.: Inhibition of hepatic drug metabolism by norethindrone. Clin Pharmacol Ther 25: 196, 1979.

Finch L: Cardiovascular effects of intraventricular dihydroxytriptamine in the conscious hypertensive rat. Clin Exp Pharmacol Physiol 2: 503, 1975.

Folks D: Monoamine oxidase inhibitors: reappraisal of dietary considerations. J Clin Psychopharmacol 3: 249, 1983.

Forster PL et al.: The efffects of sertraline on plasma concentration and renal clearance of digoxin. Biol Psychiatry 29: 355, 1991.

Frazer A et al.: The effect of triiodothyronine in combination with imipramine on [³H]-cyclic AMP production in slices of rate cerebral cortex. Neuropharmacology 13: 1131, 1974.

Fritze J et al.: Interaction between carbamazepine and fluvoxamine. Acta Psychiatr Scan 84: 583, 1991.

Fuller RW et al.: Inhibition of drug metabolism by fluoxetine. Res Commun Chem Pathol Pharmacol 13: 353, 1976.

Fuller RW et al.: Antihypertensive effects of fluoxetine and L-5-hydroxytryptophan in rats. Life Sci 25: 1237, 1979.

Gammon G et al.: Fluoxetine and methylphenidate in combination for treatment of attention deficit disorder and comorbid depressive disorder. J Child Adol Psychopharmacol 3: 1, 1993.

Gander DR: Treatment of depressive illnesses with combined antidepressants. Lancet 1: 107, 1965.

Gannon RH et al.: Fluconazole nortriptyline drug interaction. Ann Pharmacother 26: 1456, 1992.

Gatto GJ et al.: Effects of fluoxetine and desipramine on palatability-induced ethanol consumption in the alcohol-nonpreferring (NP) lines of rats. Alcohol 7: 531, 1990.

Gelenberg AJ: Can MAO inhibitor drugs be taken with analgesics? J Clin Psychopharmacol 1: 160, 1981.

Gelenberg AJ: MAOI inhibitors in sickness and in health. Biol Ther Psychiatry 5: 25, 1982.

Gelenberg AJ: Adverse reactions to MAOIs. Biol Ther Psychiatry 8: 4, 1985.

Gidal BE et al.: Evaluation of the effect of fluoxetine on the formation of carbamazepine epoxide. Ther Drug Monit 14: 405, 1993.

Gill K et al.: Serotonin uptake blockers and voluntary alcohol consumption: a review of recent studies. Recent Dev Alcohol 7: 225, 1989.

Gitlin MJ et al.: Failure of T₃ to potentiate tricyclic antidepressant response. J Affect Disord 13: 267, 1987.

Glassman AH et al.: Potentiation of a monoamine oxidase inhibitor by tryptophan. J Psychiatr Res 7: 83, 1969.

Goff D: Two cases of hypomania following the addition of L-tryptophan to a monoamine oxidase inhibitor. Am J Psychiatry 142: 1487, 1985.

Goldbloom DS et al.: Adverse interaction of fluoxetine and cyproheptadine in two patients with bulimia nervosa. J Clin Psychiatry 52: 261, 1991.

Goldstein FJ et al.: Elevation in analgesic effect and plasma levels of morphine by desipramine in rats. Pain 14: 279, 1982.

Goodnick PJ: Influence of fluoxetine on plasma levels of desipramine. Am J Psychiatry 146: 552, 1989.

Goodwin FK et al.: Potentiation of antidepressant effects by L-triiodothyronine in tricyclic non-responders. Am J Psychiatry 139: 34, 1982.

Goonewardene A: Gross oedema occurring during treatment for depression. Br Med J 1: 879, 1977.

Gorelick DA: Serotonin uptake blockers and the treatment of alcoholism. Recent Dev Alcohol 7: 267, 1989.

Gorelick DA et al.: Effect of fluoxetine on alcohol consumption in male alcoholics. Alcohol Clin Exp Res 16: 261, 1992.

Goulet JP et al.: Contraindications to vasoconstrictors in dentistry. Oral Surg Oral Med Oral Pathol 74: 692, 1992.

Gradwell BG: Psychotic reactions and phenelzine. Br Med J 2: 1018, 1960.

Grady TA et al.: Seizure associated with fluoxetine and adjuvant buspirone therapy (letter). J Clin Psychopharmacol 12: 70, 1992.

Graham PM et al.: Danger of MAOI therapy after fluoxetine withdrawal (letter). Lancet 2: 1255, 1988.

Gram LF et al.: Imipramine metabolism: pH dependent distribution and urinary excretion. Clin Pharmacol Ther 12: 239, 1971.

Gratz SS et al.: MAOI-narcotic interactions (letter). J Clin Psychiatry 54: 439, 1993.

Greb WH et al.: Absorption of paroxetine under various dietary conditions and following antacid intake. Acta Psychiatr Scand 80(suppl): 99, 1989a.

Greb WH et al.: The effect of liver enzyme inhibition by cimetidine and enzyme induction by phenobarbitone on the pharmacokinetics of paroxetine. Acta Psychiatr Scand 80: 95, 1989b.

Grimsley SR et al.: Increased carbamazepine plasma concentrations after fluoxetine coadministration. Clin Pharmacol Ther 50: 10, 1991.

Grimsley SR et al.: Paroxetine, sertraline, and fluvoxamine: new selective serotonin reuptake inhibitors. Clin Pharm 11: 930, 1992.

Grof E et al.: Effects of lithium, nortriptyline and desamethasone on insulin sensitivity. Prog Neuropsychopharmacol Biol Psychiatry 8: 687, 1984.

Grupp LA et al.: Attenuation of alcohol intake by a serotonin uptake inhibitor: evidence for mediation through the renin angiotensin system. Pharmacol Biochem Behav 30: 823, 1988.

Gulati OD et al.: Antagonism of adrenergic neuron blockade in hypertensive subjects. Clin Pharmacol Ther 7: 510, 1966.

Gundert-Remy U: Lack of interaction between the tetracyclic antidepressant maprotiline and the centrally acting antihypertensive drug clonidine. Eur J Clin Pharmacol 25: 595, 1983.

Hall RC et al.: The effect of desmethylimipramine on the absorption of alcohol and paracetamol. Postgrad Med J 52: 139, 1976.

Hamilton MJ et al.: The effect of bupropion, a new antidepressant drug, and alcohol and their interaction in man. Eur J Clin Pharmacol 25: 75, 1984.

Hammer W et al.: Antidepressant drugs. Garattini S, Dukes M (ed.). *Proceedings from the First International Symposium, Milan (1967)*. International Congress Series No. 122, Amsterdam, Excerpta Medica, 1967, p. 301.

Hansen TE et al.: Interaction of fluoxetine and pentazocine. Am J Psychiatry 147: 949, 1990.

Hansten PD: Clonidine and tricyclic antidepressants. Drug Inter Newsl 4: 13, 1984.

Haraguchi M et al.: Reduction in oral ethanol self-administration in the rat by 5-HT uptake blocker fluoxetine. Pharmacol Biochem Behav 35: 259, 1990.

Hardy JL et al.: Reduction of prothrombin and partial thromboplastin times with trazodone. Can Med Assoc J 135: 1372, 1986.

Harvey AT et al.: Cytochrome P450 enzymes: interpretation of their interactions with selective serotonin reuptake inhibitors. J Clin Psychopharmacol (in press), 1995.

Haskovec L et al.: The action of reserpine in imipramine-resistant depressive patients: A clinical and biochemical study. Psychopharmacologia 11: 18, 1967.

Hedberg DL et al.: Tranylcypromine-trifluoperazine combination in the treatment of schizophrenia. Am J Psychiatry 127: 1141, 1971.

Henauer SA et al.: Cimetidine interaction with imipramine and nortriptyline. Clin Pharmacol Ther 35: 183, 1984.

Hermann DJ et al.: Comparison of verapamil, diltiazem, and labetalol on the bioavailability and metabolism of imipramine. J Clin Pharmacol 32: 176, 1992.

Hindmarch I et al.: The effects of paroxetine and other antidepressants in combination with alcohol on psychomotor activity related to car driving. Acta Psychiatr Scand 80(suppl): 45, 1989.

Hindmarch I et al.: The effects of sertraline on psychomotor performance in elderly volunteers. J Clin Psychiatry 51: 34, 1990.

Hirsch MS et al.: Subarachnoid hemorrhage following ephedrine and MAO inhibitor. JAMA 194: 201, 1965.

Houghton GW et al.: Inhibition of phenytoin metabolism by other drugs used in epilepsy. Int J Clin Pharmacol 12: 210, 1975.

Hubbell CL et al.: Opioidergic, serotonergic, and dopaminergic manipulations and rats' intake of a sweetened alcoholic beverage. Alcohol 8: 355, 1991.

Hughes FW et al.: Delayed audiofeedback (DAF) for induction of anxiety. Effect of nortriptyline, ethanol or nortriptyline-ethanol combinations on performance with DAF. JAMA 185: 556, 1963.

Hui KK: Hypertensive crisis induced by interaction of clonidine with imipramine. J Am Geriatr Soc 31: 164, 1983.

Hullett FJ et al.: Depression associated with nifedipine-induced calcium channel blockade. Am J Psychiatry 145: 1277, 1988.

Hyatt MC et al.: Amitriptyline augments and prolongs ethanol induced euphoria. J Clin Psychopharmacol 7: 277, 1987.

Hyttel J et al.: Neuropharmacological mechanisms of serotonin reuptake inhibitors. In: Research Advances in New Psychopharmacological Treatment for Alcoholism, Amsterdam, Excerpta Medica, Elsevier, 1985, p. 107.

Iruela LM: Toxic interaction of S-adenosylmethionine and clomipramine. Am J Psychiatry 150: 522, 1993.

Jack RA et al.: Possible interaction between phenelzine and amantadine. Arch Gen Psychiatry 41: 726, 1984.

Jalil P: Toxic reactions following the combined administration of fluoxetine and phenytoin: two case reports. J Neurol Neurosurg Psychiatry 55: 412, 1992.

Janowsky EC et al.: Effects of anesthesia on patients taking psychotropic drugs. J Clin Psychopharmacol 1: 14, 1981.

Janowsky EC et al.: What precautions should be taken if a patient on a MAOI is scheduled to undergo anesthesia? J Clin Psychopharmacol 5: 128, 1985.

Jenike MA: Alcohol and antihistamines not contraindicated with MAOIs? Am J Psychiatry 140: 1107, 1983.

Jenike MA et al.: Buspirone augmentation of fluoxetine in patients with obsessive-compulsive disorder. J Clin Psychiatry 52:13, 1991.

Jerling M et al.: The use of therapeutic drug monitoring data to document kinetic drug interactions: an example with amitriptyline and nortriptyline. Ther Drug Monit 16: 1, 1994.

Jermain DM et al.: Potential fluoxetine-selegiline interaction (letter). Ann Pharmacother 26: 1300, 1992.

Joffe RT et al.: Lack of pharmacokinetic interaction of carbamazepine with tranylcypromine. Arch Gen Psychiatry 42: 738, 1985.

Joffe RT et al.: A comparison of triiodothyronine and thyroxine in the potentiation of tricyclic antidepressants. Psychiatry Res 32: 241, 1990.

Joffe RT et al.: Triiodothyronine potentiation of fluoxetine in depressed patients. Can J Psychiatry 37: 48, 1992.

Joffe RT et al.: A placebo-controlled comparison of lithium and triiodothyronine augmentation of tricyclic antidepressants in unipolar refractory depression. Arch Gen Psychiatry 50: 387, 1993a.

Joffe RT et al.: An open study of buspirone augmentation of serotonin reuptake inhibitors in refractory depression. J Clin Psychiatry 54: 269, 1993b.

Jones BD et al.: Interaction of ginseng with phenelzine. J Clin Psychopharmacol 7: 201, 1987.

Joseph AB et al.: Potentially toxic serum concentrations of desipramine after discontinuation of valproic acid. Brain Inj 7: 463, 1993.

Kaskey GB: Possible interaction between MAOI and "ecstasy." Am J Psychiatry 149: 411, 1992.

Katz MR: Raised serum levels of desipramine with the antiarrhythmic propafenone (letter). J Clin Psychiatry 52: 432, 1991.

Kaye CM et al.: A review of the metabolism and pharmacokinetics of paroxetine in man. Acta Psychiatr Scand 80(suppl): 60, 1989.

Kellstein DE et al.: Contrasting effects of acute vs. chronic tricyclic antidepressant treatment on central morphine analgesia. Pain 20: 323, 1984.

Kellstein DE et al.: Effect of chronic treatment with tricyclic antidepressants upon antinociception induced by intrathecal injection of morphine and monoamines. Neuropharmacology 27: 1, 1988.

Khurana RC: Estrogen-imipramine interaction. JAMA 222: 702, 1972.

Kincaid RL et al.: Report of a fluoxetine fatality. J Anal Toxicol 14: 327, 1990.

Kline NS et al.: Protection of patients on MAOIs against hypertensive crises. J Clin Psychopharmacol 1: 410, 1981.

Koch-Weser J: Hemorrhagic reactions and drug interactions in 500 warfarin-treated patients. Clin Pharmacol Ther 14: 139, 1973.

Koe BK et al.: Marked depletion of brain serotonin by p-chlorophenylalanine. Fed Proc 25: 452, 1966.

Kostowski W et al.: A study of the effects of clonidine on the EEG in rats treated with single and multiple doses of antidepressant. Psychopharmacology 84: 85, 1984.

Kostowski W et al.: Activity of diltiazem and nifedipine in some animal models of depression. Pol J Pharmacol Pharm 42: 121, 1990.

Kranzler HR et al.: Placebo-controlled trial of fluoxetine as an adjunct to relapse prevention in alcoholics. Am J Psychiatry 152: 391, 1995.

Krisko I et al.: Severe hyperpyrexia due to tranylcypromine-amphetamine toxicity. Ann Intern Med 70: 559, 1969.

Landauer AA et al.: Alcohol and amitriptyline effects on skills related to driving behavior. Science 163: 1467, 1969.

Larochelle P et al.: Responses to tyramine and norepinephrine after imipramine and trazodone. Clin Pharmacol Ther 26: 24, 1979.

Larson AA et al.: Effect of fluoxetine hydrochloride (Lilly 110140), a specific inhibitor of serotonin uptake, on morphine analgesia and the development of tolerance. Life Sci 2: 1807, 1977.

Lazarus A: Rhabdomyolysis in a depressed patient following overdose with combined drug therapy and alcohol (letter). J Clin Psychopharmacol 10: 154, 1990.

Lee RL et al.: Effect of tricyclic antidepressants on analgesic activity in laboratory animals. Postgrad Med J 56: 19, 1980.

Leishman AWD et al.: Antagonism of guanethidine by imipramine. Lancet 1: 112, 1963.

Lejoyeux M et al.: The serotonin syndrome (letter). Am J Psychiatry 149: 1410, 1992.

Lejoyeux M et al.: Prospective evaluation of the syndrome in depressed inpatients treated with clomipramine. Acta Psychiatr Scan 88: 369, 1993.

Lemberger L et al.: Effect of fluoxetine on psychomotor performance, physiologic response, and kinetics of ethanol. Clin Pharmacol Ther 37: 658, 1985.

Levy AB et al.: Myoclonus, hyperreflexia, and diaphoresis in patients on phenelzine-tryptophan combination treatment. Can J Psychiatry 30: 434, 1985.

Liberzon I et al.: Bupropion and delirium (letter). Am J Psychiatry 147: 1689, 1990.

Linet LS: Treatment of a refractory depression with a combination of fluoxetine and d-amphetamine. Am J Psychiatry 146: 803, 1989.

Linnoila M et al.: Effect of chronic zimelidine and ethanol on psychomotor performance. J Clin Psychopharmacol 5: 148, 1985.

Linnoila M et al.: Effects of fluvoxamine, alone and in combination with ethanol, on psychomotor and cognitive performance and on autonomic nervous system reactivity in healthy volunteers. J Clin Psychopharmacol 13: 175, 1993.

Liu SJ et al.: Increased analgesia and alteration in distribution and metabolism of methadone by desipramine in the rat. J Pharmacol Exp Ther 195: 94, 1975.

Liu SJ et al.: Enhanced development of dispositional tolerance to methadone by desipramine given together with methadone. Life Sci 36: 745, 1985.

Loomis CW et al.: Drug interactions of amitriptyline and nortriptyline with warfarin in the rat. Res Commun Chem Pathol Pharmacol 30: 41, 1980.

Lu MR et al.: Ethanol intake of chickens treated with fenfluramine, fluoxetine, and dietary tryptophan. Alcohol Clin Exp Res 16: 852, 1992.

Lu MR et al.: Ethanol consumption following acute fenfluramine, fluoxetine, and dietary tryptophan. Pharmacol Biochem Behav 44: 931, 1993.

Lydiard RB et al.: Interactions between sertraline and tricyclic antidepressants (letter). Am J Psychiatry 150: 1125, 1993.

Lyness WH et al.: Influence of dopaminergic and serotonergic neurons on intravenous ethanol self-administration in the rat. Pharmacol Biochem Behav 42: 187, 1992.

Maany I: Increase in desipramine serum levels associated with methadone treatment. Am J Psychiatry 146: 1611, 1989.

MacLeod DM: Chorea induced by tranquilizers. Lancet 1: 388, 1964.

Malec D et al.: Effect of quizapine and fluoxetine on analgesic-induced catalepsy and antinociception in the rat. J Pharm Pharmacol 32: 71, 1980.

Marathe PH et al.: Metabolic kinetics of pseudoracemic propranolol in human liver microsomes. Drug Metab Disp 22: 237, 1994.

Markel H et al.: LSD flashback syndrome exacerbated by selective serotonin reuptake inhibitor antidepressants in adolescents. J Pediatr 125: 817, 1994.

Markovitz P et al.: Busipirone augmentation of fluoxetine in obsessive-compulsive disorder. Am J Psychiatry 147: 798, 1990.

Marley E et al.: Interactions of a non-selective monoamine oxidase inhibitor, phenelzine with inhibitors of 5-hydroxytryptamine, dopamine or noradrenaline re-intake. J Psychiatr Res 18: 173, 1984.

Maskall DD et al.: Increased plasma concentration of imipramine following augmentation with fluvoxamine (letter). Am J Psychiatry 150: 1566, 1993.

Mason BJ et al.: Desipramine treatment of alcoholism. Psychopharmacol Bull 27: 155, 1991.

McBride WJ et al.: Effects of Ro 15-4513, fluoxetine and desipramine on the intake of ethanol, water and food by the alcohol-preferring (P) and nonpreferring (NP) lines of rats. Pharmacol Biochem Behav 30: 1045, 1988.

McCormick S et al.: Reversal of fluoxetine-induced anorgasmia by cyproheptadine in two patients. J Clin Psychiatry 51: 383, 1990.

Meert TF: Effects of various serotonergic agents on alcohol intake and alcohol preference in Wistar rats selected at two different levels of alcohol preference. Alcohol Alcohol 28: 157, 1993.

Metz A et al.: Combination of fluoxetine with pemoline in the treatment of major depressive disorder. Int J Clin Psychopharm 6: 93, 1991.

Meyer JF et al.: Insidious and prolonged antagonism of guanethidine by amitriptyline. JAMA 213: 1487, 1970.

Meyer JF et al.: Toxicity secondary to meperidine in patients on monoamine oxidase inhibitors: a case report and critical review. J Clin Psychopharmacol 1: 319, 1981.

Miller DD et al.: Cimetidine-imipramine interaction: a case report. Am J Psychiatry 140: 351, 1983a.

Miller DD et al.: Cimetidine's effect on steady-state serum nortriptyline concentrations. Drug Intell Clin Pharm 17: 904, 1983b.

Miller FP et al.: Comparative effects of p-chlorophenylalanine, p-chloramphetamine and p-chloro-N-methylamphetamine on rat brain norepinephrine, serotonin, 5-hydroxyindole-3-acetic acid. Biochem Pharmacol 19: 435, 1970.

Milner G et al.: The effects of doxepin alone and together with alcohol in relation to driving safety. Med J Aust 1: 837, 1978.

Mindham RHS: Psychiatric symptoms in Parkinsonism. J Neurol Neurosurg Psychiatry 33: 180, 1970.

Mirchandani H et al.: Fatal malignant hyperthermia as a result of ingestion of tranylcypromine (Parnate) combined with white wine and cheese. J Forensic Sci 30: 217, 1985.

Mitchell JR et al.: Guanethidine and related agents. III. Antagonism by drugs which inhibit the norepinephrine pump in man. J Clin Invest 49: 1596, 1970.

Montastruc JL et al.: Pseudophaeochromocytoma in parkinsonian patient treated with fluoxetine plus selegiline (letter). Lancet 341: 555, 1993.

Moody JP et al.: Pharmacokinetic aspects of protriptyline plasma levels. Eur J Clin Pharmacol 11: 51, 1977.

Morgan JP et al.: Imipramine-mediated interference with levodopa absorption from the gastrointestinal tract in man. Neurology 25: 1029, 1975.

Muller N et al.: Extremely long plasma half-life of amitriptyline in a woman with cytochrome P4502D6 29/29 wild-type allele—a slowly reversible interaction with fluoxetine. Ther Drug Monit 13: 533, 1991.

Murphy DL et al.: Monoamine oxidase-inhibiting antidepressants: a clinical update. Psychiatr Clin North Am 7: 549, 1984.

Murphy JM et al.: Monoamine uptake inhibitors attenuate ethanol intake in alcohol-preferring (P) rats. Alcohol 2: 349, 1985.

Murphy JM et al.: Effects of fluoxetine on the intragastric self-administration of ethanol in the alcohol preferring P line of rats. Alcohol 5: 283, 1988.

Naranjo CA et al.: Zimelidine-induced variations in alcohol intake by nondepressed heavy drinkers. Clin Pharmacol Ther 35: 374, 1984a.

Naranjo CA et al.: Acute pharmacokinetic and pharmacodynamic interactions of zimelidine and ethanol. Clin Pharmacol Ther 35: 362, 1984b.

Naranjo CA et al.: Serotonin uptake inhibitors attenuate ethanol intake in problem drinkers. Recent Dev Alcohol 7: 255, 1989.

Naranjo CA et al.: Fluoxetine differentially alters alcohol intake and other consummatory behaviors in problem drinkers. Clin Pharmacol Ther 47: 490, 1990.

Nelson JC et al.: A preliminary, open study of the combination of fluoxetine and desipramine for rapid treatment of major depression. Arch Gen Psychiatry 48: 303, 1991.

Nierenberg AA et al.: One antidepressant fails: What next? A survey of northeastern psychiatrists. J Clin Psychiatry 52: 383, 1991.

Nierenberg DW et al.: The central nervous system serotonin syndrome. Clin Pharmacol Ther 53: 84, 1993.

Nies A, Robinson DS: Monoamine oxidase inhibitors. In: Paykel ES (ed.): Handbook of Affective Disorders, New York, Guilford, 1982, p. 245.

Nunes EV et al.: Imipramine treatment of alcoholism with comorbid depression. Am J Psychiatry 151: 963, 1993.

Ober KF et al.: Drug interactions with guanethidine. Clin Pharmacol Ther 14: 190, 1973.

Ochs JR et al.: Chronic treatment with fluvoxamine, clovoxamine, and placebo: interaction with digoxin and effects on sleep and alertness. J Clin Pharmacol 29: 91, 1989.

Ogura C et al.: Combined thyroid (triiodothyronine)-tricyclic antidepressant treatment in depressive states. Folia Psychiatr Neurol Jpn 28: 179, 1974.

Ossipov MH et al.: Augmentation of central and peripheral morphine analgesia by desipramine. Arch Int Pharmacodyn Ther 259: 222, 1982.

Pataki C et al.: Side effects of methylphenidate and desipramine alone and in combination in children. J Am Acad Child Adolesc Psychiatry 32: 1065, 1993.

Pathak SK: Gross oedema during treatment for depression (letter). Br Med J 2: 1220, 1977.

Patman J et al.: The combined effect of alcohol and amitriptyline on skills similar to motor car driving. Med J Aust 8: 946, 1969.

Paykel ES: Hallucinosis on combined methyldopa and pargyline. Br Med J 1: 803, 1966.

Pearson HJ: Interaction of fluoxetine with carbamazepine. J Clin Psychiatry 51: 126, 1990.

Perel JM et al.: Inhibition of imipramine metabolism by methylphenidate. Fed Proc 28: 418, 1969.

Perucca E et al.: Interaction between phenytoin and imipramine. Br J Clin Pharmacol 4: 485, 1977.

Pick CG et al.: Potentiation of opioid analgesia by the antidepressant nefazodone. Eur J Pharmacol 211: 375, 1992.

Picker W et al.: Potential interaction of LSD and fluoxetine (letter). Am J Psychiatry 149: 843, 1992.

Poldinger W: Combined administration of desipramine and reserpine or tetrabenazine in depressive patients. Psychopharmacologia 4: 308, 1963.

Pond SM et al.: Effects of tricyclic antidepressants on drug metabolism. Clin Pharmacol Ther 18: 191, 1975.

Pope HG et al.: Toxic reaction to the combination of monoamine oxidase inhibitors and tryptophan. Am J Psychiatry 142: 491, 1985.

Prange AJ Jr. et al.: Enhancement of imipramine antidepressant activity by thyroid hormone. Am J Psychiatry 126: 457, 1969.

Prange AJ Jr. et al.: Hormonal alteration of imipramine response: a review. In: Sachar EJ (ed.): Hormones, Behavior, and Psychopathology, New York, Raven, 1976, p. 41.

Preskorn SH: Should bupropion dosage be adjusted based upon therapeutic drug monitoring? Psychopharmacol Bull 27: 637, 1991.

Preskorn SH et al.: Pharmacokinetics of desipramine coadministered with sertraline or fluoxetine. J Clin Psychopharmacol 14: 90, 1994.

Preskorn SH et al.: Serious adverse effects of combining fluoxetine and tricyclic antidepressants. Am J Psychiatry 147: 532, 1990.

Rabkin JG et al.: Adverse reactions to monoamine oxidase inhibitors. Part I. A comparative study. J Clin Psychopharmacol 4: 270, 1984.

Rabkin JG et al.: Adverse reactions to monoamine oxidase inhibitors. Part II. Treatment correlates and clinical management. J Clin Psychopharmacol 5: 2, 1985.

Randell J: Combining the antidepressant drugs. Br Med J 1: 521, 1965.

Raskin DE: Dangers of monoamine oxidase inhibitors (letter). J Clin Psychopharmacol 4: 238, 1984.

Rauch PK et al.: Digoxin toxicity possibly precipitated by trazodone. Psychosomatics 25: 334, 1984.

Reggev A et al.: Bradycardia induced by an interaction between phenelzine and beta blockers. Psychosomatics 30: 106, 1989.

Richelson E et al.: Antagonism by antidepressants of neurotransmitter receptors of normal human brain in vitro. J Pharmacol Exp Ther 230: 94, 1984.

Risch SC et al.: The effects of psychotropic drugs on the cardiovascular system. J Clin Psychiatry 43: 16, 1982.

Rivera-Calimlim L et al.: L-Dopa absorption and metabolism by the human stomach. J Clin Invest 49: 79, 1970.

Rohrig TP et al.: Fluoxetine overdose: a case report. J Anal Toxicol 13: 305, 1989.

Roth A et al.: Delirium associated with the combination of a neuroleptic, an SSRI, and benztropine. J Clin Psychiatry 55: 492, 1994.

Rothschild BS: Fluoxetine-nortriptyline therapy of treatment-resistant major depression in a geriatric patient. J Geriatr Psychiatry Neurol 7: 137, 1994.

Rowe H et al.: The effect of fluoxetine on warfarin metabolism in the rat and man. 23: 807, 1978.

Sandoz M et al.: Biotransformation of amitriptyline in alcoholic depressive patients. Eur J Clin Pharmacol 24: 615, 1983.

Sargent W: Combining the antidepressant drugs (letter). Br Med J 1: 251, 1965.

Sargent W: Safety of combined antidepressive drugs. Br Med J 1: 555, 1971.

Schenker S et al.: Fluoxetine disposition and elimination in cirrhosis. Clin Pharmacol Ther 44: 353, 1988.

Schuckit M et al.: Tricyclic antidepressant and monoamine oxidase inhibitors. Combination therapy in the treatment of depression. Arch Gen Psychiatry 24: 509, 1971.

Seifritz E et al.: Increased triimipramine plasma levels during fluvoxamine comedication. Eur Neuropsychopharmacol 4: 15, 1994.

Seppala T et al.: Effect of tricyclic antidepressants and alcohol on psychomotor skills related to driving. Clin Pharmacol Ther 17: 515, 1975.

Sethna ER: A study of depressive illness and the response to combined antidepressive treatment. Br J Psychiatry 124: 265, 1974.

Shader RI et al.: MAOIs and drug interactions—a proposal for a clearinghouse. J Clin Psychopharmacol 5: A17, 1985.

Shader RI: Can patients on MAOIs safely drinking white wine? J Clin Psychopharmacol 6: 254, 1986.

Sherman KE et al.: Amitriptyline and asymptomatic hypoglycemia. Ann Intern Med 109: 683, 1988.

Shrivastava RK et al.: Hypoglycemia associated with imipramine. Biol Psychiatry 18: 1509, 1983.

Shulman KI et al.: Dietary restriction, tyramine, and the use of monoamine oxidase inhibitors. J Clin Psychopharmacol 9: 397, 1989.

Sides CA: Hypertension during anaesthesia with monoamine oxidase inhibitors. Anaesthesia 42: 633, 1987.

Silverman G et al.: Interaction of benzodiazepines and tricyclic antidepressants (letter). Br Med J 14: 111, 1972.

Sjoqvist F: The pH-dependent excretion of monomethylated tricyclic antidepressants in dogs and man. Clin Pharmacol Ther 10: 826, 1969.

Skjelbo E et al.: Inhibitors of imipramine metabolism by human liver microsomes. Br J Clin Pharmacol 34: 256, 1992.

Skop BP et al.: The serotonin syndrome associated with paroxetine, and over-the-counter cold remedy, and vascular disease. Am J Emerg Med 12: 642, 1994.

Smilkstein MJ et al.: A case of MAO inhibitor/MDMA interaction: agony after ecstasy. J Toxicol Clin Toxicol 25: 149, 1987.

Smookler S et al.: Hypertensive crisis resulting from an MAO inhibitor and an over-the-counter appetite suppressant. Ann Emerg Med 11: 482, 1982.

Sovner R et al.: A potential drug interaction between fluoxetine and valproic acid (letter). J Clin Psychopharmacol 11: 389, 1991.

Sperber AD: Toxic interaction between fluvoxamine and sustained release theophylline in an 11-year-old boy. Drug Safety 6: 460, 1991.

Spigset O et al.: Serotonin syndrome caused by a moclobemide-clomipramine interaction. Br Med J 306: 248, 1993.

Spina E et al.: Interaction between fluvoxamine and imipramine/desipramine in four patients. Therapeutic Drug Monitoring 14: 194, 1992.

Spina E et al.: Fluvoxamine-induced alterations in plasma concentrations of imipramine and desipramine in depressed patients. Int J Clin Pharmacol Res 13: 167, 1993a.

Spina E et al.: Carbamazepine coadministration with fluoxetine or fluvoxamine. Ther Drug Monit 15: 247, 1993b.

Spina E et al.: Effect of fluvoxamine on the pharmacokinetics of imipramine and desipramine in healthy subjects. Ther Drug Monit 15: 243, 1993c.

Staufenberg EF et al.: Malignant hyperpyrexia syndrome in combined treatment. Br J Psychiatry 154: 577, 1989.

Steiner E et al.: Inhibition of desipramine 2-hydroxylation by quinidine and quinine. Clin Pharmacol Ther 43: 577, 1988.

Steiner W et al.: Toxic reaction following the combined administration of fluoxetine and L-tryptophan: five case reports. Biol Psychiatry 21: 1067, 1986.

Sternbach H: Danger of MAOI therapy after fluoxetine withdrawal. Lancet 2: 850, 1988.

Sternbach H: The serotonin syndrome. Am J Psychiatry 148: 705, 1991a.

Sternbach H: Fluoxetine-associated potentiation of calcium channel blockers (letter). J Clin Psychopharmacol 11: 390, 1991b.

Stiff JL et al.: Clonidine withdrawal complicated by amitriptyline therapy. Anesthesiology 59: 73, 1983.

Suchowersky O et al.: Interaction of fluoxetine and selegiline. Can J Psychiatry 35: 571, 1990.

Sullivan EA et al.: Diet and monoamine oxidase inhibitors: a re-examination. Can J Psychopharmacol 3: 249, 1983.

Sutherland DL et al.: The influence of cimetidine versus ranitidine on doxepin pharmacokinetics. Eur J Clin Pharmacol 32: 159, 1987.

Sved AF et al.: Studies on the antihypertensive action of L-tryptophan. J Pharmacol Exp Ther 221: 329, 1982.

Svedmyr N: The influence of tricyclic antidepressive agent (protriptyline) on some circulatory effects of noradrenaline and adrenaline in man. Life Sci 7: 77, 1968.

Swims MP: Potential terfenadine-fluoxetine interaction. Ann Pharmacother 27: 1404, 1993.

Tackley R et al.: Fatal disseminated intravascular coagulation following monoamine oxidase inhibitor/tricyclic interaction. Anaesthesia 42: 760, 1987.

Taiwo YO et al.: Potentiation of morphine antinociception by monamine reuptake inhibitors in the rat spinal cord. Pain 21: 329, 1985.

Tanquary J et al.: Paradoxical reaction to buspirone augmentation of fluoxetine. J Clin Psychopharmacol 10: 377, 1990.

Targurn SD et al.: Thyroid hormone and the TRH test in refractory depression. J Clin Psychiatry 45: 346, 1984.

Tephly TR et al.: Inhibition of drug metabolism vs. inhibition of drug metabolism by steroids. Mol Pharmacol 4: 10, 1968.

Teychenne PF et al.: Interactions of levodopa with inhibitors of monoamine oxidase and L-aromatic amino acid decarboxylase. Clin Pharmacol Ther 18: 273, 1975.

Thase ME et al.: Treatment of imipramine-resistant recurrent depression: I. An open clinical trial of adjunctive L-triiodothyronine. J Clin Psychiatry 50: 385, 1989.

Thomas JM et al.: Case report of a toxic reaction from a combination of tryptophan and phenelzine. Am J Psychiatry 141: 281, 1984.

Thomson AH et al.: Interaction between fluvoxamine and theophylline. Pharm J 249: 137, 1992.

Tollefson GD: Monoamine oxidase inhibitors: a review. J Clin Psychiatry 44: 280, 1983.

Toyama S et al.: Is it safe to combine a selective serotonin reuptake inhibitor with selegeline? Ann Pharmacotherapy 28: 405, 1994.

True B et al.: Profound hypoglycemia with the addition of a tricyclic antidepressant to maintenance sulfonylurea therapy. Am J Psychiatry 144: 1220, 1987.

Tsutsui S et al.: Combined therapy of T3 and antidepressants in depression. J Int Med Res 7: 138, 1979.

Van den Brekel AM et al.: Toxic effects of theophylline caused by fluvoxamine. Can Med Assoc J 151: 1289, 1994.

van Harten J: Clinical pharmacokinetics of selective serotonin reuptake inhibitors. Clin Pharmacokinet 24: 203, 1993.

van Harten J et al.: Fluvoxamine does not interact with alcohol or potentiate alcohol-related impairment of cognitive function. Clin Pharmacol Ther 52: 427, 1992.

van Putten T et al.: Delirium associated with bupropion. J Clin Psychopharmacol 10: 234, 1990.

Van Zwieten PA: Interaction between centrally acting hypotensive drugs and tricyclic antidepressants. Arch Int Pharmacodyn Ther 214: 12, 1975.

Vandel S et al.: Valpromide increases the plasma concentrations of amitriptyline and its metabolite nortriptyline in depressive patients. Ther Drug Monit 10: 386, 1988.

Vaughan DA: Interaction of fluoxetine with tricyclic antidepressants. Am J Psychiatry 145: 1478, 1988.

Vessell ES: Impairment of drug metabolism in man by allopurinol and nortriptyline. N Engl J Med 283: 1484, 1970.

Vigran IM: Dangerous potentiation of meperidine hydrochloride by pargyline hydrochloride. JAMA 187: 163, 1964.

von Moltke LL et al.: Inhibition of desipramine hydroxylation in vitro by serotonin-reuptake-inhibitor antidepressants, and by quinidine and ketoconazole: a model system to predict drug interactions in vivo. J Pharmacol Exp Ther 268: 1278, 1994.

Walker JI: Patient compliance with MAO inhibitor therapy. J Clin Psychiatry 45: 78, 1984.

Walley T et al.: Interaction of metoprolol and fluoxetine (letter). Lancet 341: 967, 1993.

Warrington SJ et al.: Evaluation of possible interactions between ethanol and trazodone or amitriptyline. Neuropsychobiology 15: 31, 1986.

Weller RA et al.: Psychotropic drugs and alcohol: pharmacokinetic and pharmacodynamic interactions. Psychosomatics 25: 301, 1984.

Wharton RN et al.: A potential use for the interaction of methylphenidate with tricyclic antidepressants. Am J Psychiatry 127: 1619, 1971.

Wheatley D: Potentiation of amitriptyline by thyroid hormone. Arch Gen Psychiatry 26: 229, 1972.

White K et al.: Combined monoamine oxidase inhibitor-tricyclic antidepressant treatment: a pilot study. Am J Psychiatry 37: 1422, 1980.

White K et al.: Combined MAOI-tricyclic antidepressant treatment: a reply to Dr. Davidson. J Clin Psychopharmacol 2: 287, 1982.

Whybrow PC et al.: Thyroid function and the response to L-triiodothyronine in depression. Arch Gen Psychiatry 26: 242, 1972.

Williams LT et al.: Thyroid hormone regulation of beta-adrenergic receptor number. J Biol Chem 252: 2787, 1977.

Wilner KD et al.: The effects of sertraline on the pharmacodynamics of warfarin in healthy volunteers. Biol Psychiatry 29: 354, 1991.

Winston F et al.: Combined antidepressant therapy. Br J Psychiatry 118: 301, 1971.

Woods DJ et al.: Interaction of phenytoin and fluoxetine. NZ Med J 107: 19, 1994.

Woolfrey S et al.: Fluoxetine-warfarin interaction. Br Med J 307: 241, 1993.

Wright JM et al.: Isoniazid-induced carbamazepine toxicity and vice versa. N Engl J Med 18: 1325, 1982.

Yagiela JA: Drug interactions and vasoconstrictors used in local anesthetic solutions. Oral Surg Oral Med Oral Pathol 59: 565, 1985.

Yaryura-Tobias JA et al.: Fluoxetine and bleeding in obsessive compulsive disorder (letter). Am J Psychiatry 148: 949, 1991.

Young JPR et al.: Controlled trial of trimipramine, monoamine oxidase inhibitor and combined treatment in depressed outpatients. Br Med J 2: 1315, 1979.

Zabik JE et al.: Serotonin and ethanol aversion in the rat. In: *Research Advances in New Psychopharmacological Treatment for Alcoholism*, Amsterdam, Excerpta Medica, Elsevier, 1985, p. 87.

Zeidenberg P et al.: Clinical and metabolic studies with imipramine in man. J Clin Psychiatry 127: 1321, 1971.

Zetin M: Combined use of trazodone and phenelzine in depression: case report. J Clin Psychiatry 45: 182, 1984.

Zetin M et al.: MAOI reaction with powdered protein dietary supplement. J Clin Psychiatry 48: 499, 1987.

Zornberg GL et al.: Severe adverse interaction between pethidine and selegiline. Lancet 337: 246, 1991.

3

Antipsychotics

DONALD C. GOFF, ROSS J. BALDESSARINI

Pharmacology of Antipsychotic Agents

Antipsychotic (neuroleptic) agents can interact with several classes of drugs, resulting in a wide range of potential clinical effects. Pharmacokinetic interactions may result from alterations in absorption, hepatic metabolism, or binding to plasma proteins, whereas pharmacodynamic interactions may arise from effects on central dopaminergic systems or effects on noradrenergic, muscarinic, or histaminergic receptors. Because the therapeutic index (risk ratio) is very large for antipsychotic agents with respect to lethal versus therapeutic doses, most interactions are not life-threatening, although they may adversely affect clinical outcome if not recognized and managed appropriately. The increasingly common practice of prescribing low doses of antipsychotic drugs makes certain drug interactions particularly likely to impair therapeutic efficacy.

Conventional antipsychotic agents comprise a chemically diverse collection of compounds that have in common antagonism of dopamine D_2 and related "D_2-like" (D_3, D_4) receptors, with variable interactions with D_1 or D_5 receptors. With the exception of the atypical agent clozapine, D_2 receptor affinity correlates highly with antipsychotic clinical potency (Creese et al. 1976). Recent studies based on positron emission tomography (PET) brain scanning methods with D_2-selective radioligands indicate that maximal D_2 receptor occupancy of approximately 80 to 85% occurs at daily doses of 10 to 15 mg and plasma concentrations of about 15 to 20 ng/ml of haloperidol or at commonly employed doses of other typical neuroleptics, and probably corresponds with maximal antipsychotic effects in many

129

patients (Farde et al. 1988, 1989a). Higher doses or plasma concentrations evidently produce no appreciable therapeutic gain and may be associated with worsening of side effects. Clozapine is considered an "atypical" antipsychotic because it produces minimal extrapyramidal side effects or hyperprolactinemia. Clozapine produces a substantial reduction in symptom severity (by 20%) in 30 to 60% of patients resistant to conventional antipsychotic therapy (Baldessarini and Frankenburg 1991). Clozapine does not follow the same dose-response relationship with regard to D_2 receptor occupancy, as it produces optimal therapeutic effects at occupancy levels of only 40 to 60%, reached at daily doses of about 300 to 500 mg (Farde et al. 1992). Risperidone is the first of several new antipsychotic agents that combine dopamine D_2 receptor antagonism with serotonin $5HT_2$ receptor antagonism. Preliminary evidence suggests that such D_2-S_2 agents may produce fewer extrapyramidal symptoms (EPS) than conventional neuroleptics, at least within a limited range of doses, and may be more effective for negative symptoms and depression (Borison 1995, Chouinard et al. 1993, Leysen et al. 1993, Marder and Meibach 1994).

Virtually all antipsychotic agents are rapidly absorbed after oral administration (peak plasma concentrations in 2–4 hours), are relatively lipophilic, and have correspondingly large apparent volumes of distribution (V_d = 8–30 L/kg). The "depot" decanoate esters of fluphenazine and haloperidol are injected intramuscularly in an oil vehicle and then slowly converted to the free active drug by esterases in muscle, blood, and other tissues (Marder et al. 1989). Diffusion of the esterified drug from the oil depot is the rate-limiting factor in absorption of these preparations (Dreyfuss et al. 1976a,b). With the exception of molindone, antipsychotic agents are highly protein bound. The proportion of free drug typically is less than 10% of total plasma concentration and may closely approximate concentrations in the cerebral spinal fluid (CSF); in some studies the plasma-free fraction has correlated reasonably well with therapeutic outcome (Farde et al. 1989b, Forsman and Ohman 1977b, Garver 1989, Rimon et al. 1981, Wode-Helgodt et al. 1978). Although the unbound fraction may theoretically be expected to represent the concentration of drug available to critical brain receptor sites, this fraction is technically difficult to measure, may vary as much as 10-fold among individuals, and generally is proportional to plasma drug levels (Curry 1970). In addition, some highly lipophilic antipsychotic agents (such as the butyrophenones) concentrate 10- to 20-fold in brain tissue, so that levels of antipsychotic agents in the proximity of relevant drug receptor sites may be much higher than levels found in plasma or CSF (Sunderland and Cohen 1987). It is therefore not suprising that measurement of unbound concentrations in plasma has not replaced conventional assays of total serum concentration of antipsychotic drugs. At typical clinical doses, the high-potency agents (such as haloperidol or fluphenazine) generally produce plasma concentrations in the range of 1 to 25 ng/ml, whereas low potency agents (such as chlorpromazine, clozapine, or thioridazine) produce levels of parent compound typically between 100 and 500 ng/ml (Cohen et al. 1979).

Most antipsychotic drugs are extensively metabolized by the liver, primarily through enzyme-mediated microsomal oxidation and conjugation reactions. Haloperidol and other butyrophenones are metabolized primarily by N-dealkylation that separates the side chain from the phenylpiperidine moiety, yielding two inactive fragments. Many drugs increase or decrease activity of the microsomal cytochrome P450 oxidative enzymes of the liver responsible for much of the metabolic clearance of common drug molecules, and therefore may produce potentially important alterations in metabolism of antipsychotic drugs. The magnitude of such effects varies markedly among individuals. Ereshefsky and colleagues (1991) compared clearance rates of thiothixene between patients coadministered hepatic oxidase enzyme-inducing drugs (e.g. anticonvulsants) and enzyme inhibitors (e.g. cimetidine) and found a greater than 10-fold difference between the two groups. A specific P450 enzyme isoform (CYP-2D6), which is located in human liver and brain, metabolizes the phenothiazines, thioridazine and perphenazine, resperidone, and the dibenzodiazepines, clozapine and fluperlapine, although the importance of this metabolic pathway for clozapine *in vivo* is unclear (Fischer et al. 1992, Heykants et al. 1994). In addition, CYP-2D6 metabolizes the antidepressants nortriptyline, desipramine, and clomipramine and other agents (Jerling et al. 1994b). Although not metabolized by CYP-2D6, haloperidol and fluphenazine display high affinities for this enzyme (inhibitory constant, K_i of about 1 μM) and therefore may inhibit the metabolism of other drugs by this enzyme (Fischer et al. 1992, Fonne-Pfister and Meyer 1988). A genetically determined deficiency of CYP-2D6, characterized by slowed metabolism of standard test agents such as debrisoquine and sparteine, is found in 7% of whites and probably is responsible for markedly slowed metabolism of certain antipsychotic agents in a small minority of patients (Steiner et al. 1988, Zanger et al. 1988). Brosen and Gram (1989) estimated that 20 to 30% of the general population fall at the extremes of the normal distribution of CYP-2D6 activity, and so are either unusually rapid or poor metabolizers of many drugs. Von Bahr and colleagues (1991) studied plasma concentrations of thioridazine in slow and rapid metabolizers of debrisoquin and found a 2.4-fold higher maximum concentration in slow metabolizers. Kalow and colleagues (1991) reported that Asians have low activity levels of CYP-2D6, which can result in slower clearance of perphenazine, clozapine, and thioridazine. However, Bertilsson and colleagues (1991) found fewer poor metabolizers of debrisoquine among Chinese compared to Swedish subjects (1% vs. 7%). Asians do not differ from whites in their rate of clearance of haloperidol (Lin et al. 1989).

Because all antipsychotic agents are subject to considerable first-pass enterohepatic metabolism when administered orally, their bioavailability is increased substantially following parenteral administration (Jorgensen 1986). For example, the bioavailability of the oral form of haloperidol has been calculated between 60 and 70%, and virtually 100% with intramuscularly injected haloperidol or its decanoate as compared with intravenous injection (Forsman and Ohman 1977a, Verghese et al. 1991). Phenothiazines produce many metabolites of varying biologic activity (Jorgensen 1986); for example, about 75 metabolites of chlorpromazine have been identified (Turano et al. 1973). The large number of potentially active metabolites may limit the clinical relevance of assays of plasma concentrations of a parent tricyclic antipsychotic compound. Activity of drug at D_2 receptors using radioreceptor competition assays that measure the ability of a drug and its metabolites to displace a radiolabeled receptor ligand from homogenates of animal basal ganglia would seem to represent a means of assaying all neuropharmacologically active molecular species in a clinical serum sample. Nevertheless, such assays have proved to be no better than chemical assays of parent drugs in predicting antipsychotic responses or extrapyramidal side effects (Baldessarini et al. 1988, Cohen et al. 1980, Cooper 1985, Creese and Snyder 1977, Van Putten et al. 1991). In contrast to the complex array of active metabolites produced by the phenothiazines, thioxanthenes, and other tricyclic antipsychotic agents, only the reduced metabolite of haloperidol, hydroxy-haloperidol, yields antipsychotic activity. However, it remains uncertain whether this metabolite possesses intrinsic antipsychotic activity in addition to its potential to be oxidized back to the ketone haloperidol (Ereshefsky et al. 1984, Ko et al. 1989, Korpi and Wyatt 1984, Straw et al. 1989, Verghese et al. 1991). Clozapine is almost entirely metabolized by the liver, producing a prominent, active N-desmethyl metabolite, norclozapine, and several relatively inactive and less prevalent N-oxide and ring hydroxy metabolites (Centorrino et al. 1994, in press, Lieberman et al. 1989).

Great individual variability exists in the metabolism of neuroleptic and other psychotropic agents, such that mean plasma concentrations may not correlate closely with oral dose, and may vary by more than 10-fold among patients receiving the same dose (Dahl 1986, Midha et al. 1988c). Dysken and colleagues (1981) found a 40-fold variation in steady-state plasma concentrations of fluphenazine during treatment with an oral daily dose of 20 mg. Reported nominal plasma elimination half-lives for most antipsychotic agents fall in the range of 10 to 30 hours, but may be misleading for some agents, particularly the butyrophenones. Increasingly sensitive assay methods have revealed complex, multicompartmental half-lives for haloperidol, with near-terminal elimination half-life values of 1 week or more (Hubbard et al. 1987, Khot et al. 1993, Midha et al. 1989). Neuroleptic levels routinely can be detected in blood, urine, and feces for many months after prolonged exposure to relatively large oral clinical doses (Sramek et al. 1987). Moreover, some clinical PET D_2 ligand-binding studies suggest that washout of haloperidol from human brain may be even slower than the rate of disappearance of the drug from plasma (Farde et al. 1989b). Slowly turning over pools also have been described for total body elimination of promazine (Curry and Hu 1990) and haloperidol (Khot et al. 1993), presumably representing very gradual release of drug from fat- and tissue-binding sites. The half-life for recovery of behavioral response to the dopamine agonist apomorphine was found to be more than 1 week in the rat following acute injection of an ED_{50} dose of haloperidol with residual antagonism persisting for up to 6 weeks (Campbell et al. 1985). Even a single ED_{50} dose of fluphenazine, which follows a simpler, more monophasic tissue elimination half-life in rat brain (Cohen et al. 1992) and human plasma (Midha et al. 1988a) than does haloperidol, can induce complex late *functional* changes in response to the dopamine agonist indicative of acute supersensitivity that requires several weeks to normalize (Cohen et al. 1992). These findings further emphasize the difficulties in predicting the impact of changes in peripheral drug metabolism on antipsychotic activity at brain receptor sites.

The following sections summarize current knowledge of interactions of neuroleptic agents with other classes of substances (*see* Table 3.1).

Table 3.1.
Interactions with Antipsychotic Agents[a]

Drug	Interaction
Alcohol	Additive sedation, incoordination
	HAL increases alcohol levels
	Alcohol may worsen EPS
Antacids	Impair absorption of CPZ
Anticholinergics	Additive anticholinergic effects
	Inconsistent effects on APD levels
	Inconsistent effects on APD efficacy
	Cognitive impairment, especially in the elderly
Anticonvulsants	
Carbamazepine	Decreases HAL and CLZ levels (ca. 50%)
	May induce delirium
Phenytoin	May decrease HAL, CPZ & CLZ levels (ca. 50%)
Phenobarbital	Lowers CPZ, TDZ & HAL levels (ca. 50%)
	TDZ lowers phenobarbital levels
	Additive sedative effects
Valproic Acid	Levels increased by CPZ
	Minor increase of CLZ levels (ca. 6%)
Antidepressants	
Tricyclics	Increase levels of CPZ, PPZ, HAL (ca. 50%)
	Nortriptyline levels increased by HAL & PPZ (ca. 10–30%)
	Desipramine levels increased by APDs (ca. 100%)
	Inconsistent effects on APD efficacy
Fluoxetine	Increases HAL levels (ca. 20%)
	Increases CLZ levels (ca. 76%)
	May cause or worsen EPS
Fluvoxamine	Increases CLZ levels
Other SSRIs	Not adequately evaluated
Anxiolytics	
Alprazolam	Increases levels of HAL and FPZ
Buspirone	Increases HAL levels (ca. 26%)
Antidiarrheals	
Attapulgite	Impairs absorbtion of promazine
Aluminum salts	May lower CPZ levels
CARDIAC AGENTS	
Antiarrhythmics	
Quinidine and	Additive cardiac depression and impaired conduction
Procainamide	when added to low-potency APDs (CLZ, CPZ, TDZ)
Antihypertensives	
Alpha methyldopa	CPZ & HAL may increase hypotension
	Added to APDs may cause confusion & behavioral deterioration
Guanethidine	APDs (except molindone) reverse antihypertensive effect
Propranolol	Levels increased by CPZ
	Increases CPZ & TDZ levels

(continued)

Interactions with Antipsychotic Agents[a]

Drug	Interaction
Pressors	
Epinephrine	Severe hypotension
Cimetidine	Lowers CPZ levels (ca. 33%)
	May inhibit metabolism of some APDs (CLZ)
Disulfiram	Lowers levels of PPZ
Lithium	May increase CPZ levels
	May cause or worsen EPS
	May cause neurotoxicity; effect on NMS not established
Orphenadrine	May cause hypoglycemia with CPZ
Stimulants	May impair APD efficacy
Amphetamine	Metabolism delayed by CPZ
Tobacco	Decreases levels of CPZ, FPZ, HAL (ca. 10–50%)
	Decreases parkinsonism

[a] APDs = antipsychotic drugs; CLZ = clozapine; CPZ = chlorpromazine; EPS = extrapyramidal symptoms; FPZ = fluphenazine; HAL = haloperidol; PMZ = promazine; PPZ = perphenazine; TDZ = thioridazine.

Alcohol

Evidence of Interaction

Alcohol alters the disposition (pharmacokinetics) and action (pharmacodynamics) of many drugs, yet its potential interactions with antipsychotic medications have received little attention. On repeated administration, alcohol induces synthesis and thus activity of enzymes of the hepatic cytochrome P450-2E family, and also may act acutely as a competitive inhibitor against drugs metabolized by these enzymes (Shoaf and Linnoila 1991). When a patient is actively drinking alcohol, metabolism of certain drugs may be competitively inhibited, whereas during periods of abstinence, metabolism may be enhanced (Lieber 1990). These effects may be further complicated by the strong association between alcohol consumption and cigarette smoking, since tobacco smoke is a potent inducer of several hepatic microsomal enzymes. Alcohol can affect the rate and extent of absorption of other drugs (Mezey 1976) and chronic alcohol use may reduce levels of plasma proteins, resulting in a higher free fraction of some highly bound drugs (Lieber 1988). Focal application of alcohol in rat brain increases release of dopamine, suggesting a potential pharmacodynamic interaction between alcohol and dopaminergic systems (Matilla 1990, Wozniak et al. 1991).

Despite the high frequency with which alcohol is consumed by patients treated with antipsychotic medication, interactions between these two drugs rarely have been reported. Morselli and colleagues (1971) measured blood alcohol levels and dexterity in 16 normal subjects after administration of alcohol, then repeated this procedure after the subjects had received chlorpromazine 200 mg/day or haloperidol 6 mg/day for 10 days. Blood levels of alcohol were significantly elevated in subjects receiving haloperidol but not in subjects receiving chlorpromazine. Although dexterity and alertness were impaired to the greatest degree by alcohol in subjects pretreated with haloperidol, it is unclear if this effect represents a drug interaction, since the effect of haloperidol alone on these measures was not determined. Seppala (1976) clarified this issue by performing a 14-day, double-blind, crossover study of the combination of chlorpromazine (30 mg daily for 7 days and 690 mg daily for 7 days) or the benzamide D_2 antagonist sulpiride (150 mg daily) with alcohol in 20 healthy volunteers. Chlorpromazine alone significantly impaired reaction time and coordination; the combination of chlorpromazine and alcohol produced impairments of reaction time, coordination, and proprioception more severe than the two neuroleptics alone or the combination of alcohol and sulpiride. Lack of an effect of sulpiride may reflect its limited access to the central nervous system (CNS) at such moderate doses. Chlorpromazine did not affect ethanol blood concentrations.

Lutz (1976) observed that akathisia and dystonic reactions occurred in 7 patients receiving stable, previously well-tolerated doses of antipsychotic medication when they started drinking alcohol. The EPS quickly subsided when patients ceased drinking alcohol or when an anticholinergic agent was added.

Mechanism

Haloperidol may increase blood alcohol concentrations by inhibiting hepatic enzymes. Sedation and incoordination are additive when antipsychotic agents are combined with alcohol and may be further intensified by pharmacokinetic interactions that may raise plasma concentrations of each drug. Potential pharmacodynamic interactions mediated by alcohol's effect on dopaminergic systems have not been studied.

Clinical Implications

Patients taking antipsychotic agents should be advised that consuming alcohol can result in potentially dangerous sedation and incoordination and may increase risk for extrapyramidal reactions such as dystonia and akathisia. Haloperidol also may interfere with the metabolism of alcohol, so that patients may become intoxicated after consuming alcohol at previously tolerated levels. Chronic alcohol use can be expected to complicate antipsychotic therapy and is associated with poorer outcome, although probably due to complex effects of comorbidity rather than a simple pharmacologic interaction. The sudden appearance of extrapyramidal symptoms in patients treated with a stable dose of antipsychotic medication might raise the question of acute alcohol use, although this possible interaction has not been firmly established.

Antacids

Evidence of Interaction

Antacids may impair absorption of antipsychotic agents. Forrest and colleagues (1970) administered a suspension of aluminum and magnesium hydroxide for 2 to 7 days to 10 patients who had been receiving chlorpromazine at daily doses of 400 to 1,200 mg for at least 12 weeks. The antacid decreased urinary excretion of chlorpromazine by 10 to 45%. Fann and colleagues (1973) measured plasma concentrations before and 2 hours after administration of a liquid suspension of chlorpromazine to 6 patients who had been medication-free for 7 days. Two days later, this procedure was repeated, but with the added administration of 30 ml of a gel of magnesium trisilicate with aluminum hydroxide immediately before, plus 10 minutes after administration of chlorpromazine. Plasma chlorpromazine concentrations were lower in all 6 patients when the neuroleptic was coadministered with the antacid. While this study demonstrated impaired absorption, it is not possible to determine whether the antacid decreased bioavailability or merely delayed complete absorption. In a similar study, Pinell and colleagues (1978) did not find a decrease in plasma concentrations of chlorpromazine after its administration with two forms of gel antacids (magnesium hydroxide with aluminum hydrochloride and calcium carbonate with glycine). Finally, a case of clinical worsening was associated with administration of aluminum hydroxide gel to a schizophrenic patient previously stabilized on haloperidol (Goldstein 1982).

Mechanism

It is assumed that chlorpromazine, and possibly other antipsychotic drugs, become bound to the gel-type antacids, reducing or delaying drug absorption (Forrest et al. 1970). Alterations of urinary pH as a result of antacid therapy also might affect the urinary excretion of metabolites of chlorpromazine, although such an effect is probably minor.

Clinical Implications

Intestinal absorption of chlorpromazine is impaired when administered with gel-type antacids composed of magnesium or aluminum hydroxide. This potential interaction has not been studied systematically with other psychotropic compounds, although a case report by Goldstein and colleagues (1982) suggests it may occur with haloperidol as well. The clinical significance of such an interaction is difficult to estimate, since it depends in part on plasma concentrations achieved prior to addition of the antacid, and on the temporal relation between administration of the two drugs. Patients treated with a relatively low dose of antipsychotic medication given within 2 hours of a gel antacid may experience clinically significant loss of antipsychotic efficacy. This problem is best avoided by administering the drugs separately—for example, the neuroleptic at bedtime, at least 4 hours after the last daily dose of antacid, or by use of parenteral (depot) forms of neuroleptic.

Anticonvulsants

Evidence of Interaction

With the exception of valproate and felbamate, most anticonvulsants induce hepatic microsomal enzymes and can lower plasma concentrations of many other drugs, including coumadin, steroids, phenytoin, and antidepressants, as well as neuroleptics (Faigle et al. 1976, Hansen et al. 1971, Ketter et al. 1991). Barbiturates significantly lower plasma concentrations of chlorpromazine and haloperidol when given repeatedly with these agents (Forrest et al. 1970, Linnoila et al. 1980). The combination of phenobarbital and thioridazine resulted in decreased concentrations of both phenobarbital and mesoridazine (a prominent active metabolite of thioridazine) (Ellenor et al. 1978, Gay and Marsden 1983, Linnoila et al. 1980). Phenytoin similarly decreases plasma concentrations of chlorpromazine, clozapine and haloperidol (Haidvkewycz and Rodin 1985, Linnoila et al. 1980, Miller 1991). Its combination with thioridazine has resulted in decreased levels of mesoridazine, but variably increased or decreased levels of phenytoin (Gay and Marsden 1983, Vincent 1980).

Unlike other anticonvulsants, valproic acid *inhibits* hepatic enzymes (Bourgeois 1988). It may elevate plasma concentrations of tricyclic antidepressants (Bertschy et al. 1990) but produces only minor increases in circulating levels of clozapine (Centorrino et al. 1994).

Best studied is carbamazepine, a powerful inducer of hepatic microsomal enzymes that increases its own metabolism and that of many other drugs. Induction of hepatic oxidases occurs over several weeks of treatment with carbamazepine. Addition of carbamazepine to haloperidol can reduce plasma concentrations of haloperidol by more than half (Arana et al. 1986b, Jann et al. 1985, Kahn et al. 1990, Kidron et al. 1985). This combination has resulted in clinical worsening of patients receiving typical, moderate doses of haloperidol (10–15 mg daily) (Arana et al. 1986b, Fast et al. 1986) but not at higher daily doses above 20 mg (Ereshefsky et al. 1984, Jann et al. 1985, Kidron et al. 1985). Carbamazepine is also reported to decrease levels of clozapine by 50% (Jerling et al. 1994a).

In addition to effects of lowering levels of haloperidol, the combination of haloperidol with carbamazepine was associated with delirium in 2 patients; 1 patient had tolerated each drug administered separately (Kanter et al. 1984, Yerevanian and Hodgman 1985). This interaction suggests a pharmacodynamically based form of intoxication.

Mechanism

Most anticonvulsants can significantly lower plasma concentrations of antipsychotic drugs by inducing the activity of hepatic microsomal enzymes.

Clinical Implications

Clinicians should monitor for emergence of psychotic symptoms and be prepared to increase the dose of antipsychotic after addition of carbamazepine, phenytoin, or a barbiturate. Since induction of hepatic metabolism may require several weeks, clinical deterioration can be gradual or delayed. Similarly, clinicians should monitor for extrapyramidal symptoms or other signs of antipsychotic toxicity following discontinuation of anticonvulsants. Addition of an anticonvulsant is most likely to result in clinical worsening if a low dose of antipsychotic is being used. Clinicians can anticipate drug interactions by increasing the antipsychotic dose by 30 to 50% when adding an anticonvulsant and similarly decrease the dose when stopping an anticonvulsant. However, these are clinical situations in which measurement of antipsychotic plasma concentrations can be useful.

Combination of an anticonvulsant and antipsychotic agent can occasionally induce delirious intoxication, even at doses that are tolerated when each agent is given individually. Valproate does not enhance clearance of antipsychotic drugs and may even increase drug levels slightly. It can be combined safely with clozapine—for example, for prophylaxis against seizures at high doses of clozapine.

Anticholinergic Agents

Evidence for Interaction

Anticholinergic agents are widely prescribed with antipsychotic agents to prevent or treat extrapyramidal symptoms. They are very effective in reducing the incidence of dystonic reactions when administered prophylactically during the first weeks of antipsychotic administration. In several placebo-controlled trials, anticholinergic prophylaxis reduced the rate of dystonia by half overall, but by 5- to 8-fold with high-potency neuroleptics (Arana et al. 1988). Because risk for dystonia is inversely correlated with age, elderly patients probably do not require prophylactic treatment with an anticholinergic agent and indeed are at increased risk of drug-induced delirium (Arana et al. 1988).

Studies of the addition or withdrawal of anticholinergic agents in patients treated for prolonged periods with antipsychotic agents have produced mixed results. Several investigators found that most patients did not experience a clinically significant worsening of extrapyramidal symptoms when these agents are withdrawn (Comaty et al. 1990, Klett et al. 1972, McEvoy 1983, Orlov et al. 1971). However, Manos and colleagues (Manos et al. 1981a, 1986) found substantial worsening of extrapyramidal symptoms in up to 68% of patients, as well as a deterioration in psychiatric symptomatology when an anticholinergic agent was withdrawn under placebo-controlled conditions from patients receiving long-term treatment with relatively high doses of high-potency antipsychotic agents. Prolonged treatment with anticholinergic agents may be necessary in some patients who suffer from persistent parkinsonism, although some patients may experience partial attenuation of bradykinesia over time or with reduction of antipsychotic dose (World Health Organization 1990). Rapid withdrawal of an anticholinergic antiparkinsonism agent also may precipitate worsening of extrapyramidal symptoms (Goff et al. 1991a), presumably by transiently elevated central cholinergic activity (Tandon et al. 1989a). While gradual discontinuation may avoid this reaction, it may not prevent emergence of parkinsonism and, in some cases, worsening of psychiatric symptoms (Manos et al. 1981b).

The continued use of anticholinergic agents beyond early prophylaxis for dystonia may have important negative consequences, particularly in the elderly. Several studies have demonstrated substantial impairment of memory and cognitive functioning at typical clinical doses of these agents (Baker et al. 1983, McEvoy and Freter 1989, Strauss et al. 1990, Tune et al. 1982). Tune and colleagues (1982) demonstrated that memory impairment in stabilized schizophrenic patients was significantly correlated with anticholinergic drug activity in serum as detected by radioreceptor competition assay, but was unrelated to similarly measured serum neuroleptic levels. Cognitive impairment may be sufficiently severe as to interfere with efforts at rehabilitation. Use of the catecholamine-enhancing agent amantadine (at daily doses below 300 mg) for neuroleptic-induced parkinsonism may carry less risk of cognitive impairment than anticholinergic agents, particularly in the elderly (Gelenberg et al. 1989, McEvoy et al. 1987).

The impact of anticholinergic agents on plasma concentrations and efficacy of antipsychotic agents has been a subject of disagreement. Some early studies indicated that trihexyphenidyl lowered plasma concentrations of chlorpromazine by as much as 45% (Rivera-Calimlim et al. 1973, 1976, Gautier et al. 1977). However, better-designed trials did not confirm this observation (Simpson et al. 1980) and found no evidence of appreciable pharmacokinetic interactions between benztropine and haloperidol (Goff et al. 1991a), biperiden and haloperidol or thioridazine (Linnoila et al. 1980), biperiden and perphenazine (Hansen et al. 1979), biperiden and remoxipride (Yisak et al. 1993), or with other comparable drug combinations (Goff and Baldessarini 1993, Hansen et al. 1979, Hitri et al. 1987, Otani et al. 1990). Simpson and colleagues (1980) added trihexylphenidyl or a placebo to chlorpromazine in middle-aged patients with chronic schizophrenia and found no effect on chlorpromazine levels, whereas Rockland and colleagues (1990) reported a 41% mean *elevation* of chlorpromazine levels in young adult patients.

Whether anticholinergic agents may affect antipsychotic efficacy through pharmacodynamic interactions also has been debated (Ziemba et al. 1978). Singh and colleagues (1973, 1975a,b) reported that addition of benztropine to haloperidol or chlorpromazine produced clinical worsening, consisting of increased hostility, belligerence, suspiciousness, and uncooperativeness. These results are difficult to interpret, however, since the specific clinical features that were affected were not consistent between or within trials. Two uncontrolled trials by other investigators also reported clinical worsening associated with addition of an anticholinergic agent (Johnstone et al. 1988, Tandon et al. 1990). In a well-designed placebo-controlled trial, Johnstone and colleagues (1983) added the anticholinergic agent procyclidine to the thioxanthene neuroleptic, flupenthixol, and found an increase in ratings of psychosis, flat affect and depression in the group receiving the anticholinergic agent. Conversely, the majority of trials did not find adverse effects on any clinical ratings when anticholinergic agents were added to an antipsychotic agent (Chien et al. 1979, Gardos et al. 1984, Gerlach et al. 1977, Goff et al. 1991a, Hanlon et al. 1966, Johnson 1975, Otani et al. 1990, Simpson et al. 1980).

In a series of studies, Tandon and colleagues (1988, 1989b, 1990, 1991, Tandon and Greden 1989) reported that anticholinergic agents improved negative symptoms of schizophrenia when added to antipsychotic agents or given alone, and suggested that a relative excess of central cholinergic function may contribute to emotional withdrawal in schizophrenia. This hypothesis further proposed a reciprocal relationship between negative and positive symptoms, so that anticholinergic agents are expected to worsen positive psychotic symptoms (agitation, hallucinations, delusions) while improving negative symptoms. However, a recent placebo-controlled trial of trihexylphenidyl in otherwise medication-free chronic schizophrenic patients failed to detect any effect of this anticholinergic agent on psychotic or negative symptoms (Goff et al. 1994).

Finally, combining an anticholinergic agent with a low-potency antipsychotic agent may produce additive anticholinergic adverse effects. Cases have been reported of fatal paralytic ileus and hyperpyrexia associated with combined treatment with a phenothiazine and an anticholinergic agent, although the same adverse reactions also have been reported with phenothiazines alone (Evans et al. 1979, Giordano et al. 1975, Mann and Bolger 1978, Zelman and Guillan 1970). Two placebo-controlled trials detected only minimal peripheral anticholinergic side effects associated with the addition of benztropine mesylate (4 mg daily) to typical clinical doses of haloperidol (Goff et al. 1991a, Winslow et al. 1986), suggesting that additive toxicity is more probable when the antipsychotic itself is appreciably anticholinergic (particularly clozapine, thioridazine, mesoridazine).

Mechanism of Interaction

Anticholinergic antiparkinson agents act by blocking central muscarinic acetylcholine receptors in the basal ganglia; presumably, toxic effects arise from similar actions at central cognitive centers or in peripheral parasympathetically innervated tissues. Because low potency antipsychotic agents also antagonize these receptors, anticholinergic side effects may be additive when such drugs are combined. Although it has been suggested that anticholinergic agents may reduce gastric motility and alter absorption of antipsychotic agents, controlled trials have not demonstrated such an interaction consistently. In addition, cholinergic receptors are known to modulate dopaminergic activity, and an inverse relationship may exist between cholinergic and dopaminergic activity levels.

Clinical Implications

Pharmacokinetic interactions between anticholinergic and antipsychotic agents, if they occur, appear to be inconsistent and generally of small magnitude. More important is the potential for cognitive impairment caused by additive anticholinergic activity, particularly in elderly patients given a low-potency antipsychotic drug. When an anticholinergic agent is combined with a low-potency antipsychotic agent, serious adverse effects may be produced, such as delirium, paralytic ileus, or hyperthermia.

Antidepressants

Evidence of Interaction

Several studies have indicated that tricyclic antidepressants and antipsychotic agents may interact by inhibiting the hepatic metabolism of both agents. Gram and colleagues (Brosen and Gram 1989, Gram et al. 1974, Gram and Overo 1972) reported that urinary excretion of nortriptyline and imipramine decreased by as much as 50% following addition of haloperidol, chlorpromazine, or perphenazine, although plasma concentrations of nortriptyline increased by only 10 to 30%. Flupenthixol did not affect antidepressant metabolism (Gram et al. 1974). In additional studies (Gram et al. 1973, Overo et al. 1977), this group determined that the clearance of tricyclic antidepressants was reduced in some patients by 50% following addition of antipsychotic agents, primarily as a result of inhibiting hepatic ring-hydroxylation of the tricyclic. However, Kragh-Sorenson and colleagues (1977) found no effect of perphenazine on nortriptyline metabolism. Vandel and colleagues (1979) observed that addition of phenothiazine to amitriptyline produced significant elevations of nortriptyline plasma concentrations but not of amitriptyline concentrations. Nelson and Jatlow (1980) compared plasma concentrations of desipramine in 15 depressed patients receiving 2.5 mg/kg of desipramine daily versus 15 delusionally depressed patients receiving an antipsychotic agent with the same weight-adjusted dose of desipramine. Patients receiving the combination had a mean desipramine plasma concentration twice that of patients given desipramine alone (225 vs. 110 ng/ml). Toxic reactions, including urinary retention, generalized seizures, and delirium, developed in several patients receiving desipramine plus an antipsychotic agent. This group replicated this finding in 82 depressed inpatients treated with desipramine, 35 of whom were concurrently receiving a phenothiazine or butyrophenone neuroleptic added to their antidepressant (Bock et al. 1983). Desipramine plasma concentrations were twice as high in patients treated with an antipsychotic drug (233 vs. 166 ng/ml) and the ratios of plasma concentrations of the hydroxymetabolite to desipramine were significantly decreased (0.29 vs. 0.49). Similarly, Siris and colleagues (1982a) warned of potentially dangerous elevations of tricyclic antidepressant plasma concentrations in patients treated with fluphenazine decanoate. These authors reported a mean imipramine plus desipramine plasma concentration of 850 ng/ml in 4 patients treated with imipramine 300 mg/day added to fluphenazine decanoate.

Tricyclic antidepressants may, in turn, elevate plasma concentrations of antipsychotic agents. Mean plasma concentrations of chlorpromazine (300 mg daily) measured by gas-liquid chromatography increased by approximately 50% in 7 schizophrenic patients 1 week after nortriptyline was added at a daily dose of 150 mg, and was associated with sufficient increases in agitation to cause premature termination of the study (Loga et al. 1981). Plasma concentrations of nortriptyline were not measured. El-Yousef and Manier (1974) studied the effect of treatment with desipramine (75–300 mg daily) added for 3 weeks to the phenothiazine, butaperazine, in a crossover study of 8 male schizophenic patients. Butaperazine plasma concentrations were significantly elevated by coadministration of desipramine, but only at daily doses of 150 mg or more of the antidepressant. Jerling and colleagues (1994) found that addition of fluvoxamine increased clozapine levels by 5- to 10-fold, which they attributed to inhibition of CYP1A2 activity by fluvoxamine.

Several cases have been reported of extrapyramidal symptoms

associated with addition of the serotonin reuptake inhibitor, fluoxetine, to antipsychotic agents (Ciraulo and Shader 1990). Adverse reactions have included dystonia (Lock et al. 1990, Meltzer et al. 1979), parkinsonism (Bouchard et al. 1989, Brod 1989, Meltzer et al. 1979, Tate 1989), dyskinesias (Budman and Bruun 1991, Fallon and Liebowitz 1991, Stein 1991) and neuroleptic malignant syndrome (Halman and Goldbloom 1990). When administered alone in some depressed patients, fluoxetine is reported to produce a syndrome that is clinically indistinguishable from neuroleptic-induced akathisia and which responds to propranolol (Lipinski et al. 1989). Extrapyramidal symptoms also have been observed in depressed patients following discontinuation of fluoxetine monotherapy (Stoukides and Stoukides 1991). Pretreatment with serotonin reuptake blockers potentiates neuroleptic-induced catalepsy in rats (Balsara et al. 1979) and dystonia and parkinsonism in monkeys (Korsgaard et al. 1985). Several serotonin reuptake blockers, including fluoxetine, paroxetine, and sertraline, are potent inhibitors of CYP-2D6-catalyzed oxidation of sparteine, and may also interact with other hepatic enzymes, suggesting that these agents may reduce clearance of antipsychotic agents, which are metabolized by these pathways (e.g., thioridazine, clozapine, and perphenazine) (Crewe et al. 1992). Addition of fluoxetine was associated with a mean increase of 20% in plasma concentrations of haloperidol in 8 patients receiving stable doses of oral haloperidol (Goff et al. 1991c) and even greater increases in levels of clozapine (Centorrino et al. 1994). In a placebo-controlled trial, addition of fluoxetine 20 mg daily to stable doses of fluphenazine decanoate increased serum concentrations of fluphenazine by an average of 65% (Goff et al. in press). Considerable variability was found between individuals in the degree of these interactions and, surprisingly, measures of extrapyramidal symptoms were not increased. It has been suggested that fluoxetine-induced extrapyramidal symptoms may be more likely to occur early in the course of neuroleptic treatment when serotonergic modulation of dopamine activity may be more prominent (Goff et al. 1991c, Korsgaard et al. 1985). The effects of fluoxetine on dopamine activity are complex and incompletely understood, but probably do not include a reduction of release of dopamine from nerve terminals (Baldessarini et al. 1992).

Several cases have been reported of adverse interactions between monoamine oxidase inhibitors (MAOIs) and antipsychotic drugs, including worsening of orthostatic hypotension, extrapyramidal signs, and anticholinergic symptoms (Sjoqvist 1965). However, this potential interaction has not been studied systematically. In a patient treated with pargyline for 2 months, a fever of 106°F developed, with coma and death following addition of the phenothiazine antipsychotic agent methotrimeprazine (Barsa and Saunders 1964). It should be emphasized that this fatality may have represented neuroleptic malignant syndrome (NMS) rather than an interaction between the MAOI and antipsychotic agent. No systematic evidence has implicated MAOIs as a risk factor for NMS, but it may be relevant that interactions of MAOIs with tricyclic antidepressants, rarely, and serotonin reuptake inhibitors, more commonly, also produce severe neurotoxic reactions with similarities to NMS, save for catatonia.

Apart from potential pharmacokinetic interactions between antidepressant and antipsychotic agents, the possible therapeutic efficacy of this combination for patients with schizophrenia remains unclear (Plasky 1991). Combining an antipsychotic agent with an antidepressant is more effective for major depression with psychotic features than either drug type used alone (Kocsis et al. 1990, Spiker 1985). However, Kramer and colleagues (1989) reported that addition of desipramine or amitriptyline in recently admitted depressed schizophrenic patients treated for 5 weeks with haloperidol failed to improve measures of depression and impaired the response of some psychotic symptoms compared with placebo. In contrast, Siris and colleagues reported that addition of high doses of imipramine (ca. 200 mg daily) to an antipsychotic agent in stable, depressed outpatients with schizophrenia improved symptoms of depression (Siris et al. 1982b, 1987a,b) and, in one study, also improved negative symptoms (Siris et al. 1991). Other investigators have found inconsistent results with the combination of an antidepressant with an antipsychotic in schizophrenic patients, with one study finding improvement of depressive symptoms but worsening of psychosis (Prusoff et al. 1979), and two others reporting no improvement of depressive symptoms (Becker 1983, Waehrens and Gerlach 1980). Chouinard (1975) studied the combination of amitriptyline and perphenazine in schizophrenic patients not selected for depressive symptoms and found no therapeutic benefit over that of the phenothiazine alone. Plasky (1991) concluded that tricyclic antidepressants may exert a destabilizing effect when administered with antipsychotic agents during acute psychotic episodes, whereas this combination may be beneficial when administered to chronic, stable schizophrenic patients with depressive or anhedonic features. The serotonin reuptake inhibitor fluvoxamine improved negative symptoms without affecting psychotic or extrapyramidal symptoms when added to antipsychotic agents in a placebo-controlled trial (Silver and Nassar 1992).

Mechanism

The tricyclic antidepressants and, particularly fluoxetine and perhaps other serotonin reuptake inhibitors, can elevate plasma concentrations of antipsychotic agents presumably by inhibiting hepatic drug metabolism. The serotonin reuptake inhibitors are potent inhibitors of hepatic cytochrome 2D6 (von Moltke 1994). Some evidence suggests that impairment of hepatic metabolism of antipsychotic agents is more obvious at higher plasma concentrations of tricyclic antidepressant, which can be encountered at typical antidepressant doses. Haloperidol and phenothiazines may elevate plasma concentrations of tricyclic antidepressants moderately, apparently by inhibiting hepatic cytochrome 2D6 metabolism by aromatic ring-hydroxylation (Brosen and Gram 1989). The moderate (20%) elevation of haloperidol plasma concentrations by fluoxetine may reflect inhibition of hepatic CYP-2D6 activity, although the clinical importance of this metabolic pathway for haloperidol remains uncertain (Brosen and Gram 1989, Jerling et al. 1994). The enhanced therapeutic efficacy of combined treatment with an antidepressant and antipsychotic agent in delusional depression presumably reflects a pharmacodynamic interaction, as may the apparent countertherapeutic effect in acutely psychotic schizophrenic patients.

Clinical Implications

The combination of an antipsychotic agent with an antidepressant is a more effective treatment for delusional depression than either agent given alone. Plasma concentrations of tricyclic antidepressants should be monitored, as well as clinical signs of toxicity, when an antipsychotic agent is added, as toxic plasma tricyclic antidepressant concentrations may develop at standard doses that are well tolerated when given alone. It is less clear whether antidepressant-induced elevation of antipsychotic levels in plasma are likely to produce clinically significant effects. Despite several reports of fluoxetine-induced extrapyramidal symptoms, controlled trials have not demonstrated an increase in extrapyramidal symptoms when fluoxetine is added to a stable, long-term antipsychotic regimen. Precipitation of extrapyramidal symptoms may be more likely if a serotonin reuptake inhibitor is added early in the course of antipsychotic therapy.

Antidiarrheal Agents

Evidence of Interaction

One study suggested that the antidiarrheal, attapulgite, may impair the absorption of neuroleptic drugs. Sorby and Liu (1966) demonstrated decreased rate and extent of urinary excretion of the phenothiazine promazine following administration of an antidiarrheal mixture of attapulgite and pectin in repeated studies in a single normal subject.

Mechanism

Attapulgite appears to decrease the rate and extent of promazine absorption from the gastrointestinal tract.

Clinical Implications

Although this finding is preliminary and has only been studied in a single-dose design with promazine, it may apply to other neuroleptics as well. It is unclear whether this pharmacokinetic interaction is likely to produce clinically significant lowering of drug plasma concentrations. Since attapulgite is contained in many over-the-counter antidiarrheal preparations, clinicians should monitor for such an interaction when patients report taking an antidiarrheal compound.

Anxiolytics

Evidence of Interaction

Combinations of benzodiazepines with antipsychotic agents have been studied in the treatment of mania or agitation in a variety of acute psychotic states, and in the treatment of chronically symptomatic schizophrenic patients (Arana et al. 1986a, Wolkowitz and Pickar 1991). The combination of lorazepam or alprazolam with a high-potency antipsychotic agent, such as haloperidol, can reduce agitation more effectively than either drug administered alone and decrease the total dose of antipsychotic agent required for behavioral control (Barbee et al. 1992, Garza-Trevino et al. 1989, Salzman et al. 1986). Parenteral administration of benzodiazepines alone also can reduce intensity of agitation and acute psychosis (Lerner et al. 1979, Salzman et al. 1991).

The value of benzodiazepines added to antipsychotic agents for nonacute schizophrenic patients is less clear. Douyon and colleagues (1989) added alprazolam to stable doses of antipsychotic agents in 9 schizophrenic patients and found a mean increase of 23% in plasma concentrations of haloperidol and fluphenazine. Patients exhibited a 20 to 30% mean reduction in psychotic and negative symptoms with the combination treatment, but there was considerable variability in response. Improvement correlated with plasma concentrations of alprazolam, but not with the amount of increase in antipsychotic plasma concentrations. Several investigators have reported significant improvement of both positive and negative symptoms of schizophrenia on addition of benzodiazepines to antipsychotic agents (Arana et al. 1986a, Cohen and Khan 1987, Pato et al. 1989, Wolkowitz et al. 1988). However benefits of benzodiazepine supplementation are most likely during acute exacerbation of illness, are found in only about 30 to 50% of chronically ill patients, and may diminish over time (Wolkowitz and Pickar 1991).

At least 6 cases of toxicity associated with addition of benzodiazepines to clozapine have been reported (Cobb et al. 1991, Friedman et al. 1991, Grohmann et al. 1989). Reports of this possible interaction have described sedation, sialorrhea, ataxia, and, in some cases, fainting, loss of consciousness, and respiratory arrest. The etiologic role of benzodiazepines in producing these reactions remains uncertain; if such an interaction does occur, it is evidently rare (Frankenburg and Baldessarini 1991, Bredbacka et al. 1993).

In an open trial, addition of buspirone at a mean daily dose of 24 mg to neuroleptics in 20 schizophrenic patients was associated with improvements in depression, tension, and Parkinsonian symptoms (Goff et al. 1991b). In the 7 patients treated with oral haloperidol, plasma concentrations of the neuroleptic were increased by 26%.

Mechanism

Alprazolam may lower antipsychotic plasma concentrations slightly, although the mechanism is not known. Enhancement of antipsychotic effects on agitation and possibly on psychotic and negative symptoms of schizophrenia may simply be the result of benzodiazepine-induced sedation, or may represent a pharmacodynamic interaction between γ-aminobutyric acid (GABA) and dopaminergic systems.

Clinical Implications

The benzodiazepines, lorazepam, alprazolam, and clonazepam are effective when combined with moderate doses of high-potency antipsychotic agents in the treatment of acute psychotic or manic agitation. During the early stages of treatment, adjuvant benzodiazepine use may allow lower doses of antipsychotic agents, and so, reduce risk of EPS. Benzodiazepines may improve psychotic and negative symptoms when combined with antipsychotics in some chronic schizophrenic patients, although this effect is variable, typically minor, and may not be sustained.

Cardiovascular Drugs

Antihypertensives

Evidence of Interaction

A variety of agents control hypertension by several differing mechanisms, and each type may interact differently with antipsychotic agents. Best studied is the β-adrenergic antagonist, propranolol, which has been reported to decrease clearance and elevate plasma levels of some phenothiazines (Ereshefsky et al. 1991). Propranolol and pindolol can increase circulating levels of chlorpromazine and thioridazine when coadministered at typical clinical doses (Greendyke and Gulya 1988, Greendyke and Kanter 1987, Peet et al. 1980, Silver et al. 1986, Vestal et al. 1979), whereas haloperidol concentrations are not affected by these agents (Greendyke and Gulya 1988, Greendyke and Kanter 1987). In turn, chlorpromazine and thioridazine, but not haloperidol, can increase plasma concentrations of propranolol and pindolol (Greendyke and Gulya 1988, Greendyke and Kanter 1987, Peet et al. 1980, Silver et al. 1986, Vestal et al. 1979). The full clinical implications of combining antipsychotics and beta blockers remain unclear, though such combinations are generally well tolerated (Yorkston et al. 1977). Vestal and colleagues (1979) described a case of orthostatic syncope after chlorpromazine 50 mg daily was added to propranolol. More ominously, Alexander and colleagues (1984) reported three episodes of severe hypotension and cardiopulmonary arrest in a 48-year-old woman with schizophrenia treated with haloperidol 10 mg and propranolol 40 mg daily; she tolerated both haloperidol and propranolol when separately combined with other psychotropic drugs.

Thioridazine and chlorpromazine frequently cause postural hypotension when administered alone (Goff and Shader 1994). Silver and colleagues (1990) measured blood pressure at rest and standing in 196 medicated schizophrenic patients and found that 77% of them displayed significant systolic hypotension after 1 minute of standing, with a mean decrease of 28 mm Hg. Thioridazine affected blood pressure significantly more than chlorpromazine or haloperidol. Although it has not been studied systematically, addition of a β-blocker might further compromise cardiovascular function by adding β-adrenergic blockade to the anti-α-adrenergic actions of chlorpromazine and thioridazine, and perhaps other low-potency antipsychotics (particularly clozapine).

Other antihypertensives also have been reported to produce hypotension when combined with low-potency antipsychotic agents. White (1986) described a patient in whom orthostatic hypotension and syncope developed when the angiotensin-converting enzyme (ACE) inhibitor captopril (12.5 mg daily) was added to chlorpromazine; the patient later tolerated each drug separately, but again became hypotensive when rechallenged with the combination. Similarly, Fruncillo (1985) reported 2 cases of severe hypotension when clonidine was added to chlorpromazine as well as other medications. Delirium occurred in a 39-year-old patient treated with fluphenazine decanoate following addition of clonidine; this reaction cleared after discontinuation of clonidine and recurred when the patient was rechallenged (Allen and Flemenbaum 1979).

The catecholamine synthesis inhibitor, α-methyldopa, also has been reported to produce hypotension and delirium when added to antipsychotic agents. Chouinard and colleagues (1973a,b) evaluated methyldopa as a possible adjuvant to antipsychotic therapy. In their first study, methyldopa was gradually increased to 1,000 mg in combination with chlorpromazine 400 mg daily. In the second study, methyldopa 500 mg was combined with haloperidol 10 mg daily. Both regimens produced substantial orthostatic hypotension with dizziness as well as reportedly impressive clinical responses, but their interpretation is limited by absence of a control group. In addition, 3 cases of cognitive or behavioral deterioration were associated with the combination of methyldopa and haloperidol. One, a 74-year-old man, tolerated 100 mg of thioridazine combined with 500 mg of methyldopa daily, but became irritable, aggressive, and assaultive when the neuroleptic was changed to haloperidol 4 mg daily (Nadel and Wallach 1979). Two other patients became confused when haloperidol was added at doses of 6 or 8 mg daily to 500 mg of methyldopa, but improved after discontinuation of haloperidol (Thornton 1976).

Finally, several studies have evaluated the effect of antipsychotic agents on blood pressure when coadministered with the peripheral antisympathetic agent guanethidine. Janowsky and colleagues

(1973) stabilized otherwise medication-free patients on guanethidine (60–150 mg daily) alone for 7 days before adding chlorpromazine, haloperidol, or thiothixine. After a delay of several days, the antipsychotic agents significantly reversed the antihypertensive effect of guanethidine and in some patients increased blood pressure; this effect was most apparent with chlorpromazine (100–400 mg daily). Blockade of the antihypertensive effect of guanethidine by chlorpromazine also was observed by Fann and colleagues (1971). Unlike chlorpromazine, molindone does not block the neuronal uptake of guanethidine in rats (Gilder et al. 1976) and, when administered at doses of 30 to 120 mg daily, molindone did not interfere with the antihypertensive effect of guanethidine in 7 hypertensive patients (Simpson 1979).

Antiarrhythmics

Evidence of Interaction

Most antipsychotic agents have direct myocardial depressant effects reflected in prolongation of the Q-T interval and nonspecific T-wave changes on the electrocardiogram (ECG) (Risch et al. 1981). Thioridazine exhibits a particularly strong myocardial depressant effect and may prolong atrial and ventricular conduction and refractory periods (Descotes et al. 1979, Yoon et al. 1979). Chlorpromazine also depresses myocardial function and can increase QT duration at daily doses as low as 150 mg (Backman and Elosuo 1964). Of great concern have been several reports of sudden death associated with antipsychotic doses of thioridazine and chlorpromazine (Aherwadker et al. 1964, Giles and Modlin 1968). Efforts to determine whether the incidence of sudden death in patients with schizophrenia increased with the introduction of neuroleptic treatment have produced conflicting results (Brill and Patton 1962, Richardson et al. 1966). Nevertheless, some cases are strongly suspected to represent heart block and ventricular arrhythmias due to cardiac actions of thioridazine or chlorpromazine (Aherwadker et al. 1964, Giles and Modlin 1968). Given the potential for additive myocardial depression, thioridazine and chlorpromazine should not be used with a direct myocardial depressant class I antiarrhythmic agent such as quinidine or procainamide. If quinidine-like agents are combined with phenothiazine antipsychotics, the ECG should be monitored for impaired conduction. The phenothiazines, pimozide, and possibly clozapine appear to be especially likely to produce ECG changes (Ban and St. Jean 1964, Risch et al. 1981). Pimozide can produce clinically significant cardiac depressant effects as a result of its calcium channel blocking action which is independent of its antagonism of dopamine receptors (Opler and Feinberg 1991). ECG conduction intervals should be monitored when pimozide is initiated, particularly in children and the elderly, and this drug should not be combined with other calcium channel blockers (e.g., nifedipine, diltiazem, and verapamil). Extremely high doses of intravenous haloperidol (up to 1,000 mg in 24 hours) have been administered safely in patients with cardiac disease in combination with antiarrhythmic agents, although rare cases of QT interval prolongation and Torsade de Pointes (a form of ventricular tachycardia with an undulating ECG baseline, often arising in the setting of prolonged QT interval) have been reported at these doses (Metzger and Friedman 1993).

Pressors

Evidence of Interaction

Because low-potency and some high potency antipsychotic agents block α- but not β-adrenergic receptors, administration of epinephrine may cause severe hypotension as a result of unopposed β-agonist activity at visceral vascular beds (Courroisier et al. 1953, Foster et al. 1954, Ginsburg and Duff 1956, Lear et al. 1957). Administration of a low-potency antipsychotic agent to a patient with a pheochromocytoma may similarly produce severe hypotension (Lund-Johnsen 1962).

Mechanism

The β-blockers propranolol and pindolol elevate circulating levels of some phenothiazines, presumably by impairing hepatic clearance. Antipsychotic agents, particularly thioridazine and chlorpromazine, also can interact with cardiovascular agents as a result of their α-adrenergic blockade, as well as mild quinidine-like direct depression of cardiac conduction. Several antipsychotic drugs (molindone is an exception) also block the uptake of guanethidine into postganglionic sympathetic neurons, and thereby reduce its antihypertensive efficacy. Pimozide has calcium channel-blocking properties that can depress cardiac conduction and produce severe additive cardiac or hypotensive effects when combined with other calcium channel blockers. The combination of low-potency antipsychotic agents with β-adrenergic agonist pressors can result in hypotension as a result of unopposed peripheral β-adrenergic agonist activity.

Clinical Implications

High-potency antipsychotic agents such as haloperidol or fluphenazine produce substantially less hypotension and cardiac depression than do thioridazine and chlorpromazine, and so are preferable for patients with cardiovascular disease and the elderly. Unlike certain phenothiazines, haloperidol plasma levels are not elevated by coadministration of propranolol or pindolol. Drugs that impair cardiac conduction (including tricyclic antidepressants) should not be added to thioridazine or chlorpromazine unless the ECG is monitored, especially in elderly or cardiac patients. Monitoring of the QT interval also is recommended when patients are started on pimozide or its dose increased, particularly in children and the elderly. Finally, pressors, such as epinephrine, which produce both α- and β-adrenergic agonist effects, should not be combined with low-potency antipsychotic agents because severe hypotension can result from excessive and unopposed β-adrenergic activity.

Cimetidine

Evidence of Interaction

Howes and colleagues (1983) reported on 8 patients receiving stable doses of chlorpromazine given the histamine H_2 antagonist cimetidine 1,200 mg daily orally; after 7 days of combined treatment, plasma concentrations of chlorpromazine fell by 33% and the ratio of hydroxy to other phenothiazines in urine fell from 2.5 to 1.7. Szymanski (1991) reported a possible interaction between the cimetidine and clozapine, characterized by severe dizziness, diaphoresis, emesis, and weakness, when 800 mg of cimetidine was added to 900 mg of clozapine daily. The patient subsequently tolerated the similar antinuclear agent ranitidine at 300 mg daily.

Mechanism

Changes in metabolite ratios in urine indicate that hepatic metabolism of chlorpromazine is inhibited by cimetidine, consistent with other drug interactions of this agent. However, the significant reduction in plasma concentrations of chlorpromazine indicates that decreased absorption is the more important mechanism responsible for this interaction. Cimetidine probably elevates plasma concentrations of clozapine by inhibiting hepatic microsomal enzymes.

Clinical Implications

Cimetidine can produce a substantial decrease in plasma concentration of chlorpromazine, which may have adverse clinical effects in patients treated with relatively low doses of the antipsychotic agent. It is not known whether other antipsychotic agents are similarly affected, but levels of clozapine may increase. Cimetidine inhibits hepatic metabolism of several drugs (Ereshefksy et al. 1991); the case reported by Szymanski (1991) of an interaction with clozapine is consistent with such an effect. Clinicians should be prepared for either an increase or decrease in antipsychotic levels when cimetidine is added.

Coffee or Tea

Evidence of Interaction

Early studies raised concern that coffee or tea may decrease bioavailability of antipsychotic agents. Kulhanek (1979) mixed tea or coffee with elixirs (alcohol solutions) of chlorpromazine, haloperidol, droperidol, fluphenazine, promethazine, or prochlorperazine *in vitro* and observed formation of insoluble precipitates. When fluphenazine was given to rats orally in a solution of coffee or tea, the degree and duration of catalepsy was decreased compared with administration of fluphenazine alone (Kulhanek and Linde 1981). Zaslove and colleagues (1991) reported that substitution of caffeinated beverages with decaffeinated beverages on an inpatient psychiatric ward resulted in a decrease in assaultive behavior. Subsequent clinical trials have not confirmed an interaction, however. Koczapski and colleagues (1989) found no effect on patients' behavior when decaffeinated coffee replaced caffeinated coffee. Bowen and colleagues (1981) compared plasma levels of chlorpromazine, haloperidol, fluphenazine, and trifluoperazine, measured by radioreceptor assay, in 16 patients given these drugs with coffee or tea versus fruit juice, and found no difference. Similarly, Wallace (1981) found no effect of coffee or tea on plasma concentrations of fluphenazine in 12 normal volunteers. Although consistent effects of consumption of caffeinated beverages have not been demonstrated in patients treated with antipsychotic drugs, acute administration of a high dose of caffeine (10 mg/kg) increased arousal and measures of psychosis in schizophrenic patients receiving oral fluphenazine (Lucas et al. 1990).

Clinical Implications

There is inadequate clinical evidence to suggest that there is a significant pharmacokinetic interaction of caffeinated beverages and antipsychotic agents. However, patients with schizophrenia commonly develop caffeinism, defined as daily consumption of 6 or more cups of coffee (ca. 600 mg of caffeine) (Goff and Ciraulo 1991). High levels of caffeine alone may cause anxiety and can exacerbate psychopathology. Caffeine withdrawal states may present with headache, lassitude, and nausea.

Disulfiram

Evidence of Interaction

Hansen and Larsen (1982) reported a case in which addition of disulfiram to perphenazine resulted in decreased plasma concentrations of perphenazine, increased concentrations of the inactive sulfoxide metabolite, and a deterioration in the patient's psychiatric condition.

Mechanism

This interaction may result from an interaction with hepatic microsomal enzymes, but remains unexplained.

Clinical Significance

In one reported case, this interaction was of a magnitude sufficient to result in clinical deterioration. Disulfiram has not been sytematically studied in relation to other antipsychotic agents, but clinicians should be aware of this potential interaction, presumed to be pharmacokinetic in nature.

Lithium

Evidence of Interaction

In one study, coadministration of lithium carbonate was associated with 40% lower peak plasma concentrations of chlorpromazine (Rivera-Calimlim et al. 1978). In rats given lithium and chlorpromazine orally, the concentrations of chlorpromazine in plasma and brain were significantly lower and the percent of chlorpromazine remaining in the stomach was significantly higher than in matched controls given chlorpromazine alone (Rivera-Calimlim 1976). These findings have not been replicated and their clinical significance is not established.

Of greater concern is the question of a potential neurotoxic reaction to the combination of lithium and antipsychotic agents. Cohen and Cohen (1974) first reported 4 cases of an irreversible neurologic reaction to the combination of lithium with haloperidol. In this and subsequent reports, a toxic interaction between lithium and antipsychotic agents was suspected and described as similar to neuroleptic malignant syndrome (NMS). It consisted of confusion, impaired consciousness, rigidity, tremor, akathisia, akinesia, dyskinesia, dystonia, and, less commonly, cerebellar signs and hyperthermia (Cohen and Cohen 1974, Jeffries et al. 1984, Louden and Waring 1976, Prakash et al. 1982, Sandyk and Hurwitz 1983, Shopsin et al. 1976, Spring and Frankel 1981). Prakash and colleagues (1982) reviewed 39 reported cases and noted that 67% involved haloperidol, whereas the other third were associated with thioridazine, perphenazine, flupenthixol, or thiothixene. It remains unclear whether this rare phenomenon is specific to an interaction of lithium with haloperidol. Haloperidol may have been implicated because it is used very commonly in combination with lithium. Parkash and colleagues (1982) also noted that in 10% of cases neurologic deficits, including dementia, persisted after discontinuation of the psychotropic agents. The early case reports emphasized high serum lithium concentrations as a risk factor, whereas a study of 22 manic patients determined that the 6 patients in whom neurotoxicity developed with the combination were receiving relatively high doses of haloperidol but did not have high serum levels of lithium (Miller and Menninger 1987).

Despite the considerable attention that this putative drug interaction has received, whether a drug interaction is in fact responsible for this neurotoxic syndrome continues to be debated. Two groups retrospectively studied a total of 494 patients treated with lithium and an antipsychotic drug and did not identify a single case of this neurotoxic reaction (Baastrup et al. 1976, Goldney and Spence 1986). Similar neurotoxicity can occur as an adverse reaction to lithium or the antipsychotic agents alone rather than as a true drug interaction. For example, lithium toxicity can manifest as confusion and ataxia, as well as cogwheel rigidity and irreversible nonspecific cerebral neurotoxicity in the absence of an antipsychotic agent (Asnis et al. 1979, Kane et al. 1978, Schou 1984). In addition, some cases of neurotoxicity attributed to the combination of lithium and antipsychotics may represent NMS. Coadministration of lithium has not been established firmly as a risk factor for NMS, although some recent evidence suggests this possibility (Addonizio et al. 1986, 1987, Deng et al. 1990, Keck et al. 1989, 1991, Pope et al. 1986, Rosebush and Stewart 1989). Interestingly, 2 cases were reported of patients who had relapses of NMS when rechallenged by lithium alone (Susman and Addonizio 1987). Finally, several reports have suggested that lithium coadministration may increase the frequency and severity of reversible extrapyramidal symptoms in patients treated with neuroleptics (Addonizio 1985, Sachdev 1986). However, Goldney and Spence (1986) found no increase in extrapyramidal symptoms in 69 manic patients treated with a combination of lithium and a neuroleptic patient compared with 60 manic patients treated with a neuroleptic alone.

Mechanism

Although lithium may elevate plasma concentrations of chlorpromazine by undetermined pharmacokinetic mechanisms, such an effect is poorly established. Rare central neurotoxic reactions, if they occur, are more likely the result of pharmacodynamic interactions. Both antipsychotics and lithium can produce extrapyramidal and neurotoxic symptoms when administered alone, so that additive toxicity remains possible. Whether coadministration may increase the risk for neuroleptic malignant syndrome remains an important question.

Clinical Implications

Reports of a potentially irreversible, though rare, neurotoxic syndrome associated with the combined use of lithium and antipsychotic agents are of great concern, but it is unclear whether this effect represents a drug interaction or neurotoxicity that can be produced by either drug administered alone. It also remains unclear whether risk of extrapyramidal symptoms is increased with this combination. Given the high morbidity of this rare syndrome, clinicians should monitor patients with particular care when administering lithium with an antipsychotic agent, and avoid high serum levels of lithium as well as high antipsychotic doses. The evidence of a greater risk of neurotoxicity associated with haloperidol than other antipsychotic agents remains unconvincing, and does not merit a specific avoidance of combined use of haloperidol and lithium, in our opinion.

Stimulants

Evidence of Interaction

Neuroleptics can counteract many of the signs of stimulant toxicity. In addition, a few studies have explored the use of stimulants to control side effects of neuroleptics, such as sedation and weight gain. Acute amphetamine toxicity can present with tachycardia, hypertension, hyperreflexia, insomnia, agitation, and psychosis. Massive overdoses may result in delirium, seizures, hyperthermia, cardiovascular collapse, and death (Goff and Ciraulo 1991). Espelin and Done (1968) were the first to evaluate chlorpromazine as a treatment for amphetamine toxicity. In a study of amphetamine intoxication in 22 children, they reported that an initial chlorpromazine dose of 1 mg/kg administered intramuscularly followed by intramuscular doses of 0.4 to 4.0 mg/kg produced sedation and resolution of amphetamine-induced agitation. Angrist and Lee (1974) demonstrated that haloperidol 5 mg produced improvement in excitement and paranoid ideation within 1 hour of intramuscular administration to 4 schizophrenic and 4 nonschizophrenic amphetamine abusers exhibiting signs of amphetamine intoxication. Both haloperidol and chlorpromazine block amphetamine toxicity in dogs administered lethal doses of amphetamine (10 mg/kg intravenously) (Catravas 1975). Surprisingly, one study suggested that low doses of chlorpromazine (1.25–2.5 mg/kg intraperitoneally) potentiated the stimulatory effects of amphetamine, whereas higher doses (10–20 mg/kg) antagonized the action of amphetamine (Sulser and Dingell 1968). In rats, metabolism of amphetamine is slowed by chlorpromazine but not by haloperidol (Lemberger et al. 1970). Because chlorpromazine may impair metabolism of amphetamine and may exacerbate amphetamine-induced cardiovascular instability, chlorpromazine is not recommended for the treatment of amphetamine toxicity (Goff and Ciraulo 1991). A high-potency agent like haloperidol is less likely to produce adverse interactions.

Chronic amphetamine abuse appears to produce sensitization, such that progressively smaller doses may produce the same level of response over time (Lieberman et al. 1990, Sato 1986). Early studies suggested that psychotic symptoms develop in many normal subjects if they are given a sufficiently large amount of amphetamine (Angrist and Gershon 1970, Goff and Ciraulo 1991, Griffith et al. 1968); this psychotogenic effect is at least partially blocked by neuroleptics. However, stimulant abuse may have long-lasting effects on dopamine systems that can interfere with antipsychotic efficacy. Bowers and colleagues (1990) reported that a past history of stimulant abuse was associated with significantly poorer response to antipsychotic treatment and with lower baseline plasma concentration of the main metabolite of dopamine, homovanillic acid (HVA). In Japan, where intravenous methamphetamine abuse was a widespread problem following World War II, Sato (1986) reported that sensitization persisted despite many years of abstinence. One study of dopamine D_2 receptor binding using positron emission tomography (PET) found a significant decrease in the D_2 receptor density of cocaine abusers after 1 week of abstinence, which returned to normal after 1 month of detoxification (Volkow et al. 1990).

The stimulants also have been evaluated as possible adjuvant treatment for control of antipsychotic side effects. In a double-blind, placebo-controlled design, Reid (1964) demonstrated that addition of phenmetrazine 50 mg daily to chlorpromazine did not produce weight loss in patients receiving a standard hospital diet. The failure of appetite suppressants to reverse neuroleptic-induced weight gain was confirmed by Modell and Hussar (1965), who added dextroamphetamine (20 mg daily) to the regimens of obese schizophrenic patients treated with a variety of neuroleptics, and by Sletten (1967), who added chlorphentermine and phenmetrazine to chlorpromazine. Burke and Sebastian (1993) recently reported that methylphenidate (5–30 mg daily) decreased clozapine-induced sedation in 2 patients without interfering with the antipsychotic effect or adding other side effects.

Finally, several studies have examined the potential benefits of adding methylphenidate or amphetamines to antipsychotic agents to treat apathy and cognitive deficits in chronically psychotic patients (Carpenter et al. 1992, Chiarello and Cole 1987, Goldberg et al. 1991, Huey et al. 1984, Sharma et al. 1991). In general, acute administration of stimulants to schizophrenic patients who are antipsychotic-free increases activation and psychosis in most but not all patients. A psychotic response to a stimulant challenge may predict a favorable response to antipsychotic medication and a shorter time to relapse after medication is discontinued (Angrist et al. 1980, Lieberman et al. 1987). Addition of low doses of stimulant to antipsychotic medication may improve some measures of cognitive function, mood, and activation in some schizophrenic patients, but psychosis may worsen in others.

Mechanism

Although only studied directly in rats, chlorpromazine may elevate amphetamine plasma concentrations by impairing hepatic metabolism. Other interactions between these two classes of drugs are most likely pharmacodynamic in nature, since the stimulants increase dopaminergic and adrenergic activity by release of catecholamines. In addition, stimulant abuse may cause enduring changes in dopamine receptor levels and function that are manifest clinically as behavioral sensitization to stimulant administration and possibly as diminished therapeutic response to antipsychotic agents.

Clinical Implications

Because of the risk of cardiovascular complications, as well as a possible interference with hepatic metabolism of amphetamine, it is best to treat amphetamine intoxication with moderate doses of a high-potency neuroleptic. Short-term treatment with daily doses of haloperidol of about 10 to 15 mg is generally safe and effective. Although a low dose of methylphenidate may improve clozapine-induced sedation, the routine use of stimulants with antipsychotic agents is not recommended because of the risk of exacerbating psychosis. Several studies have indicated that stimulants are not effective for the control of weight gain with antipsychotic agents. Finally, clinicians should be aware that stimulant abuse can significantly impair antipsychotic efficacy, and past stimulant abuse may predict subsequent poor response. This is particularly relevant in the treatment of schizophrenic patients, since this population prefers stimulants, along with alcohol and cigarettes, as substances of abuse.

Tobacco

Evidence of Interaction

Surveys of schizophrenic patients have reported rates of cigarette smoking between 74% and 92% compared with 30 to 35% for the general population (Goff et al. 1992). It has been suggested that patients with schizophrenia are more likely to smoke because of institutionalization, impaired judgment, and lack of access to other forms of recreation. However, other factors may reinforce smoking in patients with schizophrenia, including reduction of plasma neuroleptic concentrations and extrapyramidal symptoms, and partial correction of neuropsychological deficits (Adler et al. 1993, Goff et al. 1992, Shoaf and Linnoila 1991). These findings have led to a "self-medication" model for cigarette smoking in schizophrenia (Adler et al. 1993, Goff et al. 1992).

Several studies have found that schizophrenic patients who

smoke receive antipsychotic doses up to twice as high as patients who do not smoke (Decina et al. 1990, Ereshefsky et al. 1991, Goff et al. 1992, Vinarova et al. 1984, Yassa et al. 1987). This difference in clinically determined antipsychotic dose requirements may reflect in part a pharmacokinetic interaction between antipsychotic medication and one of the more than 2,000 constituents of cigarette smoke. Cigarette smoking increases clearance of haloperidol and fluphenazine by 44 to 67% and of fluphenazine decanoate by 133% (Ereshefsky et al. 1985, Jann et al. 1986). Ereshefsky and colleagues (1991) found that cigarette smoking increased clearance of thiothixene by 37%, but not when patients were also receiving hepatic enzyme inducers (e.g. anticonvulsants). Haring and colleagues (1989) reported that cigarette smoking lowered steady-state plasma concentrations of clozapine in men by 32% but did not significantly affect plasma concentrations of clozapine in women; but Centorrino and colleagues (1994) found little effect of smoking on serum levels of this agent in men or women. Midha and colleagues (1988b, 1989) reported that clearance of single doses of haloperidol and trifluoperazine were not affected by cigarette smoking status, suggesting that a pharmacokinetic interaction is likely only when plasma concentrations of the neuroleptic reach steady state (Shoaf and Linnoila 1991). Stimmel and Falloon (1983) described a patient with schizophrenia in whom extrapyramidal side effects developed in association with an elevation of serum chlorpromazine level when he stopped smoking cigarettes. The neurologic side effects returned to baseline when this patient resumed smoking.

Cigarette smoking also may affect antipsychotic efficacy and extrapyramidal symptoms by pharmacodynamic actions on brain cholinergic and dopaminergic systems. Smokers in the general population may be at lower risk for idiopathic Parkinson's disease than are nonsmokers (Barbeau et al. 1986, Baron 1986, Baumann et al. 1980, Godwin-Austen et al. 1982, Kessler and Diamond 1971, Wagner et al. 1988). Similarly, schizophrenic patients who smoke appear to be at lower risk for parkinsonian side effects of antipsychotic drugs than nonsmokers (Goff et al. 1992). Risk of neuroleptic-induced tardive dyskinesia was higher for smokers in two of three studies (Binder et al. 1987, Goff et al. 1992, Yassa et al. 1987) and, in one study, the risk for akathisia was not affected by smoking status (Goff et al. 1992). Nicotine improves attention, memory, and mood and reduces anxiety in normal subjects (Henningfield and Woodson 1989, Warburton 1989, Wesnes and Warburton 1983) and transiently may improve deficits in processing auditory stimuli that are reported to be characteristic of schizophrenic patients (Adler et al. 1993). These findings suggest that such patients may experience therapeutic benefits from cigarette smoking in addition to effects resulting from interactions between smoking and antipsychotic drugs. On the other hand, withdrawal from nicotine may produce adverse effects in some patients. Greeman and McClellan (1991) observed that attempts to ban smoking on an inpatient unit resulted in exacerbation of symptoms in schizophrenic patients.

Mechanism

As a strong inducer of hepatic microsomal enzymes, cigarette smoke can substantially lower plasma concentrations of antipsychotic agents. In addition, nicotine may have activating effects on brain dopamine systems, resulting in pharmacodynamic interactions with antipsychotic agents. Cigarette smoking may reduce extrapyramidal symptoms, improve mood, and improve attentional and neuropsychological impairments characteristic of schizophrenia. These beneficial effects may reinforce cigarette smoking, and lead patients to "self-medicate" with this agent.

Clinical Implications

Admission to a "smoke-free" inpatient unit may substantially alter a patient's metabolism of antipsychotic medication, in addition to worsening extrapyramidal symptoms and possibly exacerbating some clinical symptoms of the illness. Use of transdermal nicotine patches may reduce patients' discomfort, although nicotine patches probably do not prevent changes in antipsychotic metabolism since other constituents of cigarette smoke probably induce hepatic microsomal enzymes. Nicotine patches should be used with caution in unsupervised settings, since schizophrenic patients may continue to smoke at high levels and thereby expose themselves to toxic levels of nicotine.

REFERENCES

Addonizio G: Rapid induction of extrapyramidal side effects with combined use of lithium and neuroleptics. J Clin Psychopharmacol 5: 296, 1985.
Addonizio G et al.: Symptoms of neuroleptic malignant syndrome in 82 consecutive inpatients. Am J Psychiatry 143: 1587, 1986.
Addonizio G et al.: Neuroleptic malignant syndrome: review and analysis of 115 cases. Biol Psychiatry 22: 1004, 1987.
Adler LA et al.: Normalization of auditory physiology by cigarette smoking in schizophenic patients. Am J Psychiatry 150: 1856, 1993.
Aherwadker SJ et al.: Chlorpromazine therapy and associated acute disturbances of cardiac rhythm. Br Heart J 36: 1251, 1964.

Alexander HE et al.: Hypotension and cardiopulmonary arrest associated with concurrent haloperidol and propranolol therapy. JAMA 252: 87, 1984.

Allen RM, Flemenbaum A: Delirium associated with combined fluphenazine-clonidine therapy. J Clin Psychiatry 40: 236, 1979.

Angrist B, Gershon S: The phenomenology of experimentally induced amphetamine psychosis: preliminary observations. Biol Psychiatry 2: 95, 1970.

Angrist B, Lee HK: The antagonism of amphetamine-induced symptomatology by a neuroleptic. Am J Psychiatry 131: 817, 1974.

Angrist B et al.: Responses to apomorphine, amphetamine, and neuroleptics in schizophrenic subjects. Psychopharmacology 67: 31, 1980.

Arana GW et al.: The use of benzodiazepines for psychiatric disorders: A literature review and preliminary findings. Psychopharmacol Bull 22: 77, 1986a.

Arana GW et al.: Does carbamazepine-induced reduction of plasma haloperidol levels worsen psychotic symptoms? Am J Psychiatry 143: 650, 1986b.

Arana GW et al.: Efficacy of anticholinergic prophylaxis for uroleptic-induced acute dystonia. Am J Psychiatry 145: 993, 1988.

Asnis GM et al.: Cogwheel rigidity during chronic lithium therapy. Am J Psychiatry 136: 1225, 1979.

Baastrup PC et al.: Adverse reactions in treatment with lithium carbonate and haloperidol. JAMA 236: 2645, 1976.

Backman H, Elosuo R: Electrocardiographic findings in connection with a clinical trial of chlorpromazine: with particular references to T-wave changes and the duration of ventricular activity. Ann Med Intern Fenn 53: 1, 1964.

Baker LA et al.: The withdrawal of benztropine mesylate in chronic schizophrenic patients. Br J Psychiatry 143: 584, 1983.

Baldessarini RJ, Frankenburg R: Clozapine—a novel antipsychotic agent. New Engl J Med 324: 746, 1991.

Baldessarini RJ et al.: Significance of neuroleptic dose and plasma level in the pharmacological treatment of psychoses. Arch Gen Psychiatry 45: 79, 1988.

Baldessarini RJ et al.: Interactions of fluoxetine with metabolism of dopamine and serotonin in rat brain regions. Brain Research 579: 152, 1992.

Balsara JJ et al.: Effect of drugs influencing central serotonergic mechanisms on haloperidol-induced catalepsy. Psychopharmacology 62: 67, 1979.

Ban TA, St. Jean A: The effects of phenothiazines on the electrocardiogram. Can Med Assoc J 91: 537, 1964.

Barbeau A et al.: Smoking cancer and parkinson's disease. Ann Neurol 20: 105, 1986.

Barbee JG et al.: Alprazolam as a neuroleptic adjunct in the emergency treatment of schizophrenia. Am J Psychiatry 149: 506, 1992.

Baron JA: Cigarette smoking and Parkinson's disease. Neurology 36: 1490, 1986.

Barsa J, Saunders JC: A comparative study of tranylcypromine and pargyline. Psychopharmacologia 6: 295–298, 1964.

Baumann RJ et al.: Cigarette smoking and Parkinson's disease, 1: a comparison of cases with matched neighbors. Neurology 30: 839, 1980.

Becker RE: Implications of the efficacy of thiothixene and a chlorpromazine-imipramine combination for depression in schizophrenia. Am J Psychiatry 140: 208, 1983.

Bertilsson L et al.: Genetic regulation of the disposition of psychotropic drugs. In Meltzer HY and Nerozzi D (eds.): Current Practices and Future Developments in the Pharmacotherapy of Mental Disorders. New York, Elsevier, 1991.

Bertschy G et al.: Valpromide-amitriptyline interaction: increase in the bioavailability of amitriptyline and nortriptyline caused by valpromide. Encephale 16: 43, 1990.

Binder RL et al.: Smoking and tardive dyskinesia. Biol Psychiatry 22: 1280, 1987.

Bock JL et al.: Desipramine hydroxylation: variability and effect of antipsychotic drugs. Clin Pharmacol Ther 33:322, 1983.

Borison RL: Clinical efficacy of serotonin-dopamine antagonists relative to classical neuroleptics. J Clin Psychopharmacol 15(suppl 1): 24S–29S, 1995.

Bouchard RH et al.: Fluoxetine and extrapyramidal side effects (letter). Am J Psychiatry 146: 1352, 1989.

Bourgeois BFD: Pharmacologic interactions between valproate and other drugs. Am J Med 84: 29, 1988.

Bowen S et al.: Effect of coffee and tea on blood levels and efficacy of antipsychotic drugs (letter). Lancet 1 (8231): 1217, 1981.

Bowers MBJ et al.: Psychotogenic drug use and neuroleptic response. Schizophren Bull 16: 81, 1990.

Bredbacka PE et al.: Can severe cardiorespiratory dysregulation induced by clozapine monotherapy be predicted? Int Clin Psychopharmacol 8: 205–206, 1993.

Brill M, Patton RE: Clinical-statistical analysis of population changes in New York state mental hospitals since the introduction of psychotropic drugs. Am J Psychiatry 119: 20, 1962.

Brod TM: Fluoxetine and extrapyramidal side effects (letter). Am J Psychiatry 146: 1353, 1989.

Brosen K, Gram LF: Clinical significance of the sparteine/debrisoquine oxidation polymorphism. Eur J Clin Pharmacol 36: 537, 1989.

Budman C, Bruun R: Persistent dyskinesia in patient receiving fluoxetine (letter). Am J Psychiatry 148: 1403, 1991.

Burke M, Sebastian CS: Treatment of clozapine sedation (letter). Am J Psychiatry 150: 1900, 1993.

Campbell A et al.: Prolonged anti-dopamine actions of single doses of butyrophenones in the rat. Psychopharmacology 87: 161, 1985.

Carpenter MD et al.: Methylphenidate augmentation therapy in schizophrenia. J Clin Psychopharmacol 12: 273, 1992.

Catravas JD: Haloperidol for acute amphetamine poisoning: a study in dogs. JAMA 231: 1340, 1975.

Centorrino F et al.: Clozapine and metabolites: serum concentrations and clinical findings during treatment of chronically psychotic patients. J Clin Psychopharmacology (in press).

Centorrino F et al.: Serum concentrations of clozapine and its major metabolites: effects of cotreatment with fluoxetine or valproate. Am J Psychiatry 151: 123, 1994.

Chiarello RJ, Cole MO: The use of psychostimulants in general psychiatry. Arch Gen Psychiatry 44: 286, 1987.

Chien C-P et al.: Prophylactic usage of antiparkinsonian drugs for akinesia. Psychopharmacol Bull 15: 75, 1979.

Chouinard G: Amitriptyline-pherphenazine interaction in ambulatory schizophrenic patients. Arch Gen Psychiatry 32: 1295, 1975.

Chouinard G et al.: A Canadian multicenter placebo-controlled study of fixed doses of risperidone and haloperidol in the treatment of chronic schizophrenic patients. J Clinical Psychopharmacol 13: 25, 1993.

Chouinard G et al.: Alpha methylopa-chlorpromazine interacts in schizophrenic patients. Curr Ther Res Clin Exp 15: 60, 1973a.

Chouinard G et al.: Potentiation of haloperidol by alpha-methylopa in the treatment of schizophrenic patients. Curr Ther Res Clin Exp 15: 473, 1973b.

Ciraulo DA, Shader RI: Fluoxetine drug-drug interactions: I. Antidepressants and antipsychotics. J Clin Psychopharmacol 10: 48, 1990.

Cobb CD et al.: Possible interaction between clozapine and lorazepam (letter). Am J Psychiatry 148: 1606, 1991.

Cohen BM et al.: Neuroleptic, antimuscarinic, and antiadrenergic activity of chlorpromazine, thioridazine, and their metabolites. Psychiatry Res 1: 199, 1979.

Cohen BM et al.: Clinical use of the radioreceptor assay for neuroleptics. Psychiatry Res 2: 173, 1980.

Cohen BM et al.: Differences between antipsychotic drugs in persistence of brain levels and behavioral effects. Psychopharmacology 108: 338, 1992.

Cohen S, Khan A: Adjunctive benzodiazepines in acute schizophrenia. Neuropsychobiology 18: 9, 1987.

Cohen WJ, Cohen NH: Lithium carbonate, haloperidol, and irreversible brain damage. JAMA 230: 1283, 1974.

Comaty J et al.: Is maintenance antiparkinsonian treatment necessary? Psychopharmacol Bull 26: 267, 1990.

Cooper TB: Neuroleptic drug monitoring and radioreceptor assays. J Clin Psychopharmacol 5: A15, 1985.

Courroisier S, Fournel J, Ducrot R: Pharmacodynamic properties of 3-chloro-10 (3'-dimethylaminopropyl) phenothiazine (RP 4560). Arch Int Pharmacodyn Ther 92: 305, 1953.

Creese I, et al.: Dopamine receptor binding predicts clinical and pharmacological potencies of antischizophrenic drugs. Science 192: 481, 1976.

Creese I, Snyder SH: A novel, simple and sensitive radioreceptor assay for antischizophrenic drugs in blood. Nature 270: 180, 1977.

Crewe HK et al.: the effect of selective serotonin re-uptake inhibitors on cytochrome P450-2D6 activity in human liver. Br J Clin Pharmacol 34: 262, 1992.

Curry S: Plasma protein binding of chlorpromazine. J Pharm Psychopharmacol 22: 193, 1970.

Curry SH, Hu OYP: The third, "deep," compartment for phenothiazine drug disposition: a new look at an old problem. Psychopharmacol Bull 26: 95, 1990.

Dahl SG: Plasma level monitoring of antipsychotic drugs: clinical utility. Clin Pharmacokinet 11: 36, 1986.

Decina P et al.: Cigarette smoking and neuroleptic-induced parkinsonism. Biol Psychiatry 28: 502, 1990.

Deng MZ et al.: Neuroleptic malignant syndrome in 12 of 9,792 Chinese inpatients exposed to neuroleptics: a prospective study. Am J Psychiatry 147: 1149, 1990.

Descotes J et al.: Study of thioridazine cardiotoxic effects by means of HIS bundle activity recording. Acta Pharmacol Toxicol (Copenhagen) 44: 370, 1979.

Douyon R et al. : Neuroleptic augmentation with alprazolam: clinical effects and pharmacokinetic correlates. Am J Psychiatry 146: 231, 1989.

Dreyfuss J et al.: Release and elimination of ^{14}C-fluphenazine enanthate and decanoate ester administered in sesame oil to dogs. J Pharm Sci 65: 502, 1976a.

Dreyfuss J et al.: Fluphenazine enanthate and fluphenazine decanoate: Intramuscular injection and esterification as requirements for slow-release characteristics in man. J Pharm Sci 65: 1976b.

Dysken M et al.: Fluphenazine pharmacokinetics and therapeutic response. Psychopharmacology 73: 205, 1981.

El-Yousef MK, Manier DH: Tricyclic antidepressants and phenothiazines. (letter). JAMA 229: 1419, 1974.

Ellenor GL et al.: Phenobarbital-thioridazine interaction in man. Res Comm Chem Path Pharmacol 21: 185, 1978.

Ereshefsky L et al.: Haloperidol and reduced haloperidol plasma levels in selected schizophrenic patients. J Clin Psychopharmacol 4: 138, 1984.

Ereshefsky L et al.: Effects of smoking on fluphenazine clearance in psychiatric inpatients. Biol Psychiatry 20: 329, 1985.

Ereshefsky L et al.: Thiothixene pharmacokinetic interactions: a study of hepatic enzyme inducers, clearance inhibitors, and demographic variables. J Clin Psychopharmacol 11: 296, 1991.

Espelin DE, Done AK: Amphetamine poisoning: effectiveness of chlorpromazine. N Engl J Med 278: 1361, 1968.

Evans DL et al.: Intestinal dilatation associated with phenothiazine therapy: a case report and literature review. J Psychiatry 136: 970, 1979.

Faigle J et al.: The biotransformation of carbamazepine. In: Birkmayer B (ed.): Epileptic Seizures—Behavior—Pain, Berne, Hans Huber, 1976.

Fallon B, Liebowitz M: Fluoxetine and extrapyramidal symptoms in CNS lupus (letter). J Clin Psychopharmacol 11: 147, 1991.

Fann WE et al.: Chlorpromazine reversal of the antihypertensive action of guanethidine. (letter). Lancet 2: 436, 1971.

Fann WE et al.: Chlorpromazine: effects of antacids on gastrointestinal absorbtion. J Clin Pharmacol 13: 388, 1973.

Farde L et al.: Central D2-dopamine receptor occupancy in schizophrenic patients treated with antipsychotic drugs. Arch Gen Psychiatry 45: 71, 1988.

Farde L et al.: D1- and D2-Dopamine receptor occupancy during treatment with conventional and atypical neuroleptics. Psychopharmacology 99: S28, 1989a.

Farde L et al.: Dopamine receptor occupancy and plasma haloperidol levels. Arch Gen Psychiatry 46: 483, 1989b.

Farde L et al.: Positron emission tomographic analysis of central D1 and D2 dopamine receptor occupancy in patients treated with classical neuroleptics and clozapine: relation to extrapyramidal side effects. Arch Gen Psychiatry 49: 538, 1992.

Fast DK et al.: Effect of carbamazepine on neuroleptic plasma level and efficacy. (letter). Am J Psychiatry 143: 117, 1986.

Fischer V et al.: The antipsychotic clozapine is metabolized by the polymorphic human microsomal and recombinant cytochrome P450 2D6. J Pharm Exp Ther 260: 1355, 1992.

Fonne-Pfister R, Meyer UA: Xenobiotic and endobiotic inhibitors of cytochrome P-450dbl function, the target of the debrisoquine/sparteine type polymorphism. Biochem Biophys Pharmacol 37: 3829, 1988.

Forrest FM et al.: Modification of chlorpromazine metabolism by some other drugs frequently administered to psychiatric patients. Biol Psychiatry 2: 53, 1970.

Forsman A, Ohman R: Applied pharmacokinetics of chlorpromazine after single and chronic dosage. Curr Ther Res 21: 396, 1977a.

Forsman A, Ohman R: Studies on serum protein binding of haloperidol. Curr Ther Res 21: 245, 1977b.

Foster CA et al.: Chlorpromazine: a study of its action on the circulation in man. Lancet 2: 614, 1954.

Frankenburg F, Baldessarini RJ: Clozapine—a novel antipsychotic agent (letter). New Engl J Med 325: 518, 1991.

Friedman LJ et al.: Clozapine—a novel antipsychotic agent (letter). New Engl J Med 325: 518, 1991.

Fruncillo RJ et al.: Severe hypotension associated with concurrent clonidine and antipsychotic medication (letter). Am J Psychiatry 142: 274, 1985.

Gardos G et al.: Anticholinergic challenge and neuroleptic withdrawal. Arch Gen Psychiatry 41: 1030, 1984.

Garver DL: Neuroleptic drug levels and antipsychotic effects: a difficult correlation; potential advantage of free (or derivative) versus total plasma levels. J Clin Psychopharmacol 9: 277, 1989.

Garza-Trevino ES et al.: Efficacy of combinations of intramuscular antipsychotics and sedative-hypnotics for control of psychotic agitation. 146: 1598, 1989.

Gautier J et al.: Influence of the antiparkinsonian drugs on the plasma level of neuroleptics. Biol Psychiatry 12: 389, 1977.

Gay PE, Marsden JA: Interaction between phenobarbital and thioridazine. Neurology 33: 1631, 1983.

Gelenberg A et al.: Anticholinergic effects on memory: benztropine versus amantadine. J Clin Psychopharmacol 9: 180, 1989.

Gerlach J et al.: Antiparkinsonian agents and long-term neuroleptic treatment. Acta Psychiatr Scand 55: 251, 1977.

Gilder DA et al.: A comparison of the abilities of chlorpromazine and molindone to interact adversely with guanethidine. J Pharmacol Exp Ther 198: 255, 1976.

Giles TO, Modlin RK: Death associated with ventricular arrhythmias and thioridazine hydrochloride. JAMA 205: 108, 1968.

Ginsburg J, Duff RS: Effect of chlorpromazine on adrenaline vasoconstriction in man. Br J Pharmacol 11: 180, 1956.

Giordano J et al.: Fatal paralytic ileus complicating phenothiazine therapy. South Med J 68: 351, 1975.

Godwin-Austen RB et al.: Smoking and Parkinson's disease. J Neurol Neurosurg Psychiatry 45: 577, 1982.

Goff D, Baldessarini R: Drug interactions with antipsychotic agents. J Clin Psychopharmacol 13: 57, 1993.

Goff DC, Ciraulo DA: Stimulants. In: Ciraulo DA and Shader RI (eds.): *Clinical Manual of Chemical Dependence*, Washington, DC, American Psychiatric Press, 1991, p. 133.

Goff DC, Shader RI: Non-neurologic side effects of antipsychotic agents. In: Weinberger and Hirsch (eds.): *Schizophrenia*, Oxford, Blackwell, 1994.

Goff D et al.: The effect of benztropine on haloperidol-induced dystonia, clinical efficacy and pharmacokinetics: a prospective, double-blind trial. J Clin Psychopharmacol 11: 106, 1991a.

Goff D et al.: An open trial of buspirone added to neuroleptics in schizophrenic patients. J Clin Psychopharmacol 11: 193, 1991b.

Goff D et al.: Elevation of plasma concentrations of haloperidol after addition of fluoxetine. Am J Psychiatry 148: 790, 1991c.

Goff DC et al.: Cigarette smoking in schizophrenia: relationship to psychopathology and medication side effects. Am J Psychiatry 149: 1189, 1992.

Goff DC et al.: A placebo controlled trial of trihexyphenidyl in unmedicated schizophrenic patients. Am J Psychiatry 151: 421–429, 1994.

Goff DC et al.: A placebo controlled trial of fluoxetine added to neuroleptic in patients with schizophrenia. Psychopharmacology (in press).

Goldberg T et al.: Cognitive and behavioral effects of the coadministration of dextroamphetamine and haloperidol in schizophrenia. Am J Psychiatry 148: 78, 1991.

Goldney RD, Spence ND: Safety of the combination of lithium and neuroleptic drugs. Am J Psychiatry 143: 882, 1986.

Goldstein BJ: Interaction of antacids with psychotropics. Hosp Community Psychiatry 33: 96, 1982.

Gram LF, Christiansen J, et al.: Pharmacokinetic interaction between tricylic antidepressants and other psychopharmac. Acta Psychiatr Scand 243(suppl): 52, 1973.

Gram LF, Overo KF: Drug interaction: Inhibitory effect of neuroleptics on metabolism of tricyclic antidepressants in man. Br Med J 1: 463, 1972.

Gram LF et al.: Influence of neuroleptics and benzodiazepines on metabolism of tricyclic antidepressants in man. Am J Psychiatry 131: 863, 1974.

Greeman M, McClellan TA: Negative effects of a smoking ban on an inpatient psychiatry service. Hosp Community Psychiatry 42: 408, 1991.

Greendyke RM, Gulya A: Effect of pindolol administration on serum levels of thioridazine, haloperidol, phenytoin and phenobarbital. J Clin Psychiatry 49: 1988.

Greendyke RM, Kanter DR: Plasma propranolol levels and their effect on plasma thioridazine and haloperidol concentrations. J Clin Psychopharmacol 7: 178, 1987.

Griffith J et al.: Paranoid episodes induced by drug. JAMA 205: 39, 1968.

Grohmann R et al.: Adverse effects of clozapine. Psychopharmacology 99 (suppl): s101, 1989.

Haidvkewycz D, Rodin EA: Effect of phenothiazines on serum antiepileptic concentrations in psychiatric patients with seizure disorder. Ther Drug Monit 7: 401, 1985.

Halman M, Goldbloom DS: Fluoxetine and neuroleptic malignant syndrome. Biol Psychiatry 28: 518, 1990.

Hanlon TE et al.: Perphenazine-benztropine mesylate treatment of newly admitted psychiatric patients. Psychopharmacologia 9: 328, 1966.

Hansen J et al.: Carbamazepine-induced acceleration of diphenylhydantoin in warfarin metabolism in man. Clin Pharmacol Ther 12: 539, 1971.

Hansen LB et al.: Plasma levels of perphenazine and its major metabolites during simultaneous treatment with anticholinergic drugs. Br J Clin Pharm 7: 75, 1979.

Hansen LB, Larsen NE: Metabolic interaction between perphenazine and disulfiram. Lancet 2: 1472, 1982.

Haring C et al.: Dose-related plasma levels of clozapine. J Clin Psychopharmacol 9: 71, 1989.

Henningfield JE, Woodson PP: Dose-related actions of nicotine on behavior and physiology: review and implications for replacement therapy for nicotine dependence. J Subst Abuse Treat 1: 301, 1989.

Heykants J et al.: The pharmacokinetics of risperidone in humans: a summary. J Clin Psychiatry 55(suppl): 13–17, 1994.

Hitri A et al.: Serum neuroleptic and anticholinergic activity in relationship to cognitive toxicity of antiparkinsonian agents in schizophrenic patients. Psychopharmacol Bull 23: 33, 1987.

Howes CA et al.: Reduced steady-state plasma concentrations of chlorpromazine and indomethacin in patients receiving cimetidine. Eur J Clin Pharmacol 24: 99, 1983.

Hubbard JW et al.: Prolonged pharmacologic activity of neuroleptic drugs (letter). Arch Gen Psychiatry 44: 99, 1987.

Huey LY et al.: Effects of methylphenidate in adult psychiatric inpatients: a preliminary report. Psychopharmacol Bull 20: 10, 1984.

Jann MW et al.: Effects of carbamazepine on plasma haloperidol levels. J Clin Psychopharmacol 5: 106, 1985.

Jann MW et al.: Effects of smoking on haloperidol and reduced haloperidol plasma concentrations and haloperidol clearance. Psychopharmacology 90: 468, 1986.

Janowsky DS et al.: Antagonism of guanethidine by chlorpromazine. Am J Psychiatry 130: 808, 1973.

Jeffries J et al.: The question of lithium/neuroleptic toxicity. Can J Psychiatry 29: 601, 1984.

Jerling M et al.: Fluvoxamine inhibition and carbamazepine induction of the metabolism of clozapine: evidence from a therapeutic monitoring service. Ther Drug Monitoring 16: 368–374, 1994a.

Jerling M et al.: The use of therapeutic drug monitoring data to document kinetic drug interactions: an example with amitriptyline and nortriptyline. Ther Drug Monit 16: 1, 1994b.

Johnson DAW: Observations on the dose regime of fluphenazine decanoate in maintenance therapy of schizophrenia. Br J Psychiatry 126: 457, 1975.

Johnstone EC et al.: Adverse effects of anticholinergic medication on positive schizophrenic symptoms. Psychol Med 13: 513, 1983.

Johnstone EC et al.: The Northwick Park "functional" psychosis study: diagnosis and treatment response. Lancet 119, 1988.

Jorgensen A: Metabolism and pharmacokinetics of antipsychotic drugs. In: Bridges JW and Chasseaud LF (ed.): Progress in Drug Metabolism, Bristol, Pa., Taylor and Francis, 1986, p. 111.

Kahn EM et al.: Change in haloperidol level due to carbamazepine—a complicating factor in combined medication for schizophrenia. J Clin Psychopharmacol 10: 54, 1990.

Kalow W: Interethnic variation in drug metabolism. Trends Pharmacol Sci 12: 102, 1991.

Kane J et al.: Extrapyramidal side effects with lithium treatment. Am J Psychiatry 135: 851, 1978.

Kanter GL et al.: Case report of a possible interaction between neuroleptics and carbamazepine. Am J Psychiatry 141: 1101, 1984.

Keck PE Jr. et al.: Declining frequency of neuroleptic malignant syndrome in a hospital population. Am J Psychiatry 148: 880, 1991.

Keck PJ et al.: Risk factors for neuroleptic malignant syndrome: a case control study. Arch Gen Psychiatry 46: 914, 1989.

Kessler II, Diamond KL: Epidemiologic studies of Parkinson's disease: I. Smoking and Parkinson's disease: a survey and explanatory hypothesis. Am J Epidemiol 94: 16, 1971.

Ketter TA et al.: Principles of clinically important drug interactions with carbamazepine: Part II. J Clin Psychopharmacol 11: 306, 1991.

Khot V et al.: The assessment and clinical implications of haloperidol acute-dose, steady-state, and withdrawal pharmacokinetics. J Clin Psychopharmacol 13, 1993.

Kidron R et al.: Carbamazepine-induced reduction of blood levels of haloperidol in chronic schizophrenia. Biol Psychiatry 20: 219, 1985.

Klett CJ et al.: Evaluating the long term need for antiparkinson drugs by chronic schizophrenics. Arch Gen Psychiatry 26: 374, 1972.

Ko GN et al.: Haloperidol and reduced haloperidol concentrations in plasma and red blood cells from chronic schizophrenic patients. J Clin Psychopharmacol 9: 186, 1989.

Kocsis JH et al.: Response to treatment with antidepressants of patients with severe or moderate nonpsychotic depression and of patients with psychotic depression. Am J Psychiatry 147: 621, 1990.

Koczapski A et al.: Effects of caffeine on behavior of schizophrenic inpatients. Schizophren Bull 15: 339, 1989.

Korpi ER, Wyatt RJ: Reduced haloperidol: Effects on striatal dopamine metabolism and conversion to haloperidol in the rat. Psychopharmacology 83: 34, 1984.

Korsgaard S et al.: Behavioral aspects of serotonin-dopamine interaction in the monkey. Eur J Pharmacol 118: 245, 1985.

Kragh-Sorensen P et al.: Effect of simultaneous treatment with low doses of perphenazine on plasma and urine concentrations of nortriptyline and 10-hydroxynortriptyline. Eur J Clin Pharmacol 19: 479, 1977.

Kramer M et al.: Antidepressants in 'depressed' schizophrenic inpatients: a controlled trial. Arch Gen Psychiatry 46: 922, 1989.

Kulhanek F: Precipitation of antipsychotic drugs in interaction with coffee or tea (letter). Lancet 2: 1130, 1979.

Kulhanek F, Linde OK: Coffee and tea influence pharmacokinetics of antipsychotic drugs (letter). Lancet 2: 359, 1981.

Lear E et al.: A clinical study of mechanisms of action of chlorpromazine. JAMA 163: 30, 1957.

Lemberger L et al.: The effects of haloperidol and chlorpromazine on amphetamine metabolism and amphetamine stereotype behavior in the rat. J Pharmacol Exp Ther 174: 428, 1970.

Lerner Y et al.: Acute high-dose parenteral haloperidol treatment of psychosis. Am J Psychiatry 136: 1061, 1979.

Leysen JE et al.: Interaction of antipsychotic drugs with neurotransmitter receptor sites in vitro and in vivo in relation to pharmacological and clinical effects: role of 5HT2 receptors. Psychopharmacology 112: S40, 1993.

Lieber CS: Biochemical and molecular basis of alcohol-induced injury to liver and other tissues. N Eng J Med 319: 1639, 1988.

Lieber CS: Interaction of alcohol with other drugs and nutrients: Implications for the therapy of alcoholic liver disease. Drugs 40 (suppl): 23, 1990.

Lieberman JA et al.: Prediction of relapse in schizophrenia. Arch Gen Psychiatry 44: 597, 1987.

Lieberman JA et al.: Clozapine: guidelines for clinical management. J Clin Psychiatry 50: 329, 1989.

Lieberman JA et al.: Dopaminergic mechanisms in idiopathic and drug-induced psychoses. Schizophrenia Bull 16: 97, 1990.

Lin K-M et al.: A longitudinal assessment of haloperidol doses and serum concentrations in Asian and Caucasian schizophrenic patients. Am J Psychiatry 146: 1307, 1989.

Linnoila M et al.: Effect of anticonvulsants on plasma haloperidol and thioridazine levels. Am J Psychiatry 137: 819, 1980.

Lipinski JF et al.: Fluoxetine-induced akathisia: clinical and theoretical implications. J Clin Psychiatry 50: 339, 1989.

Lock J et al.: Possible adverse drug interactions between fluoxetine and other psychotropics (letter). J Clin Psychopharmacol 10: 383, 1990.

Loga S et al.: Interactions of orphenadrine and phenobarbitone with chlorpromazine: plasma concentrations and effects in man. Br J Clin Pharmacol 2: 197, 1975.

Loga S et al.: Interaction of chlorpromazine and nortriptyline in patients with schizophrenia. Clin Pharmacokinet 6: 454, 1981.

Loudon JB, Waring H: Toxic reactions to lithium and haloperidol (letter). Lancet 2: 1088, 1976.

Lucas PB et al.: Effects of the acute administration of caffeine in patients with schizophrenia. Biol Psychiatry 28: 35, 1990.

Lund-Johnsen P: Shock after administration of phenothiazines in patients with pheochromocytoma. Acta Med Scand 172: 525, 1962.

Lutz EG: Neuroleptic-induced akathisia and dystonia triggered by alcohol. JAMA 236: 2422, 1976.

Mann SC, Bolger WP: Psychotropic drugs, summer heat and humidity, and hyperpyrexia: a danger restated. Am J Psychiatry 135: 1097, 1978.

Manos N et al.: The need for continuous use of antiparkinsonian medication with chronic schizophrenic patients receiving long-term neuroleptic therapy. Am J Psychiatry 138: 184, 1981a.

Manos N et al.: Gradual withdrawal of antiparkinson medication in chronic schizophrenics: any better than abrupt? J Ner Ment Dis 169: 659, 1981b.

Manos N et al.: Evaluation of the need for prophylactic antiparkinsonian medication in psychotic patients treated with neuroleptics. J Clin Psychiatry 47: 114, 1986.

Marder S, Meibach RC: Risperidone in the treatment of schizophrenia. Am J Psychiatry 151: 825–835, 1994.

Marder SR et al.: Pharmacokinetics of long-acting injectable neuroleptics drugs: clinical implications. Psychopharmacology 98: 433, 1989.

Matilla MJ: Alcohol and drug interactions. Ann Med 22: 363, 1990.

McEvoy J: The clinical use of anticholinergic drugs as treatment for extrapyramidal side effects of neuroleptic drugs. J Clin Psychopharmacol 3: 288, 1983.

McEvoy J et al.: Effects of amantadine and trihexyphenidyl on memory in elderly normal volunteers. Am J Psychiatry 144: 573, 1987.

McEvoy JP, Freter S: The dose-response relationship for memory impairment by anticholinergic drugs. Compr Psychiatry 30: 135, 1989.

Meltzer HY et al.: Extrapyramidal side effects and increased serum prolactin following fluoxetine, a new antidepressant. J Neural Transm 45: 165, 1979.

Metzger E, Friedman R: Prolongation of the corrected QT and Torsades de Pointes cardiac arrhythmia associated with intravenous haloperidol in the medically ill. J Clin Psychopharmacol 13: 128, 1993.

Mezey E: Ethanol metabolism and ethanol-drug interactions. Biochem Pharmacol 25: 869, 1976.

Midha KK et al.: Variation in the single dose pharmacokinetics of fluphenazine in psychiatric patients. Psychopharmacology 96: 206, 1988a.

Midha KK et al.: A pharmacokinetic study of trifluoperazine in two ethnic populations. Psychopharmacology 95: 333, 1988b.

Midha KK et al.: The role of the analytical biochemist in resistant schizophrenia. In: Dencker SJ and Kulhanek F (eds.): Treatment Resistance in Schizophrenia, Braunschweig/Wiesbaden, Vieweg, 1988c, p. 56.

Midha KK et al.: Intersubject variation in the pharmacokinetics of haloperidol and reduced haloperidol. J Clin Psychopharmacol 9: 98, 1989.

Miller DD: Effect of phenytoin on plasma clozapine concentrations in two patients. J Clin Psychiatry 52: 23, 1991.

Miller F, Menninger J: Lithium-neuroleptic neurotoxicity is dose dependent. J Clin Psychopharmacol 7: 89, 1987.

Modell W, Hussar AE: Failure of dextroamphetamine sulfate to influence eating and sleeping patterns in obese schizophrenic patients: clinical and pharmacological significance. JAMA 193: 275, 1965.

Morselli PL et al.: Further observations on the interaction between ethanol and psychotropic drugs. Drug Res 1: 20, 1971.

Nadel I, Wallach M: Drug interactions between haloperidol and methyldopa. Br J Psychiatry 135: 484, 1979.

Nelson JC, Jatlow PI: Neuroleptic effect on desipramine steady-state plasma concentrations. Am J Psychiatry 137: 1232, 1980.

Opler LA, Feinberg SS: The role of pimozide in clinical psychiatry: a review. J Clin Psychiatry 52: 221, 1991.

Orlov P et al.: Withdrawal of antiparkinsonian drugs. Arch Gen Psychiatry 25: 410, 1971.

Otani K et al.: Biperiden and piroheptine do not affect the serum level of zotepine, a new antipsychotic drug. Br J Psychiatry 157: 128, 1990.

Overo KF et al.: Interaction of perphenazine with the kinetics of nortriptyline. Acta Pharmacol Toxicol 40: 97, 1977.

Pato CN et al.: Benzodiazepine augmentation of neuroleptic treatment in patients with schizophrenia. Psychopharmacology Bull 25: 263, 1989.

Peet M et al.: Pharmacokinetic interaction between propranolol and chlorpromazine in schizophrenic patients. Lancet 2: 978, 1980.

Pinell OC et al.: Drug-drug interaction of chlorpromazine and antacid (abstract). Clin Pharmacol Ther 23: 125, 1978.

Plasky P: Antidepressant usage in schizophrenia. Schizophren Bull 17: 649, 1991.

Pope HGJ et al.: Frequency and presentation of neuroleptic malignant syndrome in a large paychiatric hospital. Am J Psychiatry 143: 1227, 1986.

Prakash R et al.: Neurotoxicity with combined administration of lithium and a neuroleptic. Compr Psychiatry 23: 567, 1982.

Prusoff VA et al.: Treatment of secondary depression in schizophrenia. Arch Gen Psychiatry 36: 569, 1979.

Richardson HL et al.: Intramyocardial lesions in patients dying suddenly and unexpectedly. JAMA 195: 254, 1966.

Rimon R et al.: Serum and CSF levels of haloperidol by radioimmunoassay and radioreceptor assay during high-dose therapy of resistant schizophrenic patients. Psychopharmacology 73: 197, 1981.

Risch SC et al.: Interfaces of psychopharmacology and cardiology: Part 2. J Clin Psychiatry 42: 47, 1981.

Rivera-Calimlim L: Effect of lithium on gastric emptying and absorption of oral chlorpromazine. Psychopharmacol Commun 2: 263, 1976.

Rivera-Calimlim L et al.: Effects of mode of management on plasma chlorpromazine in psychiatric patients. Clin Pharmacol Ther 14: 978, 1973.

Rivera-Calimlim L et al.: Clinical response and plasma levels: Effect of dose, dosage schedules, and drug interactions on plasma chlorpromazine levels. Am J Psychiatry 133: 646, 1976.

Rivera-Calimlim L et al.: Effect of lithium of plasma chlorpromazine levels. Clin Pharmacol Ther 23: 451, 1978.

Rockland L et al.: Effects of trihexyphenidyl on plasma chlorpromazine in young schizophrenics. Can J Psychiatry 35: 604, 1990.

Rosebush P, Stewart T: A prospective analysis of 24 episodes of neuroleptic malignant syndrome. Am J Psychiatry 146: 717, 1989.

Sachdev PS: Lithium potentiation of neuroleptic-related extrapyramidal side effects (letter). Am J Psychiatry 143: 942, 1986.

Salzman C et al.: Benzodiazepines combined with neuroleptics for management of severe disruptive behavior. Psychosomatics 27 (suppl): 17, 1986.

Salzman C et al.: Parental lorazepam versus parental haloperidol for the control of psychotic disruptive behavior. J Clin Psychiatry 52: 177, 1991.

Sandyk R, Hurwitz MD: Toxic irreversible encephalopathy induced by lithium carbonate and haloperidol: a report of two cases. S Afr Med J 64: 875, 1983.

Sato M: Acute exacerbation of methamphetamine psychosis and lasting dopaminergic supersensitivity: a clinical survey. Psychopharmacol Bull 22: 751, 1986.

Schou M: Long-lasting neurological sequelae after lithium intoxication. Acta Psychiatr Scand 70: 594, 1984.

Seppala T: Effect of chlorpromazine or sulpride and alcohol on psychomotor skills related to driving. Arch Int Pharmacodyn 223: 311, 1976.

Sharma RP et al.: Behavioral and biochemical effects of methylphenidate in schizophrenic and nonschizophrenic patients. Biol Psychiatry 30: 459, 1991.

Shoaf SE, Linnoila M: Interaction of ethanol and smoking on the pharmacokinetics and pharmacodynamics of psychotropic medications. Psychopharmacol Bull 27: 577, 1991.

Shopsin B et al.: Combining lithium and neuroleptics (letter). Am J Psychiatry 133: 980, 1976.

Silver H et al.: Postural hypotension in chronically medicated schizophrenics. J Clin Psychiatry 51: 459, 1990.

Silver H, Nassar A: Fluvoxamine improves negative symptoms in treated chronic schizophrenia: an add-on double-blind, placebo-controlled study. Biol Psychiatry 31: 698, 1992.

Silver JM et al.: Elevation of thioridazine plasma levels by propranolol. Am J Psychiatry 143: 1290, 1986.

Simpson GM et al.: Effect of antiparkinsonian medication on plasma levels of chlorpromazine. Arch Gen Psychiatry 37: 205, 1980.

Simpson LL: Combined use of molindone and guanethidine in patients with schizophrenia and hypertension. Am J Psychiatry 136: 1410, 1979.

Singh MM, Kay SR: A comparative study of haloperidol and chlorpromazine in terms of clinical effects and therapeutic reversal with benztropine in schizophrenia. Psychopharmacologia 43: 103, 1975a.

Singh MM, Kay SR: Therapeutic reversal with benztropine in schizophrenics: Practical and theoretical significance. J Nerv Ment Dis 160: 258, 1975b.

Singh MM, Smith JM: Reversal of some therapeutic effects of an antipsychotic agent by an antiparkinsonism drug. J Nerv Ment Dis 157: 50, 1973.

Siris SG et al.: Plasma imipramine concentrations in patients receiving concomitant fluphenazine decanoate. Am J Psychiatry 139: 104, 1982a.

Siris SG et al.: Response of postpsychotic depression to adjunctive imipramine or amitriptyline. J Clin Psychiatry 43: 485, 1982b.

Siris SG et al.: Targeted treatment of depression-like symptoms in schizophrenia. Psychopharmacol Bull 23: 85, 1987a.

Siris SG et al.: Adjunctive imipramine in the treatment of postpsychotic depression. Arch Gen Psychiatry 44: 533, 1987b.

Siris SG et al.: The use of antidepressants for negative symptoms in a subset of schizophrenic patients. Psychopharmacol Bull 27: 331, 1991.

Sjoqvist F: Psychotropic drugs. II: interaction between monoamine oxidase (MAO) inhibitors and other substances. Proc R Soc Med 58: 967, 1965.

Sletten IW: Weight reduction with chlorpheneramine and phenmetrazine in obese psychiatric patients during chlorpromazine therapy. Curr Ther Res Clin Exp 9: 570, 1967.

Sorby DL, Liu G: Effects of absorbents on drug absorbtion: II. effect of an antidiarrheal mixture on promazine absorbtion. J Pharm Sci 55: 504, 1966.

Spiker D: The pharmacological treatment of delusional depression. Am J Psychiatry 142: 430, 1985.

Spring G, Frankel M: New data on lithium and haloperidol incompatibility. Am J Psychiatry 138: 818, 1981.

Sramek J et al.: Persistence of plasma neuroleptic levels after drug discontinuation. J Clin Psychopharmacol 7: 436, 1987.

Stein MH: Tardive dyskinesia in a patient taking haloperidol and fluoxetine (letter). Am J Psychiatry 148: 683, 1991.

Steiner E et al.: Polymorphic debrisoquine hydroxylation in 757 Swedish subjects. Clin Pharmacol Ther 44: 431, 1988.

Stimmel GL, Falloon IRH: Chlorpromazine plasma levels, adverse effects, and tobacco smoking: case report. J Clin Psychiatry 44: 420, 1983.

Stoukides JA, Stoukides CA: Extrapyramidal symptoms upon discontinuation of fluoxetine (letter). Am J Psychiatry 148: 1263, 1991.

Strauss ME et al.: Effects of anticholinergic medication on memory in schizophrenia. Schizophren Res 3: 127, 1990.

Straw GM et al.: Haloperidol and reduced haloperidol concentrations and psychiatric ratings in schizophrenic patients treated with ascorbic acid. J Clin Psychopharmacol 9: 130, 1989.

Sulser F, Dingell JV: Potentiation and blockade of the central action of ampehetamine by chlorpromazine. Biochem Pharmacol 17: 634, 1968.

Sunderland T, Cohen BM: Blood to brain distribution of neuroleptics. Psychiatry Res 20: 299, 1987.

Susman VL, Addonizio G: Reinduction of neuroleptic malignant syndrome by lithium. J Clin Psychopharmacol 7: 339, 1987.

Szymanski S: A case report of cimetidine-induced clozapine toxicity. J Clin Psychiatry 52: 21, 1991.

Tandon R et al.: Treatment of negative schizophrenic symptoms with trihexyphenidyl. J Clin Psychopharmacol 8: 212, 1988.

Tandon R et al.: Cholinergic syndrome following anticholinergic withdrawal in a schizophrenic patient abusing marijuana. Br J Psychiatry 154: 712, 1989a.

Tandon R et al.: Positive and negative symptoms in schizophrenia and the dexamethasone suppression test. Biol Psychiatry 25: 785, 1989b.

Tandon R et al.: Effect of anticholinergic medication on positive and negative symptoms in medication-free schizophrenic patients. Psychiatry Res 31: 235, 1990.

Tandon R et al.: Muscarinic cholinergic hyperactivity in schizophrenia: Relationship to positive and negative symptoms. Schizophren Res 4: 23, 1991.

Tandon R, Greden JF: Cholinergic hyperactivity and negative schizophrenic symptoms. Arch Gen Psychiatry 46: 745, 1989.

Tate JL: Extrapyramidal symptoms in a patient taking haloperidol and fluoxetine (letter). Am J Psychiatry 146: 399, 1989.

Thornton WE: Dementia induced by methyldopa with haloperidol. N Engl J Med 294: 1222, 1976.

Tune LE et al.: Serum levels of anticholinergic drugs and impaired recent memory in chronic schizophrenic patients. Am J Psychiatry 139: 1460, 1982.

Turano P et al.: Thin layer chromatography of chlorpromazine metabolites. Attempt to identify each of the metabolites appearing in blood, urine and feces of chronically medicated schizophrenics. J Chromatogr 75: 277, 1973.

Van Putten T et al.: Neuroleptic plasma levels. Schizophren Bull 17: 197, 1991.

Vandel B et al.: Interaction between amitriptyline and phenothiazine in man: effect on plasma concentration of amitriptyline and its metabolite nortriptyline and the correlation with clinical response. Psychopharmacology 65: 187, 1979.

Verghese C et al.: Pharmacokinetics of neuroleptics. Psychopharmacol Bull 27: 551, 1991.

Vestal RE et al.: Inhibition of propranolol metabolism by chlorpromazine. Clin Pharmacol Ther 25: 19, 1979.

Vinarova E et al.: Smokers need higher doses of neuroleptic drugs. Biol Psychiatry 19: 1265, 1984.

Vincent FM: Phenothiazine induced phenytoin intoxication. Ann Int Med 93: 56, 1980.

Volkow ND et al.: Effects of chronic cocaine abuse on postsynaptic dopamine receptors. Am J Psychiatry 147: 719, 1990.

von Bahr C et al.: Plasma levels of thioridazine and metabolites are influenced by the debrisoquin hydroxylation phenotype. Clin Pharmacol Ther 49: 234, 1991.

von Moltke LL et al.: Cytochromes in psychopharmacology. J Clin Psychopharmacol 14:1, 1994.

Waehrens J, Gerlach J: Antidepressant drugs in anergic schizophrenia. Acta Psychiatr Scand 61: 438, 1980.

Wagner B et al.: Does smoking reduce the risk of neuroleptic parkinsonoids? Pharmacopsychiatry 21: 301, 1988.

Wallace SM: Oral fluphenazine and tea and coffee drinking. Lancet 2: 691, 1981.

Warburton DM: Nicotine: an addictive substance or a therapeutic agent? Prog Drug Res 33: 9, 1989.

Wesnes K, Warburton DM: Nicotine, smoking and human performance. Pharmacol Ther 12: 189, 1983.

White WB: Hypotension and postural syncope secondary to the combination of chlorpromazine and captopril. Arch Int Med 146: 1833, 1986.

Winslow RS et al.: Prevention of acute dystonic reactions in patients beginning high-potency neuroleptics. Am J Psychiatry 143: 706, 1986.

Wode-Helgodt B et al.: Clinical effects and drug concentrations in plasma and cerebrospinal fluid in psychiatric patients treated with fixed doses of chlorpromazine. Acta Psychiatr Scand 58: 149, 1978.

Wolkowitz OM, Pickar D: Benzodiazepines in the treatment of schizophrenia: a review and reappraisal. Am J Psychiatry 148: 714, 1991.

Wolkowitz OM et al.: Alprazolam augmentation of the antipsychotic effects of fluphenazine in schizophrenic patients. Arch Gen Psychiatry 143: 664, 1988.

World Health Organization: Prophylactic use of anticholinergics in patients on long-term neuroleptic treatment. Br J Psychiatry 156: 412, 1990.

Wozniak KM et al.: Focal application of alcohols elevates extracellular dopamine in rat brain: a microdialysis study. Brain Res 540: 31, 1991.

Yassa R et al.: Nicotine exposure and tardive dyskinesia. Biol Psychiatry 22: 67, 1987.

Yerevanian BI, Hodgman CH: A haloperidol-carbamazepine interaction in a patient with rapid-cycling bipolar disorder. (letter). Am J Psychiatry 142: 785, 1985.

Yisak W et al.: Interaction study between remoxipride and biperiden. Psychopharmacology 111: 27, 1993.

Yoon MS et al.: Effects of thioridazine (Mellaril) on ventricular electrophysiologic properties. Am J Cardiol 43: 1155, 1979.

Yorkston NJ et al.: Propranolol as an adjunct to the treament of schizophrenia. Lancet 2: 575, 1977.

Zanger UM et al.: Absence of hepatic cytochrome P450bufl causes genetically deficient debrisoquine oxidation in man. Biochemistry 27: 5447, 1988.

Zaslove MO et al.: Changes in behaviors of inpatients after a ban on the sale of caffeinated drinks. Hosp Community Psychiatry 42: 84, 1991.

Zelman S, Guillan R: Heat stroke in phenothiazine-treated patients: A report of three fatalities. Am J Psychiatry 126: 1787, 1970.

Ziemba T et al.: Do anticholinergics antagonize antipsychotic drug action? Schizophren Bull 4: 7, 1978.

4

Lithium

OFRA SARID-SEGAL, WAYNE L. CREELMAN, DOMENIC A. CIRAULO,
RICHARD I. SHADER

Introduction

Lithium is rapidly absorbed after oral administration, with peak levels occurring 2 to 4 hours after the dose, although slow release formulations are also available. Lithium elimination is primarily through renal excretion, so that drug interactions involving hepatic metabolism do not occur. Lithium does not bind to plasma proteins. Pharmacokinetic interactions therefore usually involve altered renal clearance of lithium, with some drugs increasing clearance and lowering serum lithium (e.g. theophylline) and others drugs decreasing renal clearance, leading to toxic levels of lithium (e.g. thiazide diuretics). Lithium has a low therapeutic index, which means that there is a small difference between therapeutic and toxic levels. Symptoms and signs associated with toxic lithium levels include nausea, vomiting, diarrhea, tremor, headache, sedation, confusion, hyperreflexia, cardiac arrhythmias, hypotension, and, in the most severe cases, coma and death. Severe lithium toxicity is usually associated with serum levels above 2.5 mEq/liter; serum levels above 3.0 mEq/liter require hemodialysis, and those above 3.5 mEq/liter are life threatening. In elderly or medically compromised patients, much lower levels, even those typically considered therapeutic, may lead to toxicity.

Pharmacodynamic or receptor site interactions produce toxicity with lithium levels that are often in the therapeutic range, and the clinical presentation is usually a combination of lithium toxicity with the adverse effects of the coadministered drug. The interaction of lithium with carbamazepine and some calcium channel blockers are examples of drug interactions in which neurotoxicity develops with moderate serum lithium levels.

Aminophylline/Theophylline

Evidence of Interaction

Aminophylline and theophylline increase lithium excretion (Thomsen et al. 1968) and have been used to treat lithium toxicity. Perry et al. (1984) studied 10 normal subjects on 12 mg/kg/day of theophylline with up to 900 mg/day of lithium. The subjects received first lithium alone, then lithium with theophylline, then lithium alone, for a total of 23 days. During the intermediate period of coadministration, lithium clearance rose from 20.1 to 26.1 ml/min, with theophylline serum levels ranging from 5.4 to 12.7 μg/ml in a linear dose-dependent relationship with lithium clearance. Holstad et al. (1988) also reported enhanced clearance of lithium after theophylline infusion in normal volunteers. In a separate case report, increasing doses of theophylline led to clinical deterioration with decreased lithium levels (Cook et al. 1985).

Mechanism

Aminophylline and theophylline enhance renal excretion of lithium.

Clinical Implications

This interaction may create a problem in the treatment of manic patients who require these medications for chronic obstructive pulmonary disease. Careful titration of dosages and judicious monitoring of blood levels should permit physicians to administer aminophylline or theophylline to patients taking lithium (Sierles et al. 1982). As with any interaction of this type, the closest surveillance is required for several days after starting or stopping one of the drugs.

Antimicrobials

Evidence of Interaction

Antimicrobials (including oral tetracycline, parenteral spectinomycin, and metronidazole) may raise serum lithium levels, resulting in toxicity. These antibiotics impair renal lithium excretion (Ayd 1978, Jefferson 1987, McGennis 1978).

In an animal study, rats receiving a single dose of 10 ml/kg of lithium chloride 150 mmol combined with 33.5 mg/10 ml of tetracycline hydrochloride, 33.5 mg/10 ml ampicillin, or 15 mg/10 ml metronidazole all experienced reduced urinary lithium excretion, while renal lithium clearance remained unchanged. Tetracycline increased distal sodium reabsorption and reduced renal sodium clearance. Tetracycline and metronidazole both reduced serum lithium levels 6 hours following administration, but increased these levels 24 hours after administration (Lassen 1985). In another study evaluating the relationship of the interaction between lithium and tetracycline, Fankhauser et al. (1988) found a decrease in steady-state lithium levels, suggesting that there may be some variability in the response to coadministration of these drugs.

A number of case reports also document lithium-antibiotic reactions. A woman who had been taking lithium carbonate for 3 years took an initial 500 mg of tetracycline followed by 250 mg 3 times a day. Serum lithium concentration rose from 0.81 mmol/l to 2.75 mmol/liter over 4 days and she suffered clinical symptoms of lithium intoxication (McGennis 1978).

A 40-year-old woman taking lithium carbonate 1,800 mg, propranolol 60 mg, and levothyroxine 0.15 mg/day, took metronidazole 500 mg/day for 7 days. Serum lithium concentration rose from 1.3 to 1.9 mmol/liter (Ayd 1982a). Two other case reports of metronidazole-induced lithium toxicity have been reported (Teicher et al, 1987). In both cases serum creatinine rose concomitantly with serum lithium. In 1 case serum creatinine rose from 1.01 to 1.6 mg/dl after 2 days of metronidazole 250 mg 3 times per day, and to 1.9 mg/dl after 2 weeks. During that same period lithium level increased from 1.09 mmol/liter to 1.3 mmol/liter with symptoms of polyuria. A man taking spectinomycin to treat gonorrhea experienced a rise in serum lithium level from 0.8 to 3.2 mmol/l (Conroy 1978). Two patients taking both lithium and sulfamethoxazole-trimethoprim experienced a 30 to 40% decrease in serum lithium level in a paradoxical reaction (Desvilles 1982). Twelve patients treated with ticarcillin and lithium experienced no adverse effects.

Mechanism

Antimicrobial-induced renal impairment, reflected by a decrease in creatinine clearance, may be the mechanism responsible for increased lithium levels (Halaris 1983).

Clinical Implications

Because lithium intoxication has occurred while patients were receiving spectinomycin, tetracycline, or metronidazole, the clinician's index of suspicion should remain high when coprescribing lithium with these or other antimicrobials that affect renal function. Serial lithium levels may be helpful when antimicrobials with known renal effects are added to lithium.

Anticonvulsants

CARBAMAZEPINE

Evidence of Interaction

Carbamazepine alone and in combination with lithium may be of benefit in the treatment of mania. In 1 study 3 patients with acute mania who responded poorly to either lithium or carbamazepine alone all appeared to respond very well to a combination of the medications (Lipinski et al. 1982). Some investigators have suggested that carbamazepine used in conjunction with other medications such as neuroleptic agents or lithium affords additional benefit beyond the use of these traditional treatments alone (Ballenger et al. 1980, Okuma et al. 1973).

On the other hand, neurotoxicity may result from the combination of lithium and carbamazepine. A case has been reported involving a possible neurotoxic interaction between carbamazepine and lithium in a 22-year-old woman hospitalized for her third manic episode in 2 years (Ayd 1982b). After an unsuccessful 4-week trial of combined lithium-neuroleptic therapy, carbamazepine at a dosage of 600 mg/day was instituted. Within 72 hours the patient began to manifest signs of a severe neurotoxic reaction, with generalized truncal tremors, ataxia, horizontal nystagmus, marked hyperreflexia of both arms and legs, and occasional muscle fasciculation despite therapeutic blood levels of both drugs.

Asterixis has been reported as a result of the combination of carbamazepine and lithium treatment (Rittmannsberger et al. 1991, 1992). Since all of the patients in this series were receiving multiple medications in addition to lithium and carbamazepine, the asterixis could have been triggered by the combination of several psychotropic medications. Despite the possible induction of neutropenia by carbamazepine therapy, lithium may increase the total white blood cell (WBC) count and neutrophil count during cotreatment with carbamazepine (Brewerton 1986, Joffe 1988, Mastrosimone et al. 1979). In a placebo-controlled study of the addition of lithium carbonate to carbamazepine (Kramlinger et al. 1990) lithium reversed the leukopenia induced by carbamazepine.

Thyroid effects of both medications were observed to be additive resulting in an increase in thyrotropin (TSH) and a decrease in peripheral thyroid hormones. The increase in TSH during combination treatment of carbamazepine and lithium is less robust than with treatment with either medication alone. Vieweg and colleagues (1987) reported that lithium and carbamazepine had opposing effects in the regulation of water and electrolytes: carbamazepine can prevent the hyponatremia that occurs with abrupt discontinuation of lithium. Lithium and carbamazepine can induce sinus node dysfunction. In 5 patients who had lithium-associated sinus node dysfunction, 4 were treated with carbamazepine as well, but all had elevated or toxic lithium levels, complicating interpretation of the finding (Steckler 1994).

Mechanism

The mechanism of potentiated therapeutic effect or additive neurotoxicity is unknown. Predisposing factors to neurotoxicity may be medical or neurologic disease, or a prior history of lithium toxicity.

With respect to myelopoiesis, carbamazepine inhibits granulocyte-macrophage stem cells (Gallicchio et al. 1989). Lithium increases the production of granulocytes by stimulating the stem cells (Rossof et al. 1978, 1979, Stein et al. 1978, 1979) or by inducing the production of colony stimulating factors (Harker et al. 1977, Kramlinger et al. 1990, Richman et al. 1981).

Lithium affects thyroid function by inhibition of the release of the thyroxine and liothyronine and inhibits iodine uptake into the gland (Bakker 1977, Berens et al. 1970, Sedvall et al. 1968). Carbamazepine may increase the metabolism of thyroid hormones by induction of liver enzymes (Aanderud et al. 1981, De Luca et al. 1986, Visser et al. 1976).

The occurrence of sinus node dysfunction with combined treatment is not surprising since it is a well-recognized adverse effect of lithium (Brady et al. 1988). It is usually reversible, although the dysrhythmia may be evidence of preexisting sinus node disease (Rodney et al. 1983). Carbamazepine can prolong cardiac conduction and decrease automaticity (Stiener et al. 1970, Kasaris et al. 1992).

Clinical Implications

Combined lithium-carbamazepine treatment may enhance clinical response in acute mania. In some cases, however, their concurrent use may lead to neurotoxicity. The use of combined treatment may be considered in individuals with acute manic symptoms that remain unresponsive to either drug alone, although clinicians should remain alert for signs of neurotoxicity, including ataxia, tremors, muscle fasciculations, hyperreflexia, and nystagmus (Chaudry et al. 1983, Okuma et al. 1973).

It is not known how frequently neurotoxicity occurs with the combination. In one series, 5 of 10 unipolar and bipolar patients on carbamazepine and lithium suffered intolerable central nervous system (CNS) side effects (Ghose 1978). In another study, the 5 bipolar patients on carbamazepine and lithium who suffered neurotoxicity had a history of underlying asymptomatic CNS or systemic disease. Three had previously been neurotoxic to lithium alone, and 2 were previously neurotoxic to lithium with neuroleptics. The researchers concluded that those with underlying CNS or metabolic disorders may be predisposed to neurotoxicity and that carbamazepine could enhance this tendency (Shukla et al. 1984). Haloperidol may also interact with lithium and carbamazepine even when doses are within the normal therapeutic range, producing confusion, disorientation, visual hallucinations, other perceptual disturbances, and diplopia (Andrus 1984).

In patients with a carbamzepine-induced decrease in WBC count the addition of lithium may be of benefit (Kramlinger et al. 1990).

Periodic monitoring of the electrocardiogram (ECG) is required when using these medications alone or in combination to treat patients at risk for conduction abnormalities.

Evidence is mounting that the combination of lithium and carbamazepine is effective in both acute mania and prophylaxis (Peselow et al. 1994). The major risk of the drug combination is neurotoxicity, although cardiac effects should also be monitored.

PHENYTOIN

Evidence of Interaction

Several cases of phenytoin-induced lithium toxicity have been published in the psychiatric literature. In these cases, patients had coarse tremor, drowsiness, gastrointestinal symptoms, and coma, which in some cases persisted after lithium had been discontinued (Speirs et al. 1978). Preexisting organic brain damage may increase the susceptibility to intoxication at typically nontoxic plasma concentrations. In one case report, lithium toxicity developed during combined lithium and phenytoin treatment despite therapeutic serum concentrations of both drugs; toxic symptoms (polydipsia, polyuria, and tremor) abated when carbamazepine was substituted for phenytoin (MacCallum 1980). In another case report, in a 49-year-old man treated with phenytoin 500 mg/day for bipolar disorder, a bilateral coarse tremor of the extremities and subjective anxiety developed within 3 days of starting the medications despite therapeutic lithium and phenytoin levels. Forty-eight hours after the patient's lithium was discontinued, the symptoms disappeared (Raskin 1984).

Mechanism
The mechanism is unknown.

Clinical Implications
There are only a few reported cases of adverse interactions between lithium and phenytoin. The clinician should be aware that toxicity may occur with the combination, despite therapeutic lithium and phenytoin levels. In many, if not most cases, the drugs can be safely coadministered under careful supervision.

VALPROIC ACID

Evidence of Interaction
The combination of lithium and valproic acid may be useful in treatment-resistant bipolar patients and appears to be well tolerated (Schaff et al. 1993).

Mechanism
The mechanism is unknown.

Clinical Implication
A trial of combined treatment of treatment-resistant bipolar disorder with valproic acid and lithium may be appropriate, although data are limited.

Antidepressants
MONOAMINE OXIDASE INHIBITORS (MAOIs)

Evidence of Interactions
Several cases of individuals with depressions refractory to traditional treatment regimens have responded to the combination of lithium with tranylcypromine or phenelzine (Himmelhoch et al. 1972,

Jefferson et al. 1983, Louie et al. 1984, Nelson et al. 1982, Price et al. 1985, Zall 1971). Himmelhoch et al. (1972) reported that the addition of lithium to tranylcypromine led to "modest but definite improvement" in treatment-resistant depression. They also noted that Zall (1971) had made similar observations in 3 patients taking isocarboxazid and lithium. Price et al. (1985) studied 12 inpatients with major depression who were refractory to at least two controlled antidepressant trials. Depending on the criteria used, between 8 and 11 of 12 patients improved on a lithium-tranylcypromine combination. Louie and colleagues (1984), studying the addition of lithium to a number of antidepressants, report much less predictable results, including a manic episode in a 36-year-old man taking phenelzine 60 mg daily.

Mechanism

The mechanism of enhanced antidepressant response is unknown, although some attribute it to the fact that antidepressants normalize presynaptic serotonergic activity, whereas lithium acts via pre- and/or postsynaptic mechanisms. Phenelzine does not alter lithium influx into red blood cells or the lithium red blood cell to plasma ratio (Pandey et al. 1979).

Clinical Implications

The combination of lithium and monoamine oxidase inhibitors is one of several therapeutic regimens for depressions refractory to conventional antidepressant treatment. Adverse consequences from the combination are rare, although clinicians should be aware of a report of 2 patients taking lithium and tranylcypromine in whom tardive dyskinesia developed (Stancer 1979), and another report of an elderly man with dementia suffering significant ataxia and urinary retention while on combined therapy (Cowdry et al. 1983). Although mania has been reported with combination, and paranoid symptoms may appear in patients with a schizoaffective disorder, these all may occur with monoamine oxidase inhibitors (MAOI) alone and are quite unlikely to be attributable to a drug interaction.

CYCLIC AND RELATED ANTIDEPRESSANTS

Evidence of Interaction

A number of reports suggest that the addition of lithium to cyclic antidepressants in patients with treatment-resistant depression leads to improvement within several days. De Montigny and colleagues (1981) added lithium to tricyclic antidepressants in 8 patients with nonresponsive depressions (nonpsychotic, unipolar). Substantial decreases were seen in depression rating scale scores within 2 days, and improvement continued whether or not lithium was continued. A study comparing lithium and triiodothyronine in augmentation of tricyclic antidepressant in a placebo-controlled design found them both to be equally effective and more effective than placebo (Joffe et al. 1993). In a review of controlled trials, Austin and colleagues (1990) found a highly statistically significant effect for lithium augmentation.

Other reports described the antidepressant effect of lithium when added to a neuroleptic-desipramine combination in treatment of refractory psychotically depressed patients (Louie et al. 1984, Price et al. 1985). Louie et al. (1984) described highly variable results when adding lithium to an antidepressant in 9 patients. Two showed sustained improvement, 2 showed transient improvement and then relapse, 2 with bipolar illness became manic, and 3 did not improve.

De Montigny et al. (1983) reported that in 30 of 42 instances involving 39 unipolar depressed patients unresponsive to a 3-week trial of tricyclic antidepressants, the addition of lithium brought about a greater than 50% reduction in depression scores within 48 hours. Heninger et al. (1983) studied the addition of lithium to a tricyclic antidepressant (desipramine or amitriptyline) or mianserin in patients ($N = 15$) with major depression who had been unresponsive to a 3-week drug trial. There was a greater improvement in depression in the lithium group than the placebo group. Furthermore, subsequent substitution of lithium for placebo in the control group resulted in improvement. Rapid improvement (within 24–48 hours) was noted in 5 patients, while the remaining patients did not show a clear improvement until approximately 5 to 8 days later. Although 1 case report suggested that the combination of lithium, maprotiline 50 mg twice a day, and L-iodothyronine 25 μg was effective in a depressed 73-year-old woman (Weaver 1983), others report toxicity characterized by myoclonic jerks and tremor (Kettl et al. 1983) with the combination. Joyce et al. (1983) gave mianserin plus lithium to a 64-year-old man with a recurrent major depression that had been unresponsive to maprotiline, chlorpromazine, and electroconvulsive therapy. Within 2 days of adding lithium to mianserin, the patient improved. On the other hand, other authors have reported therapeutic failures with the combination (Graham 1984, Gray 1983).

There is 1 case report describing the effectiveness of a trazodone-lithium combination in a 45-year-old man with depression (Birkhimer et al. 1983) and another of unsuccessful treatment of a bulimic patient with the drug combination (Pope et al. 1983). Three of 6 depressed patients who failed to respond to bupropion alone improved when lithium was added (Price et al. 1985). Bupropion was observed to promote weight loss even in the presence of lithium, which when given alone leads to weight gain (Gardner 1983). Increased toxicity has been reported with the combination of antidepressants and lithium. Grand mal seizures occurred after the addition of 900 mg/day of lithium to amitriptyline 300 mg/day (Solomon 1979). Seizures recurred following rechallenge. The issue of cardiac toxicity has been raised by the report of an adolescent taking lithium and imipramine in whom cardiomyopathy and hypothyroidism developed after 6 months of treatment (Dietrich et al. 1993). After lithium and imipramine were discontinued, thyroid replacement therapy resulted in cardiac dysrhythmias.

Underactive thyroid function has been reported in 12 patients receiving lithium and tricyclic antidepressants, which led investigators to speculate that these two drugs have an additive antithyroid effect (Rogers et al. 1971).

A case report of 2 elderly patients who were treated with the combination of tricyclic antidepressant and lithium showed an increase in neurotoxicity with therapeutic doses. The symptoms experienced were tremors, severe memory difficulties, distractibility, and disorganized thinking (Austin et al. 1990).

Limited evidence suggests that the combination of lithium and tricyclic antidepressants may be of value in treating tardive dyskinesia in depressed patients as documented in 19 patients, 58% of whom experienced either moderate or marked improvement in both dyskinesia and depression with combined tricyclic antidepressant and lithium therapy (Rosenbaum et al. 1980).

Mechanism

The mechanism of lithium potentiation of antidepressant effects is unknown but may involve enhanced CNS serotonergic activity. In a study exploring the serotonergic function in lithium augmentation, McCance-Katz et al. (1992) measured the prolactin response to intravenous L-tryptophan in patients with refractory major depression. Lithium augmentation resulted in statistically significant greater increases in the prolactin response to tryptophan challenge. With regard to adverse effects, both lithium and antidepressants lower the seizure threshold, thus their combination may have had an additive effect in the occurrence of grand mal seizures as reported in the published cases. On the other hand, lithium is commonly prescribed with antidepressants without adverse consequences. Although the antithyroid effect of lithium is well known, the reported additive antithyroid effects of the combination are not proven.

Clinical Implications

In general, the combination of lithium and antidepressants appears to be well tolerated and it is an effective addition to antidepressants in the treatment of patients with refractory depression. Apparently it does not offer improved prophylaxis of recurrent manic episodes compared with lithium alone, and some have suggested that the frequency of cycling increases in bipolar patients on antidepressants. Neurotoxicity is possible when antidepressants and lithium are prescribed concurrently, and seizures have been reported. Special caution should be used in the elderly due to the increased risk of neurotoxicity, and in children and adolescents who may be more susceptible to the cardiac conduction effects of both medications. Frequent monitoring of signs of neurotoxicity such as tremors, disorientation, headaches, or confusion is necessary. Baseline and periodic ECGs are also necessary. To avoid toxicity, many experienced clinicians attempt to potentiate antidepressant response with doses of lithium that will achieve a serum level of 0.4 mEq/liter, and increase the dose only if necessary.

SELECTIVE SEROTONIN REUPTAKE INHIBITORS (SSRIs)

Evidence of Interaction

Case reports of severe lithium toxicity resulting from the combination of lithium and fluoxetine have been published. A 44-year-old woman who had been taking lithium for 20 years without problems was given fluoxetine to treat an episode of depression (Salama et al. 1989). A few days following the initiation of treatment, dizziness, unsteadiness, and stiffness of arms and legs developed. Her gait became ataxic and her speech dysarthric, with a corresponding increase in her lithium level to 1.70 mEq/liter. The patient's lithium dose was decreased and the fluoxetine was discontinued with resolution of the neurologic symptoms. In another case report, a 53-year-old woman with a major depressive episode treated with fluoxetine and lorazepam was placed on lithium augmentation, and within 48 hours she had confusion, ataxia, and inability to follow commands

(Noveske et al. 1989). She demonstrated a coarse tremor, poor coordination, and held her legs in a flexed position, extending them randomly. She could not sit, walk, or stand without help. In addition to these toxic symptoms she had a leukocyte count of 17,300/mm^3. Her symptoms improved over several days after both medications were discontinued. In another case, the serum lithium level increased to 1.38 mEq/liter in a 38-year-old woman after the addition of fluoxetine (Hadley et al. 1989). A month after her lithium dose was decreased her serum lithium level was 0.8 mEq/liter but she became acutely manic. In another report, a 36-year-old woman taking fluoxetine 40 mg/day had an exacerbation of depression and lithium was added to her treatment (Muly et al. 1993). She was given lithium 300 mg twice daily for 5 days (serum level 0.65 mEq/liter prior to increasing the lithium dose to 300 mg three times daily. Two days later signs and symptoms consistent with a serotonin syndrome developed (e.g. akathisia, myoclonus, hyperreflexia, shivering, tremor, diarrhea, and incoordination) with a serum lithium level of 0.88 mEq/liter. Lithium was discontinued and cyproheptadine 12 mg was administered. Subsequently, the patient was able to tolerate fluoxetine alone (40 mg daily) with no adverse effects.

A case has been reported of absence seizures resulting from the combination of lithium and fluoxetine (Sacristan et al. 1991). A 44-year-old man was treated with lithium for depression. Forty-two days after the addition of fluoxetine, he had discrete episodes of immobility and staring into space, which lasted a few seconds prior to resuming his previous activity. He had no recollection of these events. When his lithium dose was reduced there were no further episodes. Unfortunately, no EEG recording was done during these episodes, but a recording made later showed no seizure activity.

In another report, somnolence was observed after the addition of lithium to fluvoxamine without any other neurologic symptoms and normal laboratory results (Evans et al. 1990a). The British Committee on the Safety of Medicines has reported neurotoxicity, characterized by tremors and seizure, with the combination of fluvoxamine and lithium.

In an open, parallel randomized study, 16 volunteers received lithium 600 mg twice daily for 9 days. Ten and 20 days prior to the last lithium dose, sertraline 100 mg or placebo was administered. Sertraline did not affect the renal clearance or the serum level of lithium. The subjects who received sertraline were more likely to experience adverse events, primarily tremor (Warrington 1991). In another study of the effect of sertraline on the renal clearance of lithium, an open-label placebo-controlled study of 20 healthy subjects did not find any statistically significant changes in the clearance or serum levels of lithium. Compared with control subjects receiving placebo, subjects taking the combination experienced more adverse effects, primarily tremors (Apseloff et al. 1992). Dinan (1993) used lithium augmentation with sertraline in 11 patients with treatment-resistant depression. Seven of the patients responded within a week without significant side effects. There was no correlation of response with lithium levels.

Mechanism

The mechanism of the interaction has not been established. Some have suggested that toxicity is a consequence of altered distribution of lithium in the brain tissue as reflected by an increased ratio of erythrocyte:plasma levels or altered receptor sensitivity (Elizur et al. 1972, Francis et al. 1970, Sacristan et al. 1991, Salama et al. 1989, West et al. 1979). Concomitant use of these medications also has an additive or synergistic effect on serotonin activity, which may be responsible for both increased efficacy and neurotoxicity (Evans et al. 1990a).

Clinical Implications

Lithium is frequently given to patients taking selective serotonin reuptake inhibitors (SSRIs) to improve antidepressant response (Fava et al. 1994). The most common adverse effect appears to be tremor, which can progress in some cases to severe neurotoxicity with ataxia, confusion, and seizures. Serum lithium level may not be elevated in all cases of neurotoxicity.

CLOMIPRAMINE

Evidence of Interaction

A 59-year-old man suffered from depression and lacunar infarction of the basal ganglia. He was treated with clomipramine 25 mg/day (gradually increased to 175 mg/day), levomepromazine 25 mg/day, and flunitrazepam 2 mg/day. Since there was an incomplete response of his depression, lithium 600 mg/day was added. After lithium was increased to 1,000 mg/day, the following signs and symptoms developed: myoclonus, shivering, tremors, incoordination, and elated mood that was consistent with serotonin syndrome, with the exception of only a mild increase in temperature to 37.2°C. The lithium was stopped with a dramatic reduction of the symptoms. The clomipramine dose was later reduced with further improvement, and all symptoms abated when it was discontinued (Kojima et al. 1993).

Mechanism

Both lithium and clomipramine enhance serotonergic activity.

Clinical Implications

A serotonin syndrome may occur with the combination of lithium and clomipramine. This is a potentially serious interaction and if these drugs are used together, low doses and close monitoring are advised.

Antihypertensives (See also Calcium Channel Blockers and Diuretics, this chapter)

EVIDENCE OF INTERACTION

Methyldopa

Several case reports have documented increased toxicity when lithium is given with methyldopa (Byrd 1975, O'Regan 1976). One case report involved a 45-year-old woman with a 25-year history of manic depressive illness who, when discharged from inpatient hospitalization on a regimen of 1,800 mg of lithium carbonate and 1 g of methyldopa daily (serum lithium levels ranging between 0.5 and 0.7 mEq/liter), began to show signs of toxicity, including blurred vision, hand tremors, mild diarrhea, confusion, and slurring of speech. Ten days after discontinuation of methyldopa, the patient's serum lithium level was 1.4 mEq/liter. As lithium dosage was decreased to 900 mg/day, stable serum lithium levels were achieved (1.0 mEq/liter), with reversal of toxic symptoms (Byrd 1975). A second case report involved a 72-year-old man who also exhibited toxic symptoms as a result of the coprescription of lithium and methyldopa (Osanloo et al. 1980). In a study of 3 subjects on lithium and methyldopa, lithium levels did not change; however, confusion, sedation, and dysphoria increased (Walker et al. 1980).

Prazosin (Minipress®)

Two schizophrenics who were taking neuroleptics, lithium, and prazosin did not suffer significant adverse effects (Hommer et al. 1984). This combination may be useful when thiazides and β-blockers are not effective (Schwarcz 1982).

Propranolol (Inderal®)

Propranolol may have antimanic properties in doses considerably larger than those used in treating hypertension (Jefferson et al. 1981, Schwarcz 1982). All β-adrenergic blockers are effective in treating lithium-induced tremors. When administered with lithium, propranolol may increase lithium levels (Schou et al. 1987), although data are limited. The addition of β-blocking agents to lithium may induce bradycardia (Becker 1989).

Clonidine (Catapres®)

Bipolar patients had smaller decreases in blood pressure in response to clonidine when taking chronic doses of lithium compared with blood pressure when lithium was withdrawn (Goodnick et al. 1984). Acute doses of lithium potentiate clonidine-induced aggressive behavior in mice (Ozawa 1975).

Angiotensin-Converting Enzyme (ACE) Inhibitors

There are several reports of patients on enalapril (Vasotec®) in whom lithium intoxication developed (3.3 mmol/liter), with mild impairment of kidney function, which returned to normal after discontinuation of the medications (Douste-Blazy et al. 1986). Navis et al. (1989) reported a 65-year-old woman who was admitted after 6 months of lithium and enalapril treatment with frequent monitoring of blood levels. At the time of admission she was dehydrated, hypotensive, and oliguric, with a serum lithium level of 2.35 mmol/liter. Volume restoration resulted in eventual normalization of blood pressure and laboratory values. The authors explain the change in lithium level as resulting from volume depletion due to any cause such as gastrointestinal (GI) loss and the drug combination. Other case reports (Correa et al. 1992, Drouet et al. 1990) described toxic lithium levels that occurred when renal function was decreased. DasGupta et al. (1992) studied the drug interaction in a crossover study of 9 healthy volunteers who took lithium alone, lithium and enalapril, and lithium alone again. There were no significant differences between lithium serum levels when lithium was administered alone compared with administration with enalapril. Lisinopril (Prinivil®) 20 mg/day led to lithium toxicity in a 49-year-old woman taking lithium 1500 mg/day (Baldwin et al. 1990).

Mechanism

The mechanism of the methyldopa-lithium interaction is unclear. Methyldopa may increase serum lithium levels and thus induce toxicity; however, toxicity has been reported with normal serum lithium levels. Methyldopa may exaggerate CNS response to lithium or increase the cellular uptake of lithium. Propranolol may reduce renal clearance of lithium.

Chronic lithium treatment may decrease α_2-adrenergic receptor sensitivity, decreasing the antihypertensive response to clonidine. Lithium toxicity in the presence of enalapril, lisinopril, or other ACE inhibitors may be due to altered renal function secondary to the angiotensin-converting enzyme inhibition and/or their natriuretic effect. In DasGupta's study the dose of enalapril dose was lower than those used in the clinical cases reported. Abnormalities in hydration, renal function, and cardiovascular status may all predispose to lithium toxicity when ACE inhibitors are used concomitantly.

Clinical Implications

Signs of lithium intoxication may occur during methyldopa treatment even though lithium levels are within therapeutic range. Serum lithium levels alone, therefore, cannot be used to predict or diagnose this drug-drug interaction. Patients taking both methyldopa and lithium should be carefully monitored upon the initiation or discontinuation of methyldopa. Electroencephalograms may reflect toxicity in the presence of levels that are usually considered therapeutic.

The effectiveness of clonidine may be reduced in the presence of lithium.

Enalapril (Vasotec®) may increase serum lithium levels and lead to toxicity. Other ACE inhibitors such as ramipril (Altace®), captopril (Capoten®), lisinopril (Prinivil®, Zestril®), fosinopril (Monopril®), and benazepril (Lotensin®) have similar risk. Although some authorities have recommended against the concurrent use of lithium and enalapril (Baldwin et al. 1990), most of the evidence at this time does not support complete avoidance of lithium and ACE inhibitors. Caution should be used when treating patients with these drugs by initiating treatment with small doses of lithium (e.g. we have seen patients taking ACE inhibitors reach prophylactic lithium levels at doses as low as 300 mg/day). Lithium levels and serum creatinine should be monitored frequently.

Some authorities recommend that β-blockers are the preferred antihypertensive agents for patients taking lithium, although interactions are possible with this combination as well, with isolated reports of increased lithium levels and bradycardia.

Antiinflammatory Drugs

Evidence of Interaction

Several case reports have documented reduced renal lithium clearance, leading to 30 to 60% increases in plasma lithium levels as a result of coprescription of antiinflammatory medications that inhibit prostaglandin synthesis (Ragheb 1990, Singer et al. 1981). In 1 case report the effects of indomethacin (Indocin®) on renal lithium excretion and plasma lithium levels were studied in 4 volunteers with normal renal function. A decrease in renal lithium excretion and an increase in plasma lithium levels were found in all subjects. Increases in plasma lithium levels averaged 48% above baseline with a range of 25 to 63% (Frolich et al. 1979). In another investigation, the influence of the nonsteroidal antiinflammatory drug diclofenac (Voltaren®) on lithium kinetics was studied in 5 normal women. Diclofenac decreased lithium renal clearance by 23% and increased lithium plasma levels by 26% (Reimann et al. 1981). An interaction was also found in 3 manic patients who were given indomethacin 150 mg/day for 6 days (Ragheb et al. 1980), as were volunteers given diclofenac 150 mg/day for 8 days. In the latter study urinary clearance decreased and plasma lithium levels rose 25% (Reimann et al. 1981). Similar results have been seen with mefenamic acid (Ponstel®), clomethacin, and niflumic acid (Colonna et al. 1979, Gay et al. 1985, MacDonald et al. 1988, Shelly 1987). Another case report found that ibuprofen (Advil®, Motrin®) had inconsistent effects on plasma lithium levels and lithium clearance (Ragheb et al. 1980, 1987a). Studies on rats have documented an interaction between phenylbutazone and indomethacin and lithium urinary elimination (Imbs et al. 1980, Singer et al. 1978). Sulindac (Clinoril®) increased lithium clearance but did not affect lithium levels (Furnell et al. 1985); nor have others found any changes in lithium level when sulindac was added to treatment (Ragheb et al. 1986a,b). Ketorolac (Toradol®), a nonsteroidal antiinflammatory drug (NSAID) that is available in both oral and parenteral form and in wide clinical use for treatment of acute and chronic pain may also increase serum lithium levels. When ketorolac in oral doses of 30 mg/day was given to an 80-year-old man who had been stabilized on lithium with serum levels of 0.5 to 0.7 mEq/liter, his level rose to 1.1 mEq/liter in 6 days (Langlois et al. 1994). Piroxicam (Feldene®) also may be associated with lithium toxicity during combined therapy (Harrison et al. 1986, Kerry et al. 1983, Nadarajah et al. 1985, Walbridge et al. 1985).

Allen et al. (1989) reported successful treatment of a case of lithium-induced diabetes insipidus with indomethacin, although this is not a generally accepted treatment for the condition.

Mechanism

Nonsteroidal antiinflammatory drugs, which inhibit prostaglandin synthesis, reduce renal clearance of lithium by affecting a prostaglandin-dependent mechanism located in the renal tubule. Another possible mechanism is that NSAIDs compete with lithium for the transport mechanism at the proximal tubule (Brater 1986, 1988, Gove et al. 1983, Johnson et al. 1993, Tonkin et al. 1988).

Clinical Implications

There are many published interactions between lithium and NSAIDs that suggest the simultaneous administration of these drugs is potentially hazardous. Lithium levels should be monitored frequently when patients are taking this drug combination. Preliminary evidence suggests that sulindac (Clinoril®) and aspirin may be less likely to interact with lithium, but data are limited (Ragheb 1987b).

Antipsychotic Agents (See Chapter 3)

ANTITHYROID DRUGS

Evidence of Interaction

Hypothyroidism, and less commonly hyperthyroidism and thyrotoxicosis, have been documented in patients taking prophylactic lithium therapy for manic depressive illness (Barclay et al. 1994, Chow et al. 1993, Jefferson et al. 1994, Persad et al. 1993).

There is some evidence supporting the efficacy of lithium in thyrotoxicosis. Serum thyroid hormone levels are consistently decreased in thyrotoxic patients receiving lithium. In one study, decreases ranging from 30 to 85% of the rate of iodine and hormonal iodine secretion occurred within 12 hours of patients' reaching lithium serum levels as low as 0.5 mEq/liter. Addition of methimazole resulted in greater drops in thyroid hormone levels (Temple et al. 1972). In another study, thyrotoxic patients were treated with (1) carbimazole and lithium, (2) carbimazole and iodine, or (3) carbimazole alone. Serum thyroxine level fell almost 50% in the first 2 groups compared with 18% in group 3. Mean serum level was 0.63 mEq/liter (Turner et al. 1975, 1976). A fall of approximately 30% in serum thyroxine level in 20 thyrotoxic patients taking lithium was reported by Gerdes et al. (1973). In a comparison of lithium and methimazole, investigators found no significant difference in reduction of serum thyroxine iodine or free thyroxine index at 3 and 10 days (Kristensen et al. 1976).

Lithium has been used preoperatively to prevent thyroid storms in the surgical treatment of Graves's disease when conventional antithyroid drugs such as methimazole, propylthiouracil, or thionamide were not well tolerated (Mochinaga et al. 1994, Takami 1994).

Carbimazole treatment was effective in treating hyperthyroidism in a 68-year-old man with bipolar disorder who had been taking lithium 1,000 mg/day for 5 years (Sadoul et al. 1994). The patient developed transient hypothyroidism followed by signs and symptoms of hyperthyroidism several months later (e.g. tremor, exopthalmus, ocular muscle enlargement, increased free thyroxine, and triiodothyronine) that responded to carbimazole therapy.

Lithium has also been used as an adjunct to radioactive iodine (^{131}I) in the treatment of thyrotoxicosis (Turner et al. 1976). Patients who had been receiving lithium carbonate 400 mg for 5 days were given the standard therapeutic dose of ^{131}I and continued on lithium for another 5 days. The lithium-treated patients had increased retention of thyroidal ^{131}I compared with control subjects. The investigators suggested that this therapeutic regimen concentrates radioactive iodine in the gland and allows for a lower total body exposure to radioactivity.

Mechanism

Lithium rapidly blocks release of thyroxine and triiodothyronine from the thyroid gland, resulting in a decrease in circulating hormone.

Clinical Implications

Lithium enhances the action of thyroid suppressing drugs, and combination treatment may have some clinical value in the therapy of thyrotoxicosis, especially in individuals in whom standard therapy is contraindicated.

Benzodiazepines

Evidence of Interaction

A few anecdotal case reports describe patients who had difficulty with the combined use of lithium and a benzodiazepine. Diazepam and oxazepam in particular were reported to produce an increase in depression that was not apparent in patients receiving lithium alone. This is most probably the effect of diazepam and oxazepam alone in patients who were particularly sensitive to benzodiazepines, and no definite drug-drug interaction has been established (Rosenbaum et al. 1979). A single case report of profound hypothermia resulting from the combined use of lithium and diazepam clearly implicates lithium as the causative agent. Lithium resulted in hypothermia, a comatose state with reduced reflexes, dilated pupils, a systolic blood pressure between 40 and 60 mm Hg, pulse rate of 40 beats/min, and absence of piloerector response (Naylor et al. 1977). On the removal of lithium, the patient's temperature rose progressively to normal range and, on rechallenge with lithium, again fell to similar hypothermic levels with the above-noted symptoms.

Koczerginski et al. (1989) reported 5 cases in which the combination of lithium and clonazepam resulted in neurotoxicity, with symptoms of ataxia and dysarthria. In all of these cases lithium level was increased and the symptoms were completely reversible when lithium was stopped. All of these patients were also taking neuroleptic medications at the same time, which probably contributed to the development of the neurotoxicity (see Chapter 3). In a study of 104 outpatients taking lithium in combination with other psychoactive medications, an association was found between the use of combination treatment with lithium and benzodiazepines and sexual dysfunction (Ghadirian et al. 1992). The incidence of dysfunction was significantly higher than with any other combination or with lithium alone.

The pharmacokinetic interaction of alprazolam and lithium was studied by Evans et al. (1990b). Ten healthy volunteers were given lithium in doses of 900 to 1,500 mg/day. Although alprazolam administration (1 mg twice daily) decreased lithium clearance, steady-state lithium concentrations were increased only slightly and the change was not of clinical significance.

In one isolated case, 18 mg/day of bromazepam to a stable lithium regimen caused lithium plasma concentration to rise from 1.12 to 1.40 mmol/liter with pretoxic symptoms (Raudino et al. 1981). In another case an unspecified benzodiazepine and lithium allegedly caused neuroleptic malignant syndrome (Levenson et al. 1985).

Flumazenil, a benzodiazepine antagonist, can lead to seizures when administered to patients with a seizure disorder or on medications such as lithium that lower the seizure threshold (Spivey 1992).

Animal studies have also examined the interaction of benzodiazepines and lithium. Rats receiving lithium for 4 weeks had a 10 to 20% decrease in benzodiazepine receptor number in the frontal cortex (Hetmar et al. 1983), and another study found an 11% decrease in rat receptor binding (Kafka et al. 1982). The effect of benzodiazepine on the midbrain and cerebellum of the rat is unchanged by chronic lithium doses (Reilly et al. 1984). A combination of lithium and phenazepam caused a statistically significant increase in lithium in the liver and mesencephalon of mice, and rapid increases in lithium in the cerebral cortex, cerebellum, mesencephalon, and liver (Samoilov et al. 1980). The sedative effects of diazepam in mice were potentiated by lithium (Mannisto et al. 1976).

Mechanism

Hypothermia associated with combined lithium and diazepam treatment is most probably an idiosyncratic reaction.

It is possible that the increase in lithium level in the presence of clonazepam is a pharmacokinetic interaction involving renal excretion (Freinhar et al. 1985, Koczerginski et al. 1989), although neurotoxicity in the reported cases probably involved concurrent use of neuroleptics.

Clinical Implications

Considering the wide use of benzodiazepines to sedate acutely manic patients taking lithium and the infrequent reports of adverse consequences, the likelihood that this is a common drug-drug interaction is remote. The possibility does exist that in some patients lithium levels may be altered slightly. The clinician should be aware that more frequent serum lithium monitoring may be advisable in some cases.

Calcium Channel Blockers

Evidence of Interaction

There have been a number of case reports of interactions between verapamil (Calan®) and diltiazem (Cardizem®) with lithium (Dubovsky et al. 1987, Price et al. 1986, 1987, Valdiserri 1985, Wright et al. 1991). The primary symptoms of toxicity were ataxia, dysarthria, tremor, and nausea. In one case, rechallenge with verapamil after symptoms abated led to recurrence (Wright et al. 1991). Treatment with nifedipine, however, did not produce neurotoxicity. Neurotoxicity with psychotic symptoms were reported in a 66-year-old woman with a longstanding history of bipolar disorder who was treated with diltiazem for hypertension (Binder et al. 1991). Another case report described a reversible choreoathetosis of the neck, trunk, and all four extremities during treatment with verapamil and lithium (Helmuth et al. 1989). In another patient, stiffness and rigidity were reported during combined therapy with lithium and diltiazem (Valdiserri 1985).

Mechanism

The mechanism of the interaction in unknown; however, several possibilities have been proposed. Verapamil crosses the blood-brain barrier and there is a risk for neurotoxicity with delirium related to its use alone (Jacobson et al. 1987, Wright et al. 1991). Lithium, as well, can lead to neurotoxicity on its own, and the combination may be additive or synergistic.

In rats, verapamil increased 5HT2 receptors in the frontal cortex, whereas lithium did not (Baba et al. 1991). This animal model also suggested that lithium levels were elevated with the drug combination. Lithium increases dopamine in the striatum, where regulation of dopamine release is controlled by inhibitory D2 autoreceptors that are calcium dependent. The blockade of these receptors by verapamil can lead to increased dopamine release and result in choreoathetosis (Gudelsky et al. 1988, Helmuth et al. 1989).

Clinical Implications

The risk of neurotoxicity is increased with concurrent use of verapamil, diltiazem, and possibly other calcium channel blockers with lithium. Nifedipine did not interact in one case. Clinicians may expect to encounter this drug combination not only in lithium-treated patients with cardiovascular disease, but also in patients for whom verapamil has been prescribed as a primary or adjunctive treatment for bipolar disorder.

Digoxin

Evidence of Interaction

A single case report described a patient in whom tremulousness, confusion, and nodal bradycardia developed alternating with slow atrial fibrillation when the digoxin level was in the lower range of therapeutic effect (0.7 ng/ml) (Winters et al. 1977). Upon admission, the patient had a junctional bradycardia with a rate of 52 beats/min that fell to 30 beats/min the following day, despite discontinuation of both medications. A temporary pacemaker was required for 6 days, after which the patient reverted to normal sinus rhythm.

Mechanism

The authors of the case report suggested that the combination of lithium and digoxin lowered intracellular potassium, predisposing the patient to cardiac arrhythmias.

Clinical Implications

We are aware of only one report citing toxicity with the combination. In that case, lithium alone at a level of 2.0 mEq/liter could have resulted in toxicity. Nonetheless, this is a potentially serious interaction and close ECG monitoring may be necessary. Although one report suggested that the therapeutic response to lithium was impaired during digoxin therapy (Chambers et al. 1982), confirmatory evidence is lacking. Furthermore, a study in 6 healthy volunteers found no significant pharmacokinetic interaction between lithium and digoxin and no alterations in sodium pump activity or electrolyte concentrations (Cooper et al. 1984).

Disulfiram

Evidence of Interaction

Alcoholism is not uncommon in bipolar illness. Case reports as well as unpublished observations indicate that no clinically significant adverse interaction occurs between lithium and disulfiram (Rothstein et al. 1971, Ziegler-Driscoll et al. 1977). In one case report disulfiram appeared to precipitate hyperactive behavior that was treated very effectively with lithium at the usual therapeutic level. Although rats given lithium and disulfiram had increased mortality compared with either drug given alone, the clinical implications of this finding are unknown (Millard et al. 1969).

Clinical Implications

Lithium and disulfiram appear to be compatible medications, and there exists no theoretical or clinical reason why disulfiram administration should interfere with lithium therapy.

Diuretics

INTRODUCTION

Diuretics are generally divided into 7 classes (cf. Ciraulo et al. 1994): (1) osmotic diuretics, such as urea; (2) carbonic anhydrase inhibitors, such as aceatazolamide (Diamox®); (3) thiazide diuretics and drugs that are chemically distinct but work via similar mechanisms (e.g. the sulfonamide derivatives chlorthalidone, quinethazone [Hydromox®], metolazone [Mykrox®], and indapamide [Lozol®]); (4) loop diuretics, such as furosemide (Lasix®) and bumetanide (Bumex®); (5) aldosterone antagonists, such as ethacrynic acid (Edecrin®) and spironolactone (Aldactone®); (6) potassium-sparing diuretics, such as triamterene (Dyrenium®, or with hydrochlorthiazide, Dyazide(®); (7) methylxanthines (see Aminophylline/Theophylline, this chapter).

ACETAZOLAMIDE (DIAMOX®)

Evidence of Interaction

Renal lithium excretion was assessed in 6 healthy human subjects to determine the best methods for the treatment of lithium poisoning (Thomsen et al. 1968). Lithium excretion was not significantly affected by water diuresis or the administration of furosemide, ethacrynic acid, spironolactone, or potassium chloride. With administration of sodium bicarbonate and acetazolamide, urinary pH values rose into the 7.0 to 8.0 range, and urine flow, sodium, and potassium output were also increased, resulting in a 27 to 31% rise in lithium excretion.

Mechanism

Osmotic diuresis and administration of sodium bicarbonate or acetazolamide will produce a significant increase in lithium excretion. The increase following sodium bicarbonate and acetazolamide may be the result of increased urinary pH, but this is unlikely. It is probable that the increased lithium excretion is due to an obligatory excretion of cation with bicarbonate anion, and impairment of lithium resorption in the proximal tubule.

Clinical Implications

The clinical importance of this interaction is uncertain, although close monitoring of lithium level is advisable when adding or discontinuing acetazolamide in patients taking lithium.

ALDOSTERONE ANTAGONISTS

Summary

Ethacrynic acid and spironolactone do not usually affect serum lithium concentrations. Large doses that may cause rapid volume depletion are sometimes associated with toxic serum lithium levels.

LOOP DIURETICS

Evidence of Interaction

A 65-year-old woman who had been stable on lithium with levels of 0.7 to 0.9 mEq/liter was treated with bumetanide 0.5 mg/day for ankle edema. A month after the treatment was started, increasing tremulousness, ataxia, and confusion developed in the patient, with a lithium level of 2.3 mEq/liter (Huang 1990). Another case of an increase in lithium serum level following the addition of bumetanide was reported by Kerry et al. (1980). Previous reports exist as to the potential increase in lithium level as a result of treatment with furosemide (Hurtig et al. 1974, Thornton et al. 1975).

Other investigators, in single-dose studies, have not found that loop diuretics increase serum lithium levels (Steele et al. 1975, Thomsen et al 1968). Studies looking at the changes in lithium level as a result of an interaction with furosemide did not find significant elevation of lithium level (Jefferson et al. 1979, Safher et al. 1983). In another study comparing the effect of furosemide, hydrochlorthiazide, and placebo on lithium blood levels in 13 healthy volunteers, furosemide had no effect on serum lithium levels, whereas hydrochlorothiazide produced a small but significant elevation of the serum lithium level (Crabtree et al. 1991).

Mechanism

Loop diuretics act rapidly by inhibiting sodium reabsorption in the loop of Henle. As a consequence, there may be compensatory reabsorption of lithium. It is possible that the site of action of furosemide at the ascending limb affects both lithium and sodium transport, causing loss of lithium as well (Crabtree et al. 1991). It is possible that when used in higher doses furosemide will cause lithium retention, but the effects seem highly variable.

Clinical Implications

Although the use of loop diuretics is safe with lithium, it is important to monitor lithium levels.

POTASSIUM-SPARING DIURETICS

Evidence of an Interaction

The interaction of lithium with potassium-sparing diuretics has not been extensively studied. There is a case report of a modest elevation of lithium levels after triamterene was added (lithium levels rose from 0.65 to 0.95 mEq/liter). In a study of amiloride treatment of lithium-induced polyuria, 1 patient had an increase in lithium level from 0.8 to 2.0 mEq/liter.

Mechanism

Large-volume contractions and reduced glomerular filtration may result in impaired lithium clearance.

Clinical Implications

When potassium-sparing diuretics are used in high doses or produce large-volume contractions, close monitoring of serum lithium levels is necessary.

THIAZIDE DIURETICS

Evidence of Interaction

Some authorities believe that the lithium-thiazide combination usually leads to toxicity despite careful supervision (Coppen et al. 1982). Others suggest that with appropriate reductions in lithium doses thiazide diuretics may be safely used in the treatment of lithium-induced nephrogenic diabetes insipidus (Himmelhoch et al. 1977a, Levy et al. 1973). Several authors have documented that lithium and thiazide diuretics interact adversely, usually leading to diuretic-induced lithium retention and an increase in lithium serum levels (Himmelhoch et al. 1977b, Hurtig et al. 1974, Jefferson et al. 1979, Macfie 1975, 1980, Solomon 1980).

There is also a case report of lithium toxicity in a 64-year-old man when indapamide was added to his regular medications for the treatment of pedal edema. A week after the beginning of treatment the patient presented to the emergency room with lethargy, staggering gait, and confusion. His serum lithium level was 3.93 mEq/liter (Hanna et al. 1990).

Mechanism

Lithium is excreted by the kidneys, and significant reabsorption of lithium occurs both in the proximal tubules and probably in the loop of Henle but not at more distal areas. Thiazide diuretics block sodium reabsorption at the distal tubules, which results in sodium depletion; this in turn stimulates proximal tubular reabsorption of both sodium and lithium. As a result, renal lithium clearance decreases and lithium plasma levels increase. Treatment with thiazide diuretics results in a compensatory increase in sodium reabsorption in the proximal renal tubule. Because lithium is reabsorbed with sodium in the proximal tubule, toxicity may result. Boer et al. (1989) demonstrated that the effect of acute administration of thiazide diuretics on lithium clearance differed depending on their level of carbonic anhydrase-inhibiting activity, with the higher activity drugs increasing lithium clearance in humans.

Clinical Implications

The frequent appearance of reversible lithium toxicity emphasizes that very close monitoring must be exercised when using a thiazide-lithium combination. However, minor toxicity is clearly not a contraindication to the use of thiazides with lithium. There are two particular circumstances in which concomitant use of lithium and thiazide diuretics may actually be beneficial. The first is when moderate to large doses of lithium have induced nephrogenic diabetes insipidus, an illness in which thiazide diuretics reduce polyuria and polydipsia, thereby allowing continuation of lithium (Himmelhoch et al. 1977a, Jakobsson et al. 1994). The second circumstance involves patients in whom large doses of lithium do not produce therapeutic plasma levels and mood stabilization is not achieved. Some authorities recommend the addition of a thiazide diuretic in these patients to achieve clinically effective lithium concentrations at much lower lithium doses. A 50% reduction in lithium dosage is typical when hydrochlorothiazide 50 mg is used with lithium. Individuals vary, however, and this recommendation should serve only as a guideline. In some cases it is preferable to use furosemide instead of thiazide diuretics.

Ethanol

Evidence of Interaction

Several studies have been conducted regarding the coadministration of lithium and ethanol. One study evaluated the responses of 23 normal male subjects after pretreating these individuals with lithium prior to ethanol ingestion. Results indicated that pretreatment with lithium neither blocked nor dampened the alcohol-induced subjective "high" (Judd et al. 1977). The study did suggest that lithium may attenuate alcohol-induced cognitive inefficiency and possibly that alcohol may reverse some aspects of lithium-induced dysphoria. In a follow-up study (Judd et al. 1984) 35 male alcoholics who had been drug and alcohol free for a minimum of 21 days were studied in a repeated-measures, split-half crossover design and given lithium carbonate (mean 0.89 mEq/liter) or placebo for 14 days in a double-blind randomized fashion. Ethanol was administered in a dose of 1.32 ml/kg of 95% ethanol in 4 divided doses over 60 minutes (a mean blood alcohol concentration of 104 mg/100 ml). Lithium subjects reported less intoxication, a decreased desire to continue drinking, and less cognitive dysfunction after ethanol than placebo subjects. Other studies have evaluated lithium in the treatment of alcoholic withdrawal. In one study involving 18 hospitalized chronic alcoholics, lithium did decrease the amplitude of tremor during alcohol withdrawal but did not control the tremor or the subjective symptoms of alcohol withdrawal to a significant degree (Sellers et al. 1974). In another study lithium treatment diminished subjective symptoms of withdrawal and normalized performance on a motor-tracking task. It was also determined that lithium did not in any significant way alter patterns of catecholamine excretion, blood pressure, heart rate, serum cyclic adenosine monophosphate, serum dopamine-β-hydroxylase, sleep patterns, or tremor amplitude during withdrawal (Sellers et al. 1976).

Still other studies have investigated the efficacy of lithium in producing abstinence in alcoholics. The first study comparing lithium to placebo in alcoholics was that of Kline et al. (1974). Seventy-three male veterans with high scores on the Zung Self-Rating Scale for Depression entered the study, but at the conclusion of the 48-week double-blind period only 30 subjects remained. Lithium patients experienced significantly fewer days of pathologic drinking and hospitalization for alcoholism.

Another study of 60 male and 11 female alcoholics, 48% of whom had Beck Depression Inventory scores greater than 15 also compared lithium to placebo (Merry et al. 1976). At the end of 41 weeks of treatment, both groups had improved Beck scores, with the lithium group doing slightly better. Among those classified as depressed at the start of the study, those taking lithium had significantly fewer days drinking and fewer days of incapacitating drinking than placebo patients. The conclusions are based on a very small sample size: 9 depressed lithium patients and 7 depressed placebo patients.

A study by Pond et al. (1981) using a 3-month crossover design of lithium and placebo studied 47 alcoholic patients. Nineteen subjects completed the study. No significant differences in Minnesota Multiphasic Personality Inventory scores or drinking patterns were found.

In a double-blind placebo-controlled study, 104 men and women with alcoholism were treated with lithium or placebo and observed for 12 months (Fawcett et al., 1987). Compliance (defined as at least 15 days of compliance to the prescribed regimen for 4 months of the first 6-month follow-up) was assessed by patient self-report and interviews of significant others when possible. The lithium group was divided into high-blood level (≥0.4 mEq/liter), low-blood level (<0.4 mEq/liter), and lithium noncompliant. The placebo group was classified either as compliant or noncompliant. The high-blood level group had the highest abstinence rates: 79% at 6 months and 63% at 12 months when all dropouts were considered to have relapsed, or 79% at 6 months and 67% at 12 months by survival analysis. These findings suggest that a therapeutic lithium level is an important factor in the positive outcome, which, contrary to earlier studies, did not appear to be related to lithium's effects on affective symptoms.

Mechanism

Lithium may reduce sympathetic activity during alcoholic withdrawal. It decreases the pressor effect of infused norepinephrine and might therefore decrease catechol-mediated increases in blood pressure, thus alleviating the symptoms and clinical signs associated with alcoholic withdrawal (Sellers et al. 1976). The mechanism by which lithium may reduce ethanol consumption is unknown, although the serotonergic system has been implicated.

Clinical Implications

The implications of lithium use in alcohol withdrawal is of theoretical rather than clinical importance. Lithium-alcohol adverse interactions having clinical significance are not documented. While some alcoholics appear to benefit from lithium treatment, this has not been a consistent or robust finding. Even if some subgroup of alcoholics do benefit from lithium treatment, the clinical characteristics of responders (other than in bipolar patients) have not as yet been identified. Depressive symptoms, in most studies, do not predict response.

Levodopa

Evidence of Interaction

Lithium has been used to treat the psychiatric and dyskinetic side effects induced by levodopa. It is widely recognized that psychoses have been induced by levodopa therapy in the treatment of Parkinson's disease. One case report describes a 64-year-old man in whom a levodopa-induced psychosis developed and who responded well to treatment with lithium (Braden 1977). Another case report of a 69-year-old man suggests that lithium may be useful not only in the treatment of manic behavior but also in depressive reactions ocurring as a consequence of levodopa therapy (Ryback et al. 1971). Dalen et al. (1973) successfully treated levodopa-induced dyskinesias with lithium in 2 patients with Parkinson's disease. Another study, of 21 patients with Parkinson's disease and levodopa-induced dyskinesias, however, found lithium ineffective in all patients (McCauland et al. 1974). Five patients had adverse reactions to lithium. Poor therapeutic responses in other studies of lithium's effect on both mental and motor side effects of levodopa have led clinicians to urge caution with respect to the use of lithium in patients with Parkinson's disease (Van Woert et al. 1971, 1973).

Mechanism

Lithium and levodopa may interact by effects on noradrenergic, dopaminergic, and/or functionally related areas of the brain (Braden 1977).

Clinical Implications

Although a few case reports have found lithium to be of no value, other reports suggest that lithium may be useful in the treatment of psychiatric and motor side effects resulting from levodopa therapy.

Marijuana

Evidence of Interaction

There is one case report suggesting a possible interaction between marijuana and lithium which resulted in elevated serum lithium levels. The patient's serum lithium level was stable for a least 1 month during an inpatient hospitalization in which a dose of 2,100 mg of lithium/day was given. When the patient began to surreptitiously use marijuana, his serum lithium level rose to toxic range (Ratey et al. 1981).

Mechanism

The anticholinergic properties of marijuana may result in a decrease in gut motility, enhancing lithium absorption.

Clinical Implications

Although no additional interactions have been reported, clinicians should consider the possibility of concurrent marijuana use in patients with a history of marijuana use who have been taking regular doses of lithium but have been unable to achieve stable serum lithium levels.

Neuromuscular Blocking Agents

Evidence of Interaction

Several case reports have documented that lithium significantly prolongs both succinylcholine and pancuronium bromide neuromuscular blockade, agents used extensively in surgery and electroconvulsive treatment (Reimherr et al. 1977, Rubin et al. 1982). Neuromuscular blocking agents can be classified into two categories, the depolarizing group, including succinylcholine, and the nondepolarizing group, including pancuronium. Investigators have reported potentiation of succinylcholine by lithium carbonate (Hill et al. 1976) as well as pancuronium (Reimherr et al. 1977), resulting in prolonged recovery from anesthesia (hours). One animal study did not confirm the interaction (Waud et al. 1982).

Mechanism

It has been postulated that lithium may inhibit acetylcholine synthesis as well as the release of acetylcholine from nerve terminals, thus potentiating the neuromuscular blocking action.

Clinical Implications

Several reports have documented the fact that lithium potentiates the action of muscle relaxants; however, other studies have not found an adverse interaction. Until the matter is clarified, doses of lithium should be withheld prior to the use of these agents, or alternative relaxing agents should be used. Close monitoring of patients and appropriate ventilatory assistance should be available (Havdala et al. 1979). For therapeutic guidelines relative to electroconvulsive therapy, the reader is referred to Chapter 9.

Psyllium (Metamucil®)

Evidence of Interaction

In a study with 6 normal volunteers who received lithium alone and lithium with psyllium, urine elimination of lithium was decreased with psyllium, suggesting decreased absorption of lithium in the gut (Toutoungi et al. 1990).

Mechanism

Psyllium causes retention of water and electrolytes in the colon.

Clinical Implications

In patients taking lithium and psyllium in combination, lithium requirements may be elevated. When psyllium treatment is initiated or discontinued it is important to monitor lithium levels.

Zidovudine (AZT)

Evidence of Interaction

Lithium was used in 5 patients to reverse zidovudine-induced neutropenia (Roberts et al. 1988). Lithium levels were maintained between 0.6 and 1.2 mEq/liter. Neutrophil counts fell when lithium was discontinued in 2 patients, and in another patient, tolerance to the effect of lithium developed after 10 weeks.

Mechanism

Lithium has a myelostimulatory effect.

Clinical Implications

It is possible that lithium use will permit continued treatment with zidovudine even when neutropenia is present; however, there are insufficient studies to endorse this approach.

REFERENCES

Aanderud S et al.: The influence of carbamazepine on thyroid hormones and thyroxine-binding globulin in hypothyroid patients substituted with thyroxine. Clin Endocrinol 15: 247, 1981.
Agulnik PL et al.: Acute brain syndrome associated with lithium therapy. Am J Psychiatry 129: 621, 1973.
Allen HM et al.: Indomethacin in the treatment of lithium-induced nephrogenic diabetes insipidus. Arch Int Med 149: 1123, 1989.
Andrus PF: Lithium and carbamazepine. J Clin Psychiatry 45: 525, 1984.
Apseloff G et al.: Sertraline does not alter steady-state concentration or renal clearance of lithium in healthy volunteers. J Clin Pharmacol 32: 643, 1992.
Austin LS et al.: Toxicity resulting from lithium augmentation of antidepressant treatment in elderly patients. J Clin Psychiatry 51: 344, 1990.
Ayd FJ: Possible adverse drug-drug interaction report: lithium intoxication in a spectinomycin-treated patient. Int Drug Ther Newslett 13: 15, 1978.
Ayd FJ: Metronidazole-induced lithium intoxication. Int Drug Ther Newslett 17: 15, 1982a.
Ayd FJ: Lithium-mefenamic acid interaction. Int Drug Ther Newslett 17: 16, 1982b.
Baba S et al.: Changes in dopamine$_2$ and serotonin$_2$ receptors in rat brain after long-term verapamil treatment comparison of verapamil and lithium. Jpn J Psychiatry Neurol 45: 95, 1991.
Bakker K: The influence of lithium carbonate on the thalamo-pituitary axis: studies in

patients with affective disorders, thyrotoxicosis, and hypothyroidism (MD thesis), Groningen, The Netherlands, State University of Groningen, 1977.

Baldwin CM et al.: A case of lisinopril-induced lithium toxicity. DICP Ann Pharmacother 24: 946, 1990.

Ballenger JC et al.: Carbamazepine in manic depressive illness: a new treatment. Am J Psychiatry 137: 782, 1980.

Barclay ML: Lithium associated thyrotoxicosis: a report of 14 cases, with statistical analysis of incidence. Clin Endocrinol (Oxf) 40: 759, 1994.

Becker D: Lithium and propranolol—possible synergism (letter)? J Clin Psychiatry 50: 473, 1989.

Berens SC et al.: Antithyroid effects of lithium. J Clin Invest 49: 1357, 1970.

Binder et al.: Diltiazem induced psychosis and possible diltiazem-lithium interaction. Arch Intern Med 151: 373, 1991.

Birkhimer LJ et al.: Combined trazodone-lithium therapy for refractory depression. Am J Psychiatry 140: 1382, 1983.

Boer WH et al.: Acute effects of thiazides, with and without carbonic anhydrase activity, on lithium and free water clearance in man. Clin Sci 76: 539, 1989.

Braden W: Response to lithium in a case of L-dopa induced psychosis. Am J Psychiatry 134: 808, 1977.

Brady HR et al.: Lithium and the heart: unanswered questions. Chest 93: 166, 1988.

Brater DC: Drug-drug interaction and drug disease interaction with non-steroidal anti-inflammatory drugs. Am J Med (suppl 1A): 62, 1986.

Brater DC: Clinical pharmacology of NSAIDs. J Clin Pharmacol 28: 518, 1988.

Brewerton TD: Lithium counteracts carbamazepine-induced leukopenia while increasing its therapeutic effect. Biol Psychiatry 21: 677, 1986.

Byrd GJ: Methyldopa and lithium carbonate: suspected interaction (letter). JAMA 233: 320, 1975.

Chambers CA et al.: The effect of digoxin on the response to lithium therapy in mania. Psychol Med 12: 57, 1982.

Chaudry RP et al.: Lithium and carbamazepine interaction: possible neurotoxicity. J Clin Psychiatry 44: 30, 1983.

Chow CC et al.: Lithium associated transient thyrotoxicosis in 4 Chinese women with auto-immune thyroiditis. Aust N Z J Psychiatry 27: 246, 1993.

Ciraulo DA et al.: Drug interactions in psychopharmacology. In Shader RI (ed.): *Manual of Psychiatric Therapeutics*, 2d ed. Boston, Little, Brown, 1994.

Colonna L et al.: Association carbonate de lithium-clometacine et lithiemie. Gaz Med France 86: 4095, 1979.

Conroy RW: Possible adverse drug-drug interaction report: lithium intoxication in a spec-tinomycin-treated patient. Int Drug Ther Newslett 13: 15, 1978.

Cook BL et al.: Theophylline-lithium interaction. J Clin Psychiatry 46: 7, 1985.

Cooper SJ et al.: Pharmacodynamics and pharmacokinetics of digoxin in the presence of lithium. Br J Clin Pharmacol 18:21, 1984.

Correa FJ et al.: Angiotensin-converting enzyme inhibitors and lithium toxicity. Am J Med 93: 108, 1992.

Coppen A et al.: Lithium. In Paykel ES (ed.): *Handbook of Affective Disorders*. New York, Guilford, p. 276, 1982.

Cowdry RW et al.: Thyroid abnormalities associated with rapid cycling bipolar illness. Arch Gen Psychiatry 40: 414, 1983.

Crabtree BL et al.: Comparison of the effects of hydrochlorothiazide and furosemide on lithium disposition. Am J Psychiatry 148: 8, 1991.

Dalen P et al.: Lithium and levodopa in parkinsonism (letter). Lancet 1: 936, 1973.

DasGupta K et al.: The effect of enalapril on serum lithium levels in healthy men. J Clin Psychiatry 53: 11, 1992.

De Luca F et al.: Changes in thyroid function tests induced by 2 month carbamazepine treatment in L-thyroxine-substituted hypothyroid children. Eur J Pediatr 145: 77, 1986.

DeMontigny C et al.: Lithium induces relief of depression in tricyclic antidepressant drug non-responders. Br J Psychiatry 138: 252, 1981.

DeMontigny C et al.: Lithium carbonate addition in tricyclic antidepressant-resistant uni-polar depression. Arch Gen Psychiatry 40: 1327, 1983.

Desvilles M et al.: Effet paradoxal d l'association lithium et sulfamethoxazol-trimetroprime. Nouv Press Med 11: 3267, 1982.

Dietrich A et al.: Cardiac toxicity in an adolescent following chronic lithium and imipramine therapy. J Adolesc Health 14: 394, 1993.

Dinan TG: Lithium augmentation in sertraline resistant depression: a preliminary dose response study. Acta Psychiatry Scand 88: 300, 1993.

Douste-Blazy PH et al.: Angiotensin converting enzyme inhibitors and lithium treatment. Lancet 1: 1448, 1986.

Drouet A et al.: Lithium and converting enzyme inhibitors. Encephale 16: 51, 1990.

Dubovsky SL et al.: Verapamil a new antimanic drug with potential interaction with lithium. J Clin Psychiatry 48: 371–372, 1987.

Elizur A et al.: Intra-extracellular lithium ratio and clinical course in affective states. Clin Pharmacol Ther 13: 947, 1972.

Evans M et al.: Fluvoxamine and lithium: an unusual interaction (letter). Br J Psychiatry 156: 286, 1990a.

Evans M et al.: Evaluation of the interaction of lithium and alprazolam. J Clin Psychopharmacol 10: 355, 1990b.

Fankhauser MP et al.: Evaluation of lithium-tetracycline interaction. Clin Pharm 7: 314, 1988.

Fava M et al.: Lithium and tricyclic augmentation of fluoxetine treatment for resistant major depression: a double-blind, controlled study. Am J Psychiatry 151: 1372, 1994.

Fawcett J et al.: A double-blind placebo-controlled trial of lithium carbonate therapy for alcoholism. Arch Gen Psychiatry 44: 248, 1987.

Francis RI et al.: Lithium distribution in the brains of two manic patients. Lancet 2: 523, 1970.

Freinhar JP et al.: Use of clonazepam in two cases of acute mania. J Clin Psychiatry 46: 29, 1985.

Frolich JC et al.: Indomethacin increases plasma lithium. Br Med J 1: 1115, 1979.

Furnell MM et al.: The effect of sulindac on lithium therapy. Drug Intell Clin Pharm 19: 374, 1985.

Gallicchio VS et al.: In vitro effect of lithium on carbamazepine-induced inhibition of murine and human bone marrow-derived granulocyte-macrophage, erythroid, and megacariocyte progenitor stem cells. Proc Soc Exp Biol Med 190: 109, 1989.

Gardner EA: Long-term preventive care in depression: the use of bupropion in patients intolerant of other antidepressants. J Clin Psychiatry 44: 157, 1983.

Gay C et al.: Intoxication au lithium. Deux interaction inedities: l'acetazolamide et l'acide niflumique. Encephale 11: 261, 1985.

Gerdes H et al.: Successful treatment of thyrotoxicosis by lithium. Acta Endocrinol 173 (suppl): 23, 1973.

Ghadirian AM et al.: Lithium, benzodiazepine and sexual function in bipolar patients. Am J Psychiatry 149: 801, 1992.

Ghose K: Effect of carbamazepine in polyuria associated with lithium therapy. Pharmakopsychiat Neuro-Psychopharmakol 11: 241, 1978.

Goodnick PJ et al.: Neurochemical changes during discontinuation of lithium prophylaxis, I: increases in clonidine-induced hypotension. Biol Psychiatry 19: 883, 1984.

Gove GC et al.: Effects of indomethacin on renal concentrating capacity in lithium-treated rats. Res Commun Chem Pathol Pharmacol 39: 11, 1983.

Graham PM: Drug combination for chronic depression. Br J Psychiatry 145: 214, 1984.

Gray EG: Severe depression: a patient's thoughts. Br J Psychiatry 143: 319, 1983.

Gudelsky GA et al.: Activity of tuberoinfundibular dopaminergic neurons and concentration of serum prolactin in the rat following lithium administration. Psychopharmacology 94: 92, 1988.

Hadley A et al.: Mania resulting from lithium fluoxetine combination. Am J Psychiatry 146: 1637, 1989.

Halaris AE: The use of lithium in psychiatric practice. Psychiatr Ann 13: 53, 1983.

Hanna ME et al.: Severe lithium toxicity associated with indapamide therapy (letter). J Clin Psychopharmacol 10: 379, 1990.

Harker WG et al.: Enhancement of colony-stimulating activity production by lithium. Blood 49: 263, 1977.

Harrison TM et al.: Lithium carbonate and piroxicam. Br J Psychiatry 149: 124, 1986.
Havdala HS et al.: Potential hazards and applications of lithium in anesthesiology. Anesthesiology 50: 534, 1979.
Helmuth D et al.: Choreoathetosis induced by verapamil and lithium treatment (letter). J Clin Psychopharmacol 9: 454, 1989.
Heninger GR et al.: Lithium carbonate augmentation of antidepressant treatment. Arch Gen Psychiatry 40: 1335, 1983.
Hetmar O et al.: Decreased number of benzodiazepine receptors in frontal cortex of rat brain following long-term lithium treatment. J Neurochem 41: 217, 1983.
Hill GE et al.: Potentiation of succinylcholine neuromuscular blockade by lithium carbonate. Anesthesiology 44: 439, 1976.
Himmelhoch JM et al.: Treatment of previously intractable depressions with tranylcypromine and lithium. J Nerv Ment Dis 155: 216, 1972.
Himmelhoch JM et al.: Thiazide-lithium synergy in refractory mood swings. Am J Psychiatry 134: 149, 1977a.
Himmelhoch JM et al.: Adjustment of lithium dose during lithium-chlorothiazide therapy. Clin Pharmacol Ther 22: 225, 1977b.
Holstad SG et al.: The effects of intravenous theophylline infusion versus intravenous sodium bicarbonate infusion on lithium clearance in normal subjects. Psychiatry Res 25: 203, 1988.
Hommer DW et al.: Prazosin, a specific α1-noradrenergic receptor antagonist, has no effect on symptoms but increases autonomic arousal in schizophrenic patients. Psychiat Res 11: 193, 1984.
Huang LG: Lithium intoxication with coadministration of a loop diuretic (letter). J Clin Psychopharmacol 10: 228, 1990.
Hurtig HI et al.: Lithium toxicity enhanced by diuresis. New Engl J Med 290: 748, 1974.
Imbs JL et al.: Effects of indomethacin and methylprednisolone on renal elimination of lithium in the rat. Int Pharmacopsychiatry 15: 143, 1980.
Jacobson MJ et al.: Delirium induced by verapamil. Am J Psychiatry 144: 248, 1987.
Jakobsson B et al.: Effect of hydrochlorothiazide and indomethacin treatment on renal function in nephrogenic diabetes insipidus. Acta Paediatr 83: 522, 1994.
Jefferson JW et al.: Serum lithium levels and long-term diuretic use. JAMA 241: 1134, 1979.
Jefferson JW et al.: Lithium: interactions with other drugs. J Clin Psychopharmacol 1: 124, 1981.
Jefferson JW et al.: Combining lithium and antidepressants. J Clin Psychopharmacol 3: 303, 1983.
Jefferson JW et al.: Antibiotics: In Jefferson JW et al. (eds): Lithium Encyclopedia for Clinical Practice, 2d ed. Washington, DC, American Psychiatric Press, p. 69, 1987.
Jefferson JW et al.: Manic depressive disorder and lithium over the decades: the very educational case of Mrs. L. J. Clin Psychiatry 55: 340, 1994.
Joffe RT: Hematologic effects of lithium potentiation of carbamazepine in patients with affective illness. Int Clin Psychopharmacol 3: 53, 1988.
Joffe RT et al.: A placebo controlled comparison of lithium and triiodo thyronine augmentation of tricyclic antidepressants in unipolar refractory depression. Arch Gen Psychiatry 50: 387, 1993.
Johnson AG et al.: Adverse drug interactions with nonsteroidal anti-inflammatory drugs (NSAIDs). Recognition, management and avoidance. Drug Safety 8: 99, 1993.
Joyce PR et al.: Rapid response to lithium in treatment resistant depression. Br J Psychiatry 142: 204, 1983.
Judd LL et al.: Lithium carbonate and ethanol induced "highs" in normal subjects. Arch Gen Psychiatry 34: 463, 1977.
Judd LL et al.: Lithium antagonizes ethanol intoxication in alcoholics. Am J Psychiatry 141: 155, 1984.
Kafka M et al.: Effect of lithium on circadian neurotransmitter receptor rhythms. Neuropsychobiology 8: 41, 1982.
Kasaris EJ et al.: Carbamazepine induced cardiac dysfunction. Arch Intern Med 152: 186, 1992.
Kerry RJ et al.: Diuretics are dangerous with lithium. Br Med J 2: 371, 1980.
Kerry RJ et al.: Possible toxic interaction between lithium and piroxicam. Lancet 1: 418, 1983.

Kettl P et al.: Maprotiline-induced myoclonus. J Clin Psychopharmacol 3: 264, 1983.
Kline NS et al.: Evaluation of lithium therapy in chronic and periodic alcoholism. Am J Med Sci 268: 15, 1974.
Koczerginski D et al.: Clonazepam and lithium—a toxic combination in treatment of mania? Internat Clin Psychopharmacol 4: 195, 1989.
Kojima H et al.: Serotonin syndrome during clomipramine and lithium treatment (letter). Am J Psychiatry 150: 1897, 1993.
Kramlinger KG et al.: Addition of lithium carbonate to carbamazepine: hematologic and thyroid effects. Am J Psychiatry 147: 615, 1990.
Kristensen O, et al.: Lithium carbonate in the treatment of thyrotoxicosis: a controlled trial. Lancet 1: 603, 1976.
Langlois R et al.: Increased serum lithium levels due to ketorolac therapy. Can Med Assoc J 150: 1455, 1994.
Lassen E: Effects of acute and short-time antibiotic treatment on renal lithium elimination and serum lithium levels in the rat. Acta Pharmacol Toxicol 56: 273, 1985.
Levenson J: Neuroleptic malignant syndrome. Am J Psychiatry 142: 1137, 1985.
Levy ST et al.: Lithium-induced diabetes insipidus: manic symptoms, brain and electrolyte correlates, and chlorothiazide treatment. Am J Psychiatry 130: 1014, 1973.
Lipinski JF et al.: Possible synergistic action between carbamazepine and lithium carbonate in the treatment of three acutely manic patients. Am J Psychiatry 139: 948, 1982.
Louie AK et al.: Lithium potentiation of antidepressant treatment. J Clin Psychopharmacol 4: 316, 1984.
Louie AK et al.: Lithium potentiation of antidepressive illness. Br Med J i: 881, 1984.
MacCallum WAG: Interaction of lithium and phenytoin. Br Med J 1: 610, 1980.
MacDonald J et al.: Toxic interaction of lithium carbonate and mefenamic acid. Br Med J 297: 1339, 1988.
Macfie AC: Lithium poisoning precipitated by diuretics. Br Med J 1: 516, 1975.
Macfie AC: Lithium toxicity precipitated by a diuretic. Psychosomatics 21: 425, 1980.
Mannisto P et al.: Effect of lithium and rubidium on the sleeping time caused by various intravenous anesthetics in the mouse. Br J Anaesth 48: 185, 1976.
Mastrosimone F et al.: The use of lithium salts in trigeminal neuralgia in prevention of neutropenia due to carbamazepine preliminary consideration. Acta Neurol 39: 149, 1979.
McCance-Katz E et al.: Serotonergic function during lithium augmentation of refractory depression. Psychopharmacology (Berlin) 108: 93, 1992.
McCauland JA et al.: Lithium in Parkinson's disease (letter). Lancet 1: 1117, 1974.
McGennis AJ: Lithium carbonate and tetracycline interaction. Br Med J 1: 1183, 1978.
Merry J et al.: Prophylactic treatment of alcoholism by lithium carbonate. Lancet 2: 481, 1976.
Millard SA et al.: Biochemical effects due to interaction of lithium ions and disulfiram in rats. Proc Soc Exp Biol Med 131: 1210, 1969.
Mochinaga N et al.: Successful preoperative preparation for thyroidectomy in Graves' disease using lithium alone: report of two cases. Surg Today 24: 464, 1994.
Muly EC et al.: Serotonin syndrome produced by a combination of fluoxetine and lithium (letter). Am J Psychiatry 150: 1565, 1993.
Nadarajah J et al.: Piroxicam-induced lithium toxicity. Ann Rheum Dis 44: 502, 1985.
Navis GJ et al.: Volume homeostatsis, angiotensin-converting enzyme inhibition, and lithium therapy (letter). Am J Med 86: 621, 1989.
Naylor GJ et al.: Profound hypothermia on combined lithium carbonate and diazepam treatment. Br Med J 2: 22, 1977.
Nelson JC et al.: Rapid response to lithium in phenelzine nonresponders. Br J Psychiatry 141: 85, 1982.
Noveske FG et al.: Possible toxicity of combined fluoxetine and lithium. Am J Psychiatry 146: 1515, 1989.
O'Regan JB: Adverse interaction of lithium carbonate and methyldopa (letter). Can Med Assoc J 115: 385, 1976.
Okuma T et al.: Anti-manic and prophylactic effects of carbamazepine (Tegretol) on manic depressive psychosis: a preliminary report. Folia Psychiatr Neurol Jap 27: 283, 1973.

Osanloo E et al.: Interaction of lithium and methyldopa. Ann Int Med 92: 433, 1980.

Ozawa H et al.: Potentiating effect of lithium chloride on aggressive behavior induced in mice by nialamide plus L-dopa and by clonidine. Eur J Pharmacol 34: 169, 1975.

Pandey GN et al.: Effect of neuroleptic drugs on lithium uptake by the human erythrocyte. Clin Pharmacol Ther 26: 96, 1979.

Perry PJ et al.: Theophylline precipitated alterations of lithium clearance. Acta Psychiatr Scand 69: 528, 1984.

Persad E et al.: Hyperthyroidism after treatment with lithium. Can J Psychiatry 38: 599, 1993.

Peselow ED et al.: Lithium prophylaxis of bipolar illness: the value of combination treatment. Br J Psychiatry 164: 208, 1994.

Pond SM et al.: An evaluation of the effects of lithium in the treatment of chronic alcoholism, I: clinical results. Alcoholism 5: 247, 1981.

Pope HG et al.: Antidepressant treatment of bulimia. Preliminary experience and practical recommendation. J Clin Psychopharmacol 3: 274, 1983.

Price LH et al.: Efficacy of lithium-tranylcypromine treatment in refractory depression. Am J Psychiatry 142: 619, 1985.

Price WA et al.: Neurotoxicity caused by lithium-verapamil synergism. J Clin Psychopharmacol 26: 717, 1986.

Price WA et al.: Lithium-verapamil toxicity in the elderly. J Am Geriatr Soc 35: 177, 1987.

Ragheb MA et al.: Interaction of indomethacin and ibuprofen with lithium in manic patients under a steady-state lithium level. J Clin Psychiatry 41: 397, 1980.

Ragheb MA et al.: Failure of sulindac to increase serum lithium levels. J Clin Psychiatry 47: 33, 1986a.

Ragheb MA et al: Lithium interaction with sulindac and naproxen. J Clin Psychopharmacol 6: 150, 1986b.

Ragheb MA: Ibuprofen can increase serum lithium level in lithium-treated patients. J Clin Psychiatry 48: 161, 1987a.

Ragheb MA: Aspirin does not significantly affect patients' serum lithium levels. J Clin Psychiatry 48: 425, 1987b.

Ragheb MA: The clinical significance of lithium-nonsteroidal anti-inflammatory drug interactions. J Clin Psychopharmacol 10: 350, 1990.

Raskin DE: Lithium and phenytoin interaction (letter). J Clin Psychopharmacol 4: 120, 1984.

Ratey JJ et al.: Lithium and marijuana. J Clin Psychopharmacol 1: 32, 1981.

Raudino F: Interaction between benzodiazepines and blood levels of lithium salts. Clin Therapeutics 98: 683, 1981.

Reilly M et al.: Influence of chronic lithium administration on binding to benzodiazepine and histamine H_1 receptors in rat brain. J Recept Res 3: 703, 1983–1984.

Reimann IW et al.: Effects of diclofenac on lithium kinetics. Clin Pharmacol Ther 30: 348, 1981.

Reimherr FW et al.: Prolongation of muscle relaxant effects by lithium carbonate. Am J Psychiatry 134: 205, 1977.

Richman CM et al.: Granulopoietic effects of lithium on human bone marrow in vitro. Exp Hematol 9: 449, 1981.

Rittmannsberger H et al.: Asterixis as a side effect of carbamazepine therapy. Klin Wochenschr 69: 279, 1991.

Rittmannsberger H et al.: Asterixis induced by carbamazepine therapy. Biol Psychiatry 32: 364, 1992.

Roberts DE et al.: Effect of lithium carbonate on zidovudine-associated neutropenia in the acquired immunodeficiency syndrome. Am J Med 85: 428, 1988.

Rodney WM et al.: Lithium induced dysrhythmias as a marker for sick sinus syndrome. J Fam Pract 16: 797, 1983.

Rogers MP et al.: Clinical hypothyroidism occurring during lithium treatment: two case histories and a review of thyroid function in 19 patients. Am J Psychiatry 128: 158, 1971.

Rosenbaum AH et al.: Drugs that alter mood, II: lithium. Mayo Clin Proc 54: 401, 1979.

Rosenbaum AH et al.: Tardive dyskinesia in depressed patients: successful therapy with antidepressants and lithium. Psychosomatics 21: 715, 1980.

Rossof AH et al.: Lithium stimulation of granulopoiesis (letter). New Engl J Med 298: 280, 1978.

Rossof AH et al.: Lithium carbonate increases marrow granulocyte-committed colony-forming units and peripheral blood granulocyte in a canine model. Exp Hematol 7: 255, 1979.

Rothstein E et al.: Combined use of lithium and disulfiram (letter). New Engl J Med 285: 238, 1971.

Rubin EH et al.: Lithium-ketamine interaction: an animal study of potential clinical and theoretical interest. J Clin Psychopharmacol 2: 211, 1982.

Ryback RS et al.: Manic response to levodopa therapy: report of a case. New Engl J Med 285: 788, 1971.

Sacristan JA et al.: Absence seizures induced by lithium: possible interaction with fluoxetine (letter). Am J Psychiatry 148: 146, 1991.

Sadoul JL et al.: Lithium therapy and hyperthyroidism: disease caused or facilitated by lithium? Ann Endocrinol 54: 353, 1994.

Safher D et al.: Frusemide: a safe diuretic during lithium therapy? Affective Disord 5: 289, 1983.

Salama AA et al.: A case of severe lithium toxicity induced by combined fluoxetine and lithium carbonate. Am J Psychiatry 146: 278, 1989.

Samoilov N et al.: Effect of psychotropic drugs on the pharmacokinetics of lithium. Byull Eksp Biol Med 89: 696, 1980.

Schaff MR et al.: Divalproex sodium in the treatment of refractory affective disorders. J Clin Psychiatry 54: 380, 1993.

Schou M et al.: Use of propranolol during lithium treatment: an enquiry and suggestion. Pharmacopsychiatry 20: 131, 1987.

Schwarcz G: The problem of anti-hypertensive treatment in lithium patients. Compr Psychiatry 23: 50, 1982.

Sedvall G et al.: Effects of lithium salts on plasma protein bound iodine and uptake of 1^{131} in thyroid gland of man and rat. Life Sci 7: 1257, 1968.

Sellers EM et al.: Lithium treatment of alcoholic withdrawal. Clin Pharmacol Ther 15: 218, 1974.

Sellers EM et al.: Lithium treatment during alcoholic withdrawal. Clin Pharmacol Ther 20: 199, 1976.

Shelly RK: Lithium toxicity and mefenamic acid: a possible interaction and the role of prostaglandin inhibition. Br J Psychiatry 151: 847, 1987.

Shukla S et al.: Lithium-carbamazepine neurotoxicity and risk factors. Am J Psychiatry 141: 1604, 1984.

Sierles FS et al.: Concurrent use of theophylline and lithium in a patient with chronic obstructive lung disease and bipolar disorder. Am J Psychiatry 139: 117, 1982.

Singer L et al.: Baise de la clearance renale du lithium sous l'effet de la phenylbutazone. Encephale 4: 33, 1978.

Solomon JG: Seizures during lithium-amitriptyline therapy. Postgrad Med 66: 145, 1979.

Solomon JG: Lithium poisoning precipitated by a diuretic. Psychosomatics 21: 425, 1980.

Speirs J et al.: Severe lithium toxicity with "normal" serum concentrations. Br Med J 1: 815, 1978.

Spivey WH: Flumazenil and seizures: analysis of 43 cases. Clin Ther 14: 292, 1992.

Stancer HC: Tardive dyskinesia not associated with neuroleptics. Am J Psychiatry 135: 127, 1979.

Steele TH et al.: Renal lithium reabsorption in man: physiologic and pharmacologic determinants. Am J Med Sci 269: 349, 1975.

Stein RS et al.: Lithium induced granulocytosis. Ann Intern Med 88: 809, 1978.

Stein RS et al.: Lithium and granulocytopenia during induction therapy of acute myelogenous leukemia. Blood 54: 636, 1979.

Steckler TL: Lithium and carbamazepine associated sinus node dysfunction: nine year experience in a psychiatric hospital. J Clinical Psychopharmacology 14: 336, 1994.

Stiener C et al.: The antiarrhythmic action of carbamazepine (Tegretol). J Pharmacol Exp Ther 173: 323, 1970.

Takami H: Lithium in the preoperative preparation of Graves' disease. Int Surg 79: 89, 1994.

4 / LITHIUM   213

Teicher MH et al.: Possible nephrotoxic interaction of lithium in metronidazole (letter). JAMA 257: 3365, 1987.

Temple R et al.: The use of lithium in the treatment of thyrotoxicosis. J Clin Invest 51: 2746, 1972.

Thomsen K et al.: Renal lithium excretion in man. Am J Physiol 215: 823, 1968.

Thornton WE et al.: Lithium intoxication: a report of two cases. Can Psychiatry Assoc J 20: 281, 1975.

Tonkin AL et al.: Interaction of nonsteroidal anti-inflammatory drugs. Bailiêre Clin Rheum 2: 455, 1988.

Toutoungi M et al.: Probable interaction entre le psyllium et le lithium. Therapie 45: 357, 1990.

Turner JG et al.: Use of lithium in the treatment of thyrotoxicosis. NZ Med J 82: 57, 1975.

Turner JG et al.: Lithium and thyrotoxicosis (letter). Lancet 2: 904, 1976.

Valdiserri EV: A possible interaction between lithium and diltiazem. J Clin Psychiatry 46: 540, 1985.

Van Woert MH et al.: Manic behavior and levodopa (letter). NEJM 285: 1326, 1971.

Van Woert MH et al.: Lithium and levodopa in Parkinsonism (letter). Lancet 1: 1390, 1973.

Vieweg V et al.: Absence of carbamazepine induced heponatremia among patients also given lithium. Am J Psychiatry 144: 943, 1987.

Visser TJ et al.: Subcellular localization of rat liver enzyme converting thyroxine into triiodothyronine and possible involvement of essential thiol groups. Biochem J 157: 479, 1976.

Walbridge DG et al.: An interaction between lithium carbonate and piroxicam presenting a lithium toxicity. Br J Psychiatry 147: 206, 1985.

Walker N et al.: Lithium-methyldopa interactions in normal subjects. Drug Intell Clin Pharm 14: 638, 1980.

Warrington SJ: Clinical implications of the pharmacology of sertraline. Internat Clin Psychopharmacology 6: 11, 1991.

Waud BE et al.: Lithium and neuromuscular transmission. Anesth Analg 61: 399, 1982.

Weaver KEC: Lithium for delusional depression. Am J Psychiatry 140: 962, 1983.

West AP et al.: Paradoxical lithium neurotoxicity: a report of five cases and a hypothesis about risk for neurotoxicity. Am J Psychiatry 136: 963, 1979.

Winters WD et al.: Digoxin-lithium drug interaction. Clin Toxicol 10: 487, 1977.

Wright BA et al.: Lithium and calcium channel blockers: possible neurotoxicity. Biol Psychiatry 30: 635, 1991.

Zall H: Lithium and isocarboxazid—an effective drug approach in severe depression. Am J Psychiatry 127: 1400, 1971.

Ziegler-Driscoll G et al.: Lithium use in the treatment of affective disorders in an abstinent therapeutic community. In Seixas J (ed.), Currents in Alcoholism. New York, Grune and Stratton, 1977, vol 2, pp. 19–34.

5

Benzodiazepines

BRIAN F. SANDS, WAYNE L. CREELMAN, DOMENIC A. CIRAULO,
DAVID J. GREENBLATT and RICHARD I. SHADER

All benzodiazepines (BZDs) share 4 pharmacologic effects: anxiolysis, sedation, centrally mediated muscle relaxation, and elevation of seizure threshold. They are safe and effective drugs, with relatively few drug interactions. Most of their adverse effects are extensions of their therapeutic action (e.g. sedation). Psychomotor impairment and anterograde memory loss (to varying degrees among different BZDs) may present clinical problems especially among the elderly.

The best understood mechanism for the action of BZDs is through binding to a membrane-spanning heteromeric protein complex that gates a chloride ion channel. This structure also includes receptors for β-aminobutyric acid (GABA), barbiturates, ethanol, and neurosteroids. GABA binding results in chloride channel opening and neuronal hyperpolarization; the net result is that the neuron is less likely to fire. The binding of BZDs allosterically enhances the actions of GABA and increases the frequency of channel openings.

There are currently 14 benzodiazepines on the U.S. market that share some common structural elements but differ in others. Pharmacodynamic interactions (e.g. additive or synergistic sedation or decrements in psychomotor function when combined with other central nervous system [CNS] depressants) are the most common clinically, but recent studies have identified important pharmacokinetic interactions as well. Pharmacokinetic interactions may be divided into those that affect the rate of absorption (such as acute ethanol-BZD administration) and those that affect drug elimination (Abernethy et al. 1984). Although some interactions involving displacement from protein binding sites have also been reported, these are rarely of clinical importance.

The 3-hydroxy substituted BZDs (i.e. lorazepam [Ativan®], oxazepam [Serax®], and temazepam [Restoril®]) require only glucuronidation and are relatively unaffected by inhibition or induction of metabolism. Those drugs that require phase 1 metabolism are the 2-keto BZDs diazepam (Valium®), chlordiazepoxide (Librium®), prazepam (Centrax®), clorazepate (Tranxene®), halazepam (Paxipam®), and flurazepam (Dalmane®), the 2-nitro BZD clonazepam (Klonopin®), and the triazolo BZDs triazolam (Halcion®), alprazolam (Xanax®), and estazolam (ProSom®). All except clonazepam (which undergoes nitro reduction as its primary metabolic step) require oxidative metabolism. Both oxidation and nitro reduction are sensitive to alterations in hepatic function.

Oxidative drug metabolism is largely accomplished via microsomal cytochrome P450 pathways. It should be remembered, however, that not all oxidative reactions are microsomal (e.g. monoamine oxidation of dopamine, diamine oxidation of histamine, purine oxidation of theophylline). Nevertheless, most phase 1 oxidative metabolism is cytochrome P450 dependent, and recent advances in our understanding of these isozyme families and their preferred substrates has shed more light on the differential effects of some drugs on BZD metabolism. For example, there is considerable interindividual variation in the plasma levels for diazepam and its metabolites. Some of this variability may be attributed to the fact that diazepam N-demethylation appears to involve two pathways. One pathway involves 3A3/4 isozymes that also are responsible for the hydroxylation of diazepam (and also the formation of temazepam). The other is the N-demethylation pathway, which involves 2C19 isozymes and cosegregates with S-mephenytoin metabolism; the latter being subject to genetic polymorphism. Oxidation of alprazolam and other triazolobenzodiazepines (e.g. midazolam, triazolam) is primarily accomplished via 3A3/4 isozymes. Cytochrome P450 3A3/4 microsomal isozymes are abundantly present in hepatic and gut wall tissues as well as in brain.

Anticoagulants

Evidence of Interaction

Fourteen healthy subjects (6 men and 8 women) and 5 male patients with cirrhosis were evaluated with respect to the effect of heparin administration on plasma binding of benzodiazepines (Desmond et al. 1980b). The effects of intravenous administration of 100 units of heparin on plasma binding of diazepam, chlordiazepoxide, oxazepam, and lorazepam were assessed. Results of the study indicated that in the healthy nonfasted subjects, heparin caused a rapid 150 to 250% rise in the free fraction of diazepam, chlordiazepoxide, and oxazepam, but no change in the free fraction of lorazepam. When the subjects were fasted, the changes in free fractions were somewhat smaller but still significant. The cirrhotic subjects' responses to heparin were variable. Patients with cirrhosis often have elevated free fatty acid levels (Merli et al. 1986). Another study found substantial variability in the effect depending on the biologic activity of the heparin (which varied with the manufacturer and lot), sampling times, and fasting state of subjects (Naranjo et al. 1980c).

Mechanism

Free fraction of diazepam is influenced by serum concentration, changes in free fatty acids, heparin, and other factors (Naranjo et al. 1980a, 1982).

Clinical Implications

None.   Any increase in free benzodiazepine level would be transient and rapidly compensated for by drug metabolism.

Anesthetics and Neuromuscular Blocking Agents

Evidence of Interaction

Diazepam prolonged the duration of neuromuscular blockade induced by gallamine and reduced that produced by succinylcholine (Feldman et al. 1970). Other studies found no interaction between gallamine and diazepam (Dretchen et al. 1979, Webb et al. 1971). Another study found that diazepam prevented some adverse effects of succinylcholine (Fahmy et al. 1979). One hundred twenty adult patients (ages 18–42 years) were studied after administration of anesthesia with halothane (1%) and nitrous oxide and oxygen (4:2 liters/min). Succinylcholine was administered to facilitate endotracheal intubation. Diazepam exerted a clear protective effect against the undesirable effects of succinylcholine. Diazepam prevented fasciculations, muscle pains, and antagonized increases in serum potassium, creatinine phosphokinase, and heart rate produced by succinylcholine. In a series of 37 patients undergoing elective abdominal surgery, midazolam (0.1–0.15 mg/kg) was administered with suxamethonium or pancuronium (Tassonyi 1984). Midazolam did not affect the intensity or duration of neuromuscular blockade induced by either drug alone.

Flumazenil did not antagonize halothane anesthesia in rats (Murayama et al. 1992). Trifluroacetic acid, a metabolite of halothane, altered protein binding of diazepam and midazolam and may temporarily potentiate the pharmacologic effect of diazepam postoperatively (Suarez et al. 1991).

Mechanism

Not established. Benzodiazepines in very high concentrations can produce impairment at the neuromuscular junction but not in concentrations achieved clinically (Madan et al. 1963, Oetliker 1970, Prindle et al. 1970). Most likely, the mechanism is centrally mediated. Halothane alters protein binding of diazepam and midazolam.

Clinical Implications

Diazepam may block some of the adverse effects associated with administration of intravenous succinylcholine; however, the clinical importance of this is not well established. Evidence does not consistently support enhanced neuromuscular blockade when gallamine and diazepam are administered concurrently. Suxamethonium and pancuronium are not potentiated by midazolam.

Anesthetics (Local)

Evidence of Interaction

Diazepam 10 mg orally was randomly given to half of a group of 21 children undergoing surgery for which a combination 50% lidocaine (1%) and 50% bupivicaine (.25%) was used for a caudal block. In the diazepam-treated group, the plasma area-under-the-curve for bupivicaine but not lidocaine was significantly increased (Giaufre et al. 1988).

Mechanism and Clinical Implications

Unknown. One study examining the possible influence of diazepam on bupivicaine binding failed to demonstrate such an influence (Bruguerolle et al. 1990).

Anorectic Drugs

Evidence of Interaction

In a study (Feldman et al. 1978) of 10 male Sprague-Dawley rats, chlordiazepoxide increased food intake in free-feeding rats. By testing the effects of chlordiazepoxide alone and then in combination with fluoxetine, a specific blocker of serotonin uptake, chlordiazepoxide-induced feeding was blocked by fluoxetine in a dose-related manner. In other studies, chlordiazepoxide blocked the anorexic effect of amphetamine (Cooper et al. 1978) but increased amphetamine stereotypies (Babbini et al. 1971, Ellinwood et al. 1976).

Mechanism

Administration of combinations of chlordiazepoxide and fluoxetine to rats showed an antagonistic dose-dependent relationship, implicating a satiety of hunger mechanisms mediated by serotonin.

Clinical Implications

Based on the studies available, it is uncertain whether this interaction is of clinical importance in humans (Ellinwood et al. 1976, Svenson and Hamilton 1966).

Antacids

Evidence of Interaction

The effect of antacids on absorption of clorazepate was assessed in 15 healthy adult men between 27 and 55 years of age who participated in a 3-period, randomized, balanced, complete crossover study (Chun et al. 1977). The 15 men each ingested a 15-mg dose of clorazepate alone or with single or multiple doses of antacids. The results of this study indicated a trend of initially slower absorption and lower peak desmethyldiazepam plasma levels when clorazepate was administered with the antacid suspension. There was no significant difference among treatments, however, in the extent of absorption as measured by the area under the plasma level time curves. In a later study (Shader et al. 1982), 10 healthy volunteers each ingested single 15-mg doses of clorazepate dipotassium with 60 ml of water or with 60 ml of magnesium aluminum hydroxide (Maalox®) on 2 occasions in a randomized, 2-way crossover design. In this study, administration of single doses of clorazepate with usual doses of magnesium aluminum hydroxide reduced the rate of appearance in blood of desmethyldiazepam as it had in the previous study, but the extent of appearance of desmethyldiazepam was also decreased, as were self-rated clinical effects. Steady-state desmethyldiazepam concentrations with long-term clorazepate use were not influenced, however, by either low-dose or high-dose regimens (Shader et al. 1982).

In an additional study (Greenblatt et al. 1976), the effect on 10 healthy men of ingesting 25 mg of chlordiazepoxide with either 100 mg of water or with 100 mg of magnesium and aluminum hydroxide (Maalox) in a single-dose crossover regimen was assessed. The antacid prolonged the mean chlordiazepoxide absorption half-time from 11 to 24 minutes, and in 6 of 10 subjects, the antacid delayed the achievement of peak blood concentration by 0.5 to 43.0 hours. Desmethylchlordiazepoxide formation was slowed. The area under the 24-hour blood concentration curve for chlordiazepoxide and for its metabolite was not influenced by the antacid. The apparent elimination half-life of chlordiazepoxide (8.4 and 8.2 hours) was not significantly affected. A decreased rate but with an unaltered extent of absorption was also found with single doses of diazepam taken with magnesium aluminum hydroxide or food (Greenblatt et al. 1978). In summary, administration of chlordiazepoxide or diazepam with antacid reduced the rate but not the extent of absorption.

Mechanism

The transformation of the prodrug clorazepate to desmethyldiazepam by hydrolysis and decarboxylation *in vitro* is strongly dependent on gastric pH. Single-dose studies of desmethyldiazepam plasma levels after administration of oral clorazepate show that the clorazepate results in reduced absorption of desmethyldiazepam if gastric pH is elevated by single doses of antacid. As steady-state plasma desmethyldiazepam concentrations were not influenced by antacid regimens, the *in vivo* formation of desmethyldiazepam from clorazepate is more complex than was predicted *in vitro* and appears to depend on more than gastric acidity alone. The delay in chlordiazepoxide absorption attributable to the antacid most probably is due to gastric emptying being delayed by the antacid.

Clinical Implications

The biodegradation of clorazepate to desmethyldiazepam in humans decreased with an increase in gastric pH, since the pH of the stomach influences the formation of desmethyldiazepam from the prodrug clorazepate (Abruzzo et al. 1977). Although acute studies have indicated a delay in the formation of desmethyldiazepam with corresponding decreased clinical effect, chronic clorazepate-antacid treatment did not appear to have a significant clinical effect.

Antacid suspensions prolonged the mean benzodiazepine absorption half-life; however, the areas under the 24-hour blood concentration curves were not influenced. Even though the administration of benzodiazepine with antacid reduced the rate of absorption, since there was no alteration in the elimination half-lives or the completeness of absorption, this interaction is of clinical importance primarily for single-dose treatment. Subjective antianxiety effects are altered when absorption is slowed, and it is also possible that some decrease in efficacy results from lower peak drug levels. The delay in chlordiazepoxide absorption when administered with antacid may be undesirable in those patients who require a rapid onset of antianxiety effects during acute episodes of anxiety, although chlordiazepoxide would not be the drug of choice in these situations. The interaction will be less of a problem for patients with chronic anxiety states such as the individuals who take chlordiazepoxide on a repeated basis. Accumulation and steady-state concentrations of chlordiazepoxide and its metabolites will depend on the completeness of absorption, which is not influenced by an antacid.

Anticholinergic Agents

Evidence of Interaction

As a consequence of anticholinergic compounds slowing gastric motility, gastrointestinal absorption of benzodiazepines may be hindered by the addition of anticholinergic agents. All tricyclic antidepressants as well as maprotiline have significant anticholinergic effects (Snyder 1974). Antiparkinsonian agents, as well as some antipsychotic agents, will also increase the additive atropinic effects (Snyder 1974).

Mechanism

Anticholinergic agents slow gastric motility, altering drug absorption. For drugs metabolized in the gut or gut wall, there is the potential for both slowed rate and decreased bioavailability.

Clinical Implications

Although the coadministration of benzodiazepines and anticholinergic agents may slow time to peak absorption of benzodiazepines, elimination is not significantly altered. There is a potential for gut metabolism to reduce bioavailability (for example, cytochrome 3A3/4 is present in the gut wall), but this has not been studied.

Anticonvulsants

Evidence of Interaction

Valproic Acid. Six healthy male volunteers between 21 and 35 years of age participated in a study focusing on the interaction between valproic acid and diazepam. Oral administration of sodium valproate 1,500 mg daily affected the distribution and elimination kinetics of intravenously administered diazepam by increasing the unbound fraction of diazepam in serum approximately 2-fold. A significant increase in apparent volume of distribution and plasma clearance of diazepam was also found. A positive correlation between the change in free fraction and the increase in apparent volume of distribution of unbound diazepam in serum was significantly higher during valproate administration, and both the intrinsic clearance and volume of the distribution of unbound drug were significantly reduced. The mean serum levels of desmethyldiazepam were also significantly lower during valproate coadministration. These results suggest that valproic acid will predictably displace diazepam from plasma protein-binding sites as well as inhibit its metabolism (Dhillon et al. 1982).

Phenytoin. Although the literature documents several case reports of potentially important pharmacokinetic interactions between phenytoin and clonazepam, the data are preliminary (Shader et al. 1978). In one controlled study in which this combination was examined, substituting clonazepam for placebo in 18 patients stabilized on phenytoin resulted in a statistically significant fall in blood levels of phenytoin in 12 patients (Edwards et al. 1973). Several investigators have also claimed that other benzodiazepines (chlordiazepoxide, diazepam) may elevate blood levels of phenytoin, yet, again, solid evidence is lacking.

Carbamazepine. In a study of the influence of carbamazepine on clonazepam, 7 subjects received clonazepam 1 mg each day for 29 days and carbamazepine 200 mg on days 8 to 29 (Lai et al. 1978). After an initial steady state had been reached by day 7, the clonazepam levels declined 5 to 15 days after the addition of carbamazepine to a new steady state 19 to 37% lower than previously. In 1 case report, a patient receiving alprazolam 7.5 mg daily had greater than 50% reductions in plasma alprazolam after carbamazepine was added (Arana et al. 1988).

Mechanism

Valproic acid displaces diazepam from plasma protein-binding sites and inhibits metabolism. Carbamazepine is a potent enzyme inducer and can decrease the levels of many drugs that are metabolized by the mixed oxidase system.

Clinical Implications

The findings suggest that clinical effects may be enhanced in those individuals prescribed both valproic acid and benzodiazepines. Dose reduction may be required. Carbamazepine is a potent enzyme inducer (*see* Chapter 6) and patients who take this anticonvulsant with clonazepam, alprazolam, or other benzodiazepines may require higher doses of the benzodiazepine.

Antidepressants

CYCLIC ANTIDEPRESSANTS

Evidence of Interaction

Amitriptyline 75 mg orally was administered to 12 subjects with and without diazepam 10 mg orally. In measurements of performance such as body sway, visual reaction time, critical flicker fusion, and others, both amitriptyline and diazepam produced decrements in performance, and the combination produced the greatest decrements (Patat et al. 1988). Plasma drug levels were not reported in either of the studies.

Alprazolam 4 mg/day was administered for 7 days in 30 patients with major depressive disorder who were being treated with imipramine 100 to 300 mg/day. Imipramine and desipramine levels increased 25% (imipramine clearance decreased 20%) during alprazolam dosing (Antal et al. 1986). There was, however, no increase in side effects. In another study exploring the interaction of alprazolam with nortriptyline, a secondary amine tricyclic antidepressant, alprazolam 0.5 mg orally 3 times a day failed to significantly influence steady-state plasma concentrations of nortriptyline or its 10-hydroxy metabolite (Bertilsson et al. 1988). The same group also found that the 2-hydroxylation of desipramine was not inhibited by alprazolam in human liver microsomes.

The steady-state, peak concentration, area-under-the-curve (AUC), and elimination half-life of alprazolam were nearly doubled when it was coadministered with nefazodone (alprazolam 1 mg twice daily) and nefazodone 200 mg twice daily at steady state. Nefazodone concentrations were not affected. Effects with triazolam were even greater. When a single oral dose of triazolam 0.25 mg was coadministered with nefazodone 200 mg twice daily at steady state, triazolam half-life and AUC 4-fold and peak concentration increased by a factor of 1.7. As with triazolam, nefazodone concentrations were not affected (manufacturer's product information). Increases in benzodiazepine levels may be associated with psychomotor impairment.

Mechanism

Alprazolam-tricyclic pharmacokinetic interactions are presumed to result from competition for hepatic metabolic processing. Alprazolam along with the other triazolobenzodiazepines are oxidized mainly by the P450-3A4 subfamily (Kronbach et al. 1989). Tertiary amines and their primary metabolites are oxidized by the P450-2D6 subfamily (Llerena et al. 1993), the P450-3A subfamily (Lemoine et al. 1993, Ohmori et al. 1993), and the P450-2C subfamily (Perucca et al. 1994). Decrements in psychomotor function could be the result of both pharmacodynamic and pharmacokinetic interactions.

Clinical Implications

Clinicians may wish to more closely monitor tricyclic antidepressant levels in patients who are also on alprazolam. Amitriptyline and probably other tertiary amine tricyclics interact with diazepam to produce decrements in psychomotor function that are at least additive. Additionally, the sedating effects of benzodiazepines in combination with all tricyclic antidepressants can mask the early warning signals of antidepressant toxicity (Beresford et al. 1981). Nefazodone also inhibits metabolism of triazolobenzodiazepines.

MONOAMINE OXIDASE INHIBITORS (MAOIs)

There have been a few case reports of a benzodiazepine-monoamine oxidase inhibitor (BZD-MAOI) interaction (1 case involving edema and 2 cases involving chorea (Blackwell 1991). These do not represent enough data to influence clinical decisions (see Chapter 2).

SELECTIVE SEROTONIN REUPTAKE INHIBITORS (SSRIs)

Evidence of Interaction

Fluoxetine. In a double-blind parallel study in 80 subjects, subjects were randomly divided into 1 of 4 treatment groups: (1) alprazolam 1 mg 4 times daily; (2) alprazolam 1 mg 4 times daily plus fluoxetine 60 mg daily; (3) fluoxetine 60 mg daily; and (4) placebo 4 times daily. Combined administration of alprazolam and fluoxetine resulted in an approximate 30% increase in plasma alprazolam concentrations and increased psychomotor effects compared to those with alprazolam alone (Lasher et al. 1991). There was no effect of alprazolam on fluoxetine or norfluoxetine levels. In a double-blind crossover study alprazolam 1 mg or clonazepam 1 mg were administered with fluoxetine 40 mg daily. Coadministration of fluoxetine and alprazolam resulted in significant increases in alprazolam half-life and plasma area-under-the-curve, but there was no significant effect on clonazepam kinetics (Greenblatt et al. 1992). A significant decrease in clearance of diazepam when coadministered with fluoxetine has also been demonstrated (Lemberger et al. 1988), but not with fluoxetine and triazolam (Wright et al. 1992).

Paroxetine.   Twenty-four subjects received paroxetine 30 mg daily for 14 days. Half of the group then had diazepam 5 mg 3 times daily added to their regimen, while both groups continued to receive paroxetine for an additional 13 days. Diazepam did not affect paroxetine kinetics (Bannister et al. 1989). Although not the focus of this study, paroxetine may impair diazepam metabolism.

Fluvoxamine.   Fluvoxamine 100 to 150 mg daily reduced oral clearance and prolonged elimination half-life of diazepam (a 10-mg single oral dose) in healthy volunteers (Perucca et al. 1994). The area-under-the-curve for the major metabolite of diazepam, N-desmethyldiazepam, was increased during fluvoxamine treatment compared with diazepam administered alone.

Mechanism

All 4 of the currently available SSRIs (fluoxetine, sertraline, fluvoxamine, and paroxetine) inhibit human cytochrome isozyme activity. Differential effects on BZDs are probably due to selectivity of cytochrome P450 subfamilies (*see* Chapter 1 for discussion of drug metabolism and Chapter 2 for discussion of SSRI effects on cytochrome P450 isozymes).

Clinical Implications

Fluoxetine may cause clinically significant decreases in the clearance of diazepam and alprazolam, but not triazolam or clonazepam. Although fluoxetine and the other SSRIs exert a greater inhibitory effect on the P450-2D6 subfamily, they also inhibit the P450-3A4 subfamily (von Moltke et al. 1994a). It is not clear why fluoxetine impaired alprazolam but not triazolam metabolism, since both are metabolized by the P450-3A4 subfamily. While there are insufficient data to draw definitive conclusions, the SSRIs would not be expected to influence clearance of those BZDs that require conjugation only (e.g. lorazepam, oxazepam, temazepam). Although data published to date are limited to fluoxetine, these effects would be expected with all currently available SSRIs.

Antiinflammatory Drugs

Evidence of Interaction

A study of objective and subjective effects of single oral doses of indomethacin 50 and 100 mg, diazepam 10 to 15 mg alone and in combination found that indomethacin did not alter the performance on digit substitution, letter cancellation, tracking, and flicker-fusion tests when given alone or with diazepam (Nuotto et al. 1988). Both drugs produced complaints of dizziness that were additive in combination in subjects.

Clinical Implications

There is no clinically significant interaction between indomethacin and diazepam.

Antimicrobials

Evidence of Interaction

Antibiotics. Administration of erythromycin 333 mg 3 times daily for 3 days decreased triazolam clearance by 52% in a randomized complete crossover study with 16 subjects. As compared to a control group, the elimination half-life of triazolam 0.5 mg administered orally to subjects receiving erythromycin increased from 3.6 to 5.9 hours (Phillips et al. 1986). Troleandomycin, another macrolide antibiotic, significantly enhanced the plasma concentration area-under-the-curve for triazolam 0.25 mg in a double-blind, crossover study (Warot et al. 1987). Psychomotor impairment induced by triazolam was prolonged when administered with the antibiotic. Case reports have also shown enhanced pharmacologic effects of triazolam following josamycin (Carry et al. 1982).

Midazolam is another triazolobenzodiazepine that interacts with erythromycin. In addition to a case report and open series (Hiller et al. 1990), double-blind, randomized crossover studies also support this effect (Mattila et al. 1993, Olkkola et al. 1993). In a pair of double-blind, randomized, crossover studies, erythromycin 500 mg 3 times a day or placebo were administered to 12 healthy volunteers for 1 week. On the 6th day, midazolam 15 mg was administered to all subjects orally in the first study and midazolam 0.05 mg/kg was administered intravenously in the second study (Olkkola et al. 1993). The plasma area-under-the-curve of oral midazolam was increased 4-fold by erythromycin pretreatment, which also decreased clearance of intravenously administered midazolam by 54%.

Ciprofloxacin, a fluoroquinolone antibiotic, administered 500 mg twice daily for 3 days failed to affect half-life or total clearance of diazepam 10 mg administered intravenously (Wijnands et al. 1990).

In a controlled trial, subjects were given metronidazole 250 mg 3 times daily or placebo. On 4th day of the protocol, the subjects received alprazolam 1 mg orally, lorazepam 2 mg intravenously, or phenytoin 300 mg intravenously. This regimen had no significant effects on the pharmacokinetics of either alprazolam or lorazepam (Blyden et al. 1988).

Mechanism

Macrolide antibiotics inhibit the cytochrome P450-3A subfamily (Gonzalez 1992) which is responsible for metabolism of triazolobenzodiazepines (Kronbach et al. 1989).

Clinical Implications

Macrolide antibiotics may cause significant decreases in clearance of triazolam and midazolam, which could lead to increased clinical effects or toxicity. Prolonged sedation may occur when midazolam is used as a preanesthetic agent in patients taking macrolide antibiotics. No such interaction has been demonstrated between ciprofloxacin and diazepam, nor with metronidazole and lorazepam or alprazolam.

Evidence of Interaction

Antituberculosis Drugs. The influence of antituberculosis drugs on diazepam disposition was assessed in a series of volunteers and patients who received single intravenous doses of diazepam (Ochs et al. 1981). In the first study, 9 healthy subjects received diazepam in the drug-free control state and again during treatment with isoniazid (INH) 180 mg/day. INH did not appear to alter diazepam volume of distribution or protein binding, but did prolong the mean elimination half-life from 34 to 45 hours and reduced total clearance from 0.54 to 0.40 ml/min/kg. In the second study, diazepam disposition in a group of 7 tuberculosis patients receiving triple therapy with INH, ethambutol, and rifampin was compared with that in healthy drug-free control subjects matched for age and sex. Diazepam volume of distribution and protein binding were nearly identical among the groups, but the mean half-life was much shorter among patients (14 hours) than among control subjects (58 hours), and total clearance correspondingly increased from 0.37 to 1.5 ml/min/kg. In the third study, diazepam disposition among 6 newly diagnosed tuberculosis patients receiving initial therapy with ethambutol alone was compared with that among age- and sex-matched control subjects. The diazepam unbound fractions tended to be higher, and diazepam volume of distribution and clearance was lower in patients than in controls, but these differences were not statistically significant.

Mechanism

Diazepam is biotransformed by hepatic N-demethylation. Although INH had no effect on diazepam distribution or protein binding, it prolonged elimination half-life and reduced total clearance. Prolonged half-life was also seen in concurrent ingestion of INH and triazolam, another benzodiazepine metabolized by oxidation, while oxazepam (biotransformed by conjugation) was not so affected (Ochs et al. 1983b). INH impairs demethylation of diazepam. The markedly increased clearance and the shortened half-life of diazepam in the triple therapy study were probably due to the enzyme-inducing effects of rifampin. Rifampin stimulates demethylation of diazepam and the hydroxylation of its metabolic product, desmethyldiazepam.

Clinical Implications

The dosage of oxidatively metabolized benzodiazepines may require adjustment in patients with tuberculosis receiving chemotherapy. Results of the 3 studies described above suggest that patients receiving INH will require lower doses of such drugs, while those receiving rifampin, either alone or in combination, may require higher doses.

Evidence of Interaction

Antimycotics.   Ketoconazole decreased clearance of chlordiazepoxide (Brown et al. 1994) and midazolam (Olkkola et al. 1994). In a double-blind, randomized, crossover study conducted in 3 phases at 4-week intervals, 9 subjects were given ketoconazole 400 mg, itraconazole 200 mg, or placebo each day for 4 days. On the 4th day, subjects received an oral dose of midazolam 7.5 mg. Both antimycotics increased the plasma concentration vs. time area-under-the-curve from 10 to 15 times and resulted in significant decreases in performance of psychomotor tests.

Mechanism

Ketoconazole is a potent inhibitor of P450-3A4 and, to a lesser extent, other cytochrome P450 subfamilies.

Clinical Implications

Ketoconazole, itraconazole, and related drugs inhibit metabolism of triazolobenzodiazepines such as midazolam, alprazolam, and triazolam (von Moltke et al. 1994b). Dosage reductions or the use of benzodiazepines that are not metabolized primarily by the 3A4 subfamily are appropriate when using these antimycotics.

Evidence of Interaction

Influenza vaccine. In an open trial, 31 male and 14 female subjects were divided into groups and given on 3 separate occasions either antipyrine 1 g intravenously, alprazolam 1 mg orally, paracetamol 650 mg intravenously, or lorazepam 2 mg intravenously. For each group, the drug was administered before influenza vaccine (0.5 ml intramuscularly) and at 7 and 21 days postvaccination. No significant pharmacokinetic differences were seen for either alprazolam or lorazepam (Scavone et al. 1995).

Clinical Implications

There is no interaction between influenza vaccine and alprazolam or lorazepam. Although there have been a few clinical reports of influenza vaccine inhibiting warfarin and phenytoin metabolism, this does not appear to be a problem with benzodiazepines.

Antipsychotics/Neuroleptics (See Chapter 3)

Barbiturates

Evidence of Interaction

Barbiturates induce the metabolism of benzodiazepines. In several epileptic children receiving long-term diazepam therapy, desmethyldiazepam blood levels exceeded diazepam concentrations when phenobarbital was given concurrently, whereas diazepam levels exceeded those of its metabolite when phenobarbital was not administered (Viala et al. 1971). Overdose with benzodiazepines and barbiturates led to severe central nervous system depression in 21 of 31 patients in a case series (Greenblatt et al. 1977).

Mechanism

Phenobarbital induces microsomal enzyme activity, resulting in increased metabolism of benzodiazepines. A receptor site interaction leading to additive sedation and central nervous system depression also occurs.

Clinical Implications

The pharmacokinetic and pharmacodynamic interactions will lead to opposite effects. Dosage adjustments must be made based on clinical observation and guided by judicious use of plasma drug levels.

β-Adrenergic Blocking Agents

Evidence of Interaction

Propranolol (Inderal®). In a study of healthy volunteers, diazepam 5 to 10 mg intravenously, lorazepam 2 mg intravenously, or alprazolam 1 mg orally were given once in a control state and again with propranolol 80 mg 3 times daily. Propranolol increased diazepam elimination half-life (58 vs. 49 hours), decreased clearance, and increased the 168-hour plasma versus time area-under-the-curve for desmethyldiazepam. There was no effect on the pharmacokinetics of lorazepam or alprazolam (Ochs et al. 1984). In another study, there was no interaction between oxazepam and propranolol (Sonne et al. 1990).

Metoprolol (Lopressor®). Metoprolol had no significant effects on the pharmacokinetics of lorazepam in 12 healthy male volunteers (Scott et al. 1991), but did impair metabolism of diazepam and desmethyldiazepam in another study (Hawksworth et al. 1984), although the magnitude of the effect is variable (Klotz et al. 1984).

Labetolol (Normodyne®). Oxazepam 15 mg orally was given to 6 subjects before and after receiving a single dose of labetolol 200 mg. No pharmacokinetic differences were found (Sonne et al. 1990).

Atenolol (Tenormin®). Atenolol did not affect diazepam metabolism (Hawksworth et al. 1984).

Mechanism

Propranolol and metoprolol impair microsomal oxidation of diazepam, and although the specific subfamily has not yet been identified, etoprolol and timolol are metabolized through P-450 2D6 (von Moltke et al. 1994a).

Clinical Significance

Propranolol and metoprolol may inhibit metabolism of benzodiazepines that undergo demethylation (e.g. diazepam) but do not interfere with hydroxylation of alprazolam or glucuronidation of lorazepam, oxazepam, or probably temazepam. The combination of β-adrenergic blockers and benzodiazepines is common for the treatment of anxiety, sedative-hypnotic withdrawal, and agitated psychotic states.

Cigarette (Smoking) Interactions

Evidence of Interaction

Some early reports showed an increased clearance of diazepam and lorazepam in smokers, particularly among young subjects (Greenblatt et al. 1980a,b), while others showed that the pharmacokinetics of diazepam and chlordiazepoxide were unaffected by smoking (Desmond et al. 1980a, Klotz et al. 1975). Results of most recent studies found no pharmacokinetic effect of smoking on triazolam (Ochs et al. 1987), clorazepate (Ochs et al. 1986), diazepam, midazolam, or lorazepam (Ochs et al. 1985a).

Mechanism

Results of studies in which increased clearance had been reported suggested that cigarette smoking induced hepatic drug metabolism, resulting in a reduction in blood levels and effects of the involved drug. This is obviously open to question, given that the later studies found no pharmacokinetic effect.

Clinical Implications

Smokers should not require different dosing of benzodiazepines than nonsmokers.

Digoxin

Evidence of Interaction

Although it has been anecdotally reported that administration of diazepam increased blood levels of digoxin when the drugs were given concurrently (Castillo-Ferrando et al. 1980), a controlled study in 8 healthy men revealed that therapeutic doses of alprazolam did not significantly alter digoxin clearance (Ochs et al. 1985b). In contrast to that report, however, was an open study in which 12 subjects who were receiving chronic digoxin therapy (0.25 mg daily) received alprazolam 1.0 mg or 0.5 mg daily for 7 days; the plasma concentration versus time area-under-the-curve for digoxin was significantly increased in subjects receiving the 1.0 mg alprazolam dose. This effect was more pronounced in subjects older than 65 years of age (Guven et al. 1993). Clinical digoxin toxicity was seen in one elderly patient.

Mechanism

The mechanism of this interaction is not known.

Clinical Implications

Until the issue is further clarified, clinicians should carefully monitor plasma digoxin levels in patients concurrently receiving diazepam or alprazolam with digoxin.

Disulfiram

Evidence of Interaction

Concurrent prescribing of a benzodiazepine and disulfiram in an alcoholic patient is not uncommon. To evaluate possible drug interaction, 6 volunteers were given intravenous chlordiazepoxide before and after treatment with disulfiram at a dosage of 500 mg/day for 14 days (Sellers et al. 1976). Disulfiram prolonged the elimination half-life of chlordiazepoxide from 8.5 to 19 hours and reduced its total metabolic clearance from 0.74 to 0.24 ml/min/kg. Clearance of diazepam was also impaired by disulfiram, whereas it did not affect lorazepam or oxazepam (Mcleod et al. 1978, Sellers et al. 1976, Sellers et al. 1980). One study found no interaction between alprazolam and disulfiram, but subject compliance in that study was not optimal (Diquet et al. 1990).

Mechanism

Disulfiram inhibits the biotransformation of oxidatively metabolized benzodiazepines (e.g. chlordiazepoxide, diazepam), but does not appear to influence glucuronidated benzodiazepines (oxazepam, lorazepam, temazepam). Despite one report of noninteraction between alprazolam (which is hydroxylated) and disulfiram, this finding may be an artifact of poor subject compliance, and clinicians should be cautious when they prescribe the combination.

Clinical Implications

This potential interaction should be considered by clinicians in working with disulfiram-treated alcoholic patients who are candidates for benzodiazepine therapy. Either dose reduction or use of a benzodiazepine that undergoes glucuronidation (oxazepam, lorazepam) may be necessary.

Ethanol

Evidence of Interaction

Benzodiazepines may interact with alcohol to produce several clinically significant adverse effects. Published studies vary as to the route, dosage, and concentration of ethanol administered, the use of alcoholic or normal subjects, the accuracy of pharmacokinetic data interpretation (e.g. often in early studies the terms half-life and clearance were used interchangeably), and the relevance to clinical practice. For example, diazepam taken with a typical social cocktail slowed the rate of diazepam absorption but did not influence the completeness of absorption or the rate of elimination (Divoll et al. 1981); yet ethanol in higher concentrations increased the absorption of clobazam and chlordiazepoxide.

Sellers et al. (1980) using a balanced crossover experimental design assessed the disposition of intravenous diazepam combined with oral ethanol in 6 healthy male subjects. The patients were assigned to 2 treatment programs 28 days apart. Program 1 consisted of diazepam at 10 mg given intravenously over 29 minutes, preceded by 60 minutes of ethanol at 0.7 g/kg (diluted to 20% v/v) given orally over 15 minutes and followed by 8 hours of ethanol at 0.15 g/kg/hr to maintain the blood alcohol concentrations between 800 and 1,000 mg/liter; and program 2 consisted of diazepam at 10 mg given intravenously over 20 minutes. The area-under-the-plasma-versus-time-curve for free and bound diazepam increased in all subjects after ethanol was given, indicating an increase in the total amount of drug absorbed. Since the area-under-the-curve of free diazepam also rose in all patients and the area-under-the-curve of the metabolite N-desmethyldiazepam fell, there had been inhibition of hepatic intrinsic clearance of free drug.

Ethanol ingested orally increased the area-under-the-curve of triazolam but had no effect on the half-life in one study (Dorian et al. 1985) and had no effect on serum triazolam peak concentration, time to peak, or elimination half-life in another study (Ochs et al. 1984). These results are in contrast to those of Hayes and colleagues (1977), who found that simultaneous ingestion of alcohol and diazepam accelerated the absorption of the latter. A critical deficiency is that intertrial washout periods in this crossover study were incomplete, however. An evaluation carried out by Laisi et al. (1979) on the effect of several common alcoholic beverages on the absorption of diazepam found that alcoholic beverages, particularly beer, whiskey, and white wine, enhanced the absorption of diazepam. Diazepam in combination with ethanol resulted in more severe psychomotor impairment (tracking skills, oculomotor coordination) than that of either agent alone. Whiting et al. (1979) found that acute alcohol intoxication resulted in inhibition of the conversion of chlordiazepoxide to its major active metabolite desmethylchlordiazepoxide. The elimination half-life of desmethylchlordiazepoxide was shorter in alcoholics than in alcohol-free volunteers, possibly due to induction of the conversion of desmethylchlordiazepoxide.

Mechanism

A pharmacodynamic interaction with additive central nervous system depression is most important clinically. The mechanism for interaction is not known, but a study in which cell-free preparations of rat brain were used demonstrated that ethanol enhanced chloride uptake, an effect markedly inhibited by γ-aminobutyric acid (GABA) antagonists picrotoxin and bicuculline (Suzdak et al. 1986). While alcohol enhancement at benzodiazepine binding in the brain has been reported (Burch et al. 1980), this does not occur to a significant degree at physiologic concentrations of alcohol (Greenberg et al. 1984). Chronic ethanol consumption in mice decreased benzodiazepine binding in the cortex and diminished the effects of clonazepam (Barnhill et al. 1991). As noted above, pharmacokinetic factors of enhanced absorption, metabolism, and disposition exist but are small and inconsistent.

Clinical Implications

Ethanol and benzodiazepines produce additive central nervous system depression. Most studies of diazepam, chlordiazepoxide, lorazepam, nitrazepam, bromazepam, adinazolam, and other benzodiazepines confirm an interaction (Linnoila et al. 1990, Sands et al. 1995). Pharmacokinetic interactions produced by alcohol are highly variable and often difficult to predict, depending on the concentration of the alcohol, the extent and duration of alcohol ingestion, the health of the patient (e.g. liver and nutrition status), and the pharmacologic characteristics of the coadministered drug. Compared with these small and inconsistent pharmacokinetic effects, the pharmacodynamic interactions produced by the benzodiazepines may be large and should be emphasized to patients treated with these agents. Alcoholic liver disease may also impair metabolism of benzodiazepines (Juhl et al. 1984), but most commonly alcoholics early in abstinence have hepatic enzyme induction and cross-tolerance to benzodiazepines. Alcoholics are more likely to have positive mood responses associated with drug abuse potential after receiving certain benzodiazepines (e.g. diazepam, alprazolam) and report an increased desire to drink ethanol after a single dose of these benzodiazepines (Ciraulo et al. 1988, 1994).

Food

Evidence of Interaction

Chlordiazepoxide, diazepam, and clobazam have been shown to have delayed absorption when given with food. An early study (Yu 1976) was designed to determine the effects of food on the bioavailability of chlordiazepoxide in subjects on 3 different regimens: fasted (without breakfast), before breakfast, and after breakfast. Statistical analysis indicated that there were no significant overall differences in bioavailability between those on the fasted regimen and those on the other 2 regimens. In another study of the effect of antacids and food on diazepam absorption in 9 healthy volunteers, food reduced the rate but not the extent of absorption (Greenblatt et al. 1978). In a third study, the effect of food on clobazam absorption was evaluated in 12 healthy, male volunteers, aged 22 to 34 years (Divoll et al. 1982b). Clobazam is a 1,5-benzodiazepine derivative used in the treatment of anxiety. This study was designed to assess the effect of food on the absorption and elimination of clobazam. Clobazam was given in the fasting state on one occasion and followed a standard breakfast on another. Compared with administration of clobazam in the fasting state, administration of this agent with food reduced the mean peak plasma concentration and prolonged the time necessary to reach peak concentration. Total area-under-the-curve was not influenced, nor was the elimination half-life of clobazam. The extent of formation of desmethylclobazam, the major metabolite of clobazam, was also not influenced.

Mechanism

Food delays absorption of most substances absorbed in the small bowel, and this mechanism probably delays absorption of the benzodiazepines also. Additionally, food decreases serum free-fatty acids, which can increase serum diazepam free fraction (Naranjo et al. 1980a,b).

Clinical Implications

When rapid onset of action is needed following a single dose of benzodiazepine, it should be administered on an empty stomach.

Histamine$_2$-Antagonists and Proton Pump Inhibitors

There are now 6 drugs available on the U.S. market for decreasing gastric secretion of hydrochloric acid (HCL). Cimetidine, ranitidine, famotidine, and nizatidine all block H_2 receptors on parietal cells, while omeprazole and lansoprazole inhibit the gastric proton pump that makes HCL production possible. Where interactions between these drugs and BZDs exist, they seem to be on the basis of their effects on hepatic microsomal P450 function. Effects differ between different BZDs, with those BZDs that are oxidatively metabolized more likely to be affected, but this is not without exception.

Evidence of Interaction

Cimetidine (Tagamet®). In a study of 8 normal subjects (Desmond et al. 1980a), chlordiazepoxide disposition and elimination were evaluated before and after 1 week of cimetidine therapy (30 mg orally 4 times a day). Impaired clearance of chlordiazepoxide from plasma was found, at least in part, to be due to decreased demethylation of the drug to N-desmethylchlordiazepoxide. Although the volume of distribution of chlordiazepoxide was not altered by cimetidine, the elimination half-life of chlordiazepoxide was significantly prolonged. In another study, pretreatment of 6 healthy subjects with 5 doses (200 mg every 6 hours) of cimetidine prolonged the half-life of a single 0.1-mg/kg intravenous dose of diazepam from 33.5 to 51.3 hours and reduced the diazepam volume of distribution 0.71 to 0.51 liters/kg (Klotz et al. 1980). These findings have been extended to a number of other benzodiazepines metabolized by the mixed oxidase system, including desalkylflurazepam (Greenblatt et al. 1984a), diazepam (Greenblatt et al. 1984c), nitrazepam (Ochs et al. 1983a), the triazolobenzodiazepines alprazolam and triazolam (Abernethy et al. 1983b, Pourbaix et al. 1985), and desmethyldiazepam (Divoll et al. 1982a). The only benzodiazepine metabolized by the mixed oxidase system that has so far failed to be affected pharmacokinetically by cimetidine is midazolam (Greenblatt et al. 1986). However, in a double-blind study comparing the effect of pretreatment with cimetidine 800 mg/day, ranitidine 300 mg/day, or placebo on psychomotor performance following midazolam 0.07 mg/kg, there were significant differences in performance on the Digit Symbol Substitution Test and visual analog scales between cimetidine and placebo or ranitidine (Sanders et al. 1993). The authors did not report any kinetic data, so it is unclear from this study whether the decrements reflect cimetidine induced impairment of midazolam metabolism or a pharmacodynamic effect.

Studies with benzodiazepines metabolized primarily by conjugation reveal no interaction. Lorazepam disposition and elimination were studied in 8 healthy subjects before and after 1 week of therapy with 300 mg of cimetidine taken orally 4 times a day. In addition, in 4 of the 8 normal subjects, the disposition and elimination of oxazepam were also studied before and after similar treatment with doses of cimetidine. Results of the study indicated that cimetidine did not alter the elimination of either lorazepam or oxazepam (Patwardhan et al. 1980). These results have been confirmed (Greenblatt et al. 1984a) and extended to temazepam (Greenblatt et al. 1984b).

Ranitidine (Zantac®). Studies with ranitidine have shown no influence on the kinetics of diazepam, lorazepam (Abernethy et al. 1984), or midazolam (Greenblatt et al. 1986). However, one group has demonstrated that while the pharmacokinetics of triazolam administered intravenously were unaffected by pretreatment with ranitidine, such pretreatment resulted in a significantly increased plasma versus time area-under-the-curve after orally administered triazolam (Vanderveen et al. 1991). There was no effect on terminal elimination rate constant, and the authors concluded that ranitidine increased the absorption but not the metabolism of triazolam. In one study that directly addressed cognitive function, ranitidine 150 mg/day or placebo was administered for 1 week to 28 subjects in a double-blind study. Midazolam 0.07 mg/kg and placebo produced similar impairment in tests of cognitive function such as the Digit Symbol Substitution Test (Sanders et al. 1993).

Famotidine (Pepcid®). In an open crossover study of 11 male subjects given diazepam alone and with famotidine 40 mg twice daily, or cimetidine 300 mg 4 times daily, there were no differences between famotidine and control groups in diazepam elimination half-life (53 vs. 55 hours), total clearance (0.28 vs. 0.28 mL/min/kg), or total plasma versus time area-under-the-curve. Desmethyldiazepam 7 day plasma versus time area-under-the-curve was also unaffected (Locniskar et al. 1986b).

Nizatidine (Axid®). Nine male subjects were treated with nizatidine 300 mg/day or placebo for 6 days then crossed-over after an 8-day washout period in a double-blind study design. On day 3 of each treatment period, diazepam 10 mg orally was administered and diazepam and desmethyldiazepam were assayed at intervals of up to 84 hours (Klotz et al. 1987). No differences were found between drug and placebo in elimination half-life, or plasma clearance for diazepam (Klotz et al. 1987). In another study, metabolism of chlordiazepoxide and lorazepam were similarly unaffected by nizatidine (Secor et al. 1985).

Omeprazole (Prilosec®). Long-term treatment with omeprazole decreased diazepam clearance (Andersson et al. 1990a,b, Gugler and Jensen 1985). Interactions involving omeprazole are complicated by wide interindividual differences in omeprazole metabolism, with very slow metabolism in approximately 5% of the population (Andersson et al. 1990b). In a double-blind, crossover study where diazepam 0.1 mg/kg was administered intravenously, after 1 week of treatment with omeprazole 20 mg/day or placebo in 4 slow metabolizers and 6 rapid metabolizers, the slow metabolizers of omeprazole were also slow metabolizers of diazepam (Andersson et al. 1990b). The mean clearance of diazepam was decreased 26% after omeprazole as compared with placebo in the rapid omeprazole metabolizers, but was unchanged in the slow metabolizers.

Lansoprazole (Prevacid®). Lansoprazole is a substituted benzimidazole as is omeprazole; but unlike omeprazole, it does not appear to alter diazepam kinetics. In a double-blind, crossover study, 12 male subjects were administered lansoprazole 60 mg/day or placebo for 10 days. On day 7, 0.1 mg/kg of diazepam was administered intravenously with no significant differences in elimination half-life or clearance (Lefebvre et al. 1992).

Mechanism

Cimetidine impairs hepatic microsomal P450 oxidation across a broad range of isozymes and omeprazole more specifically inhibits the P450-2C subfamily (Andersson et al. 1990b). This subfamily is responsible for at least one pathway of diazepam metabolism (Andersson et al. 1994) and the triazolobenzodiazepines midazolam and alprazolam are oxidized by the P450-3A4 isozyme family (Kronbach et al. 1989). Since some BZDs do not require oxidative metabolism at all, and those that do utilize at least 2 different P450 isozyme subfamilies, differential effects are to be expected.

Clinical Implications

Despite clear-cut evidence for cimetidine-induced reduction in clearance of benzodiazepines metabolized by the mixed oxidase system, the actual clinical effect (at least with diazepam) is negligible (Greenblatt et al. 1984c). The only significant clinical effect appears to be increased cognitive impairment following midazolam administration in persons receiving cimetidine (Sanders et al. 1993). Despite the lack of evidence of clinical effects from the decreased clearance, prudence would dictate that in the elderly or already hepatically compromised patient taking cimetidine or omeprazole, only benzodiazepines that are eliminated by conjugation should be prescribed, or consideration should be given to substituting ranitidine, famotidine, nizatidine, or lansoprazole.

Levodopa

Evidence of Interaction

In a 66-year-old woman with parkinsonism who was under satisfactory control with levodopa, benzotropine, and diphenhydramine, an acute worsening of her disease developed after the administration of chlordiazepoxide (Yosselson-Superstine et al. 1982). Five days after the chlordiazepoxide was stopped, her parkinsonism was again under satisfactory control.

Mechanism

The reduction in levodopa efficacy probably is secondary to the GABA agonist effect of benzodiazepines, which reduces the dopaminergic enhancement of levodopa.

Clinical Implications

Anecdotal case reports (Hunter et al. 1970) have documented the ability of benzodiazepines to alter the clinical response to levodopa in several patients with parkinsonism. Although it is unnecessary to avoid prescribing both drugs concurrently, the clinician should be observant regarding any worsening of signs of parkinsonism in patients receiving this drug combination.

Lithium (See Chapter 4)

Metoclopramide (Reglan®)

In 6 subjects who received oral diazepam 0.2 mg/kg alone or with oral metoclopramide 10 mg, no difference was found in rate of absorption, despite a previous study that showed that intravenously administered metoclopramide increased oral diazepam bioavailability (Chapman et al. 1988).

Mechanism

Metoclopramide increases gastrointestinal motility. When given intravenously, but not orally, it can increase the rate of diazepam absorption (Chapman et al. 1988). The difference may reflect the fact that a single oral dose of metoclopramide might not be absorbed quickly enough to affect gut motility and thereby alter absorption of a simultaneous diazepam dose. Furthermore the effects of enhanced gut motility are quite variable. For example, if a tablet dissolves slowly, enhanced motility can decrease oral bioavailability.

Clinical Implications

None.

Opioids

Evidence of Interaction

Fourteen subjects were given single oral doses of diazepam 10 mg intravenously, alprazolam 1.0 mg orally, and lorazepam 2 mg intravenously both with and without propoxyphene 65 mg every 6 hours. Propoxyphene prolonged the half-life of alprazolam from 12 to 18 hours. Effects on diazepam and lorazepam were insignificant (Abernethy et al. 1985b).

In dogs, effects of midazolam administered intravenously at 9.6 μg/kg/min, fentanyl administered intravenously at 3 doses (0.05, 0.2, and 3.2 μg/kg/min), and combinations of midazolam with all 3 fentanyl doses on enflurane MAC were studied (Schwleger et al. 1989). MAC is a widely used term in anesthesiology which means the minimal alveolar concentration of a volatile anesthetic at 1 atmosphere that prevents response to a noxious stimulus in 50% of subjects. Effects of combining midazolam with the 2 lower doses were additive in reducing MAC and somewhat less than additive at the highest dose.

An open human study with midazolam and morphine in 90 adult female patients showed additive sedation with the combination (Tverskoy et al. 1989).

Mechanism

The propoxyphene interaction is most likely due to propoxyphene-induced inhibition of microsomal P450 oxidation. Specific studies with propoxyphene are lacking, but since alprazolam oxidation is mediated by the P450-3A4 subfamily, it is likely that propoxyphene oxidation is also mediated by this subfamily, although another narcotic, methadone, inhibits the microsomal P450-2D6 subfamily (Wu et al. 1993). Midazolam interactions with morphine and fentanyl are likely to be pharmacodynamic.

Clinical Significance

Alprazolam clearance is impaired and elimination half-life is prolonged when given concurrently with propoxyphene, which could lead to enhanced effects or toxicity. Diazepam and lorazepam metabolism are not affected by coadministration of propoxyphene.

Midazolam is additive in increasing MAC when given with morphine or fentanyl. In neither study cited was respiratory status examined and the interactions could be more than additive in this parameter, so these data should not be construed as a reason to decrease vigilance when these agents are given together for outpatient procedures.

Physostigmine

Evidence of Interaction

In the past, physostigmine was used (Avant et al. 1979) to treat the respiratory depression sometimes seen with benzodiazepine intoxication. Physostigmine can reverse diazepam-induced sleep in humans and inhibit the binding in brain homogenates in a dose-dependent manner (Speeg et al. 1980).

Mechanism

Physostigmine is a competitive inhibitor at the benzodiazepine receptor (Speeg et al. 1980).

Clinical Implications

Physostigmine is a very potent antidote for acute diazepam poisoning. Although physostigmine can reverse diazepam-induced hypnosis, the specific bezodiazepine antagonist, flumazenil, is the preferred treatment of benzodiazepine overdose.

Probenecid

Evidence of Interaction

Nine subjects received lorazepam 2 mg intravenously with and without concurrent probenecid 500 mg orally every 6 hours. Lorazepam half-life was increased during concurrent probenecid treatment from 14.3 ±1.08 hour to 33.0 ±3.9 hour (Abernethy et al. 1985a). In primate hepatic microsomes, probenecid slowed glucuronidation of lorazepam by what appeared to be competitive inhibition (von Moltke et al. 1993).

Mechanism

Probenecid impairs glucuronidation of lorazepam *in vitro* (von Moltke et al. 1993), which is probably the mechanism for increased lorazepam half-life *in vivo*.

Clinical Significance

The increase in lorazepam half-life is of potential clinical significance, and clinicians should closely monitor patients receiving both drugs for evidence of increased action of lorazepam.

Steroids

Evidence of Interaction

In one of the earliest studies of the effect of oral contraceptives on the disposition of chlordiazepoxide (Roberts et al. 1979), the elimination half-life was longer and the clearance of free chlordiazepoxide was lower in women taking oral contraceptive steroids than in those women not using them, yet the differences were not found to be statistically significant. In another study, Abernethy et al. (1982) determined that long-term use of low-dose estrogen-containing oral contraceptives impaired diazepam clearance and greatly increased the elimination half-life of diazepam. In another study, it was demonstrated that the volumes of distribution and plasma clearance of lorazepam and oxazepam were significantly increased in women taking oral contraceptive steroids (norethindrone acetate 1 mg, ethinyl estradiol 50 µg), while the plasma clearance (but not volume of distribution) of chlordiazepoxide was decreased (Patwardhan et al.

1983). Oral contraceptives did not impair clearance of a benzodiazepine metabolized by hydroxylation (alprazolam) (Locniskar et al. 1986a, Scavone et al. 1988a) or by conjugation, such as lorazepam (Locniskar et al. 1986a) or oxazepam (Abernethy et al. 1983a).

Mechanism

Oral contraceptive steroids may inhibit the biotransformation of benzodiazepines and alter plasma binding.

Clinical Implications

In patients receiving an oral contraceptive, adjustment in dose of benzodiazepines metabolized by oxidation is recommended but is probably not necessary for benzodiazepines metabolized by hydroxylation or conjugation.

Xanthines (Caffeine and Theophylline)

Evidence of Interaction

In a study of 18 normal volunteers, lorazepam 2.5 mg in comparison with a placebo significantly impaired performance skills in a verbal learning task, in the digit-symbol substitution task, and in symbol-copying and number cancellation tasks. Caffeine citrate 125 to 500 mg when given alone significantly improved performance on the digit-symbol substitution test and reduced the lorazepam impairment. In the symbol-copying test, caffeine counteracted the lorazepam impairment. Caffeine citrate 500 mg counteracted the lorazepam effects of reducing anxiety as measured by the Taylor Trait Anxiety Scale (File 1982). Caffeine also antagonized diazepam impairment of the symbol cancellation task but not other measures in a double-blind study of the effects of caffeine (0, 3, and 6 mg/kg) and diazepam (0, 0.15, and 0.30 mg/kg) on "several mood, cognitive, learning, memory, and psychomotor tasks" in 108 young healthy adults (Loke et al. 1985).

In a similar study of the interaction of diazepam and theophylline, another methylxanthine, 100 ml of physiologic sodium chloride solution, was administered without or with theophylline (4.4 mg/kg) to 8 healthy men 40 minutes after an oral dose of diazepam (0.25 mg/kg) had been administered in a single-blind method. Theophylline antagonized diazepam-induced decrements in psychomotor performance as measured by the card-sorting test and the digit-symbol substitution test (Henauer et al. 1983).

Mechanism

The antagonism of the methylxanthines theophylline and caffeine on diazepam or lorazepam-induced decrements in performance in the symbol-copying test most likely was on a pharmacodynamic rather than a pharmacokinetic basis. Recent evidence suggests that this pharmacodynamic effect is due to antagonism at the same endogenous benzodiazepine receptor sites (Paul et al. 1980). This is supported by animal evidence that benzodiazepines inhibit caffeine-induced seizures in mice with a potency that parallels their affinities for the central benzodiazepine receptor (Marangos et al. 1981).

Clinical Implications

Methylxanthines antagonize the psychomotor impairment caused by benzodiazepines, but antagonism of benzodiazepine anxiolysis has been demonstrated only inconsistently.

REFERENCES

Abernethy DR et al.: Impairment of diazepam metabolism by low-dose estrogen-containing oral contraceptive steroids. New Engl J Med 306:791, 1982.
Abernethy DR et al.: Lorazepam and oxazepam kinetics in women on low-dose oral contraceptives. Clin Pharmacol Ther 33:628, 1983a.
Abernethy DR et al.: Interaction of cimetidine with the triazolobenzodiazepines alprazolam and triazolam. Psychopharmacology (Berlin) 80: 275, 1983b.
Abernethy DR et al.: Probenecid impairment of acetaminophen and lorazepam clearance: direct inhibition of ether glucuronide formation. J Pharmacol Exp Ther 234 :345, 1985a.
Abernethy DR et al.: Interaction of propoxyphene with diazepam, alprazolam and lorazepam. Br J Clin Pharmacol 19: 51, 1985b.
Abernethy DR et al.: Ranitidine does not impair oxidative or conjugative metabolism: non-interaction with antipyrine, diazepam, and lorazepam. Clin Pharmacol Ther 35: 188, 1984.
Abruzzo CW et al.: Changes in the oral absorption characteristics in man of dipotassium clorazepate at normal and elevated gastric pH. J Pharmacokinet Biopharm 5: 377, 1977.
Andersson T et al.: Effect of omeprazole and cimetidine on plasma diazepam levels. Eur J Clin Pharmacol 39: 51, 1990a.
Andersson T et al.: Effect of omeprazole treatment on diazepam plasma levels in slow versus normal rapid metabolizers of omeprazole. Clin Pharmacol Ther 47: 79, 1990b.
Andersson T et al.: Diazepam metabolism by human liver microsomes is mediated by both S-mephenytoin hydroxylase and CYP3A isoforms. Br J Clin Pharmacol 38: 131, 1994.
Antal EJ et al.: Multicenter evaluation of the kinetic and clinical interaction of alprazolam and imipramine. Clin Pharmacol Ther 39: 178, 1986.
Arana GW et al.: Carbamazepine-induced reduction of plasma alprazolam concentrations: a clinical case report. J Clin Psychiatry 49: 448, 1988.
Avant GR et al.: Physostigmine reversal of diazepam-induced hypnosis in human volunteers. Ann Intern Med 91: 53, 1979.
Babbini MN et al.: Enhancement of amphetamine-induced stereotyped behavior by benzodiazepines. Eur J Pharmacol 13: 330, 1971.
Bannister SJ et al.: Evaluation of the potential for interactions of paroxetine with diazepam, cimetidine, warfarin, and digoxin. Acta Psychiatr Scand 350(suppl): 102, 1989.
Barnhill JG et al.: Benzodiazepine response and receptor binding after chronic ethanol ingestion in a mouse model. J Pharmacol Exp Ther 258: 812, 1991.

Beresford TP et al.: Adverse reactions to a benzodiazepine-tricyclic antidepressant compound. J Clin Psychopharmacol 1: 392, 1981.

Bertilsson L et al.: Alprazolam does not inhibit the metabolism of nortriptyline in depressed patients or inhibit the metabolism of desipramine in human liver microsomes. Ther Drug Monit 10: 231, 1988.

Blackwell B: Monoamine oxidase inihibitor interactions with other drugs. J Clin Psychopharmacol 11: 55, 1991.

Blyden GT et al.: Metronidazole impairs clearance of phenytoin but not of alprazolam or lorazepam. J Clin Pharmacol 28: 240, 1988.

Brown MW et al.: Effect of ketoconazole on hepatic oxidative drug metabolism. Clin Pharmacol Ther 55: 481, 1994.

Bruguerolle B et al.: Bupivacaine free plasma levels in children after caudal anaesthesia: influence of pretreatment with diazepam? Fundam Clin Pharmacol 4: 159, 1990.

Burch TP et al.: Ethanol enhances [3H]diazepam binding at the benzodiazepine-GABA receptor-ionophore complex. Eur J Pharmacol 67: 325, 1980.

Carry PV et al.: New interactions with macrolides. Lyon Med 248: 189, 1982.

Castillo-Ferrando JR et al.: Digoxin levels and diazepam (letter). Lancet 2: 368, 1980.

Chapman MH et al.: Co-administered oral metoclopramide does not enhance the rate of absorption of oral diazepam. Anaesth Intensive Care 16: 202, 1988.

Chun AHC et al.: Effect of antacids on absorption of clorazepate. Clin Pharmacol Ther 22: 329, 1977.

Ciraulo DA et al: Abuse liability and clinical pharmacokinetics of alprazoalm in alcoholic men. J Clin Psychiatry 49: 333, 1988.

Ciraulo DA et al: Effects of benzodiazepines, buspirone and placebo treatment on mood and EEG activity in alcoholics and normal subjects. American Psychiatric Association Annual Meeting, Philadelphia. Scientific Abstracts 159, 1994.

Cooper SJ et al: Feeding parameters in the rat: interaction of chlordiazepoxide with (+)-amphetamine or fenfluramine. Proceedings of the British Pharmacology Society. Br J Pharmacol 64: 378, 1978.

Desmond PV et al.: No effect of smoking on metabolism of chlordiazepoxide (letter). N Engl J Med 300: 199, 1979.

Desmond PV et al.: Cimetidine impairs elimination of chlordiazepoxide (Librium) in man. Ann Intern Med 93: 266, 1980a.

Desmond PV et al.: Effect of heparin administration on plasma binding of benzodiazepines. Br J Clin Pharmacol 9: 171, 1980b.

Dhillon S et al.: Valproic acid and diazepam interaction in vivo. Br J Clin Pharmacol 13: 553, 1982.

Diquet B et al.: Lack of interaction between disulfiram and alprazolam in alcoholic patients. Eur J Clin Pharmacol 38: 157, 1990.

Divoll M et al.: Alcohol does not enhance diazepam absorption. Pharmacology 22: 263, 1981.

Divoll M et al.: Cimetidine impairs clearance of antipyrine and desmethyldiazepam in the elderly. J Am Geriatr Soc 30: 684, 1982a.

Divoll M et al.: Clobazam kinetics: intrasubject variability and effect of food on absorption. J Clin Pharmacol 22: 69, 1982b.

Dorian P et al.: Triazolam and ethanol interaction: kinetic and dynamic consequences. Clin Pharmacol Ther 37: 558, 1985.

Dretchen K et al.: Diazepam prevents some adverse effects of succinylcholine. Clin Pharmacol Ther 26: 395, 1979.

Edwards VE et al.: Clonazepam—a clinical study of its effectiveness as an anticonvulsant. Proc Aust Assoc Neurol 10: 61, 1973.

Ellinwood EH et al.: Stimulants: interaction with clinically relevant drugs. Ann NY Acad Sci 281: 393, 1976.

Fahmy NR et al.: Diazepam prevents some adverse effects of succinylcholine. Clin Pharmacol Ther 26: 395, 1979.

Feldman SA et al.: Interaction of diazepam with the muscle-relaxant drugs. Brit Med J 2: 336, 1978.

File SE: Recovery from lorazepam tolerance and the effects of a benzodiazepine antagonist on the development of tolerance. Psychopharmacology 77: 284, 1982.

Giaufre E et al.: The influence of diazepam on the plasma concentrations of bupivacaine and lignocaine after caudal injection of a mixture of the local anaesthetics in children. Br J Clin Pharmacol 26: 116, 1988.

Gonzalez FJ: Human cytochrome P450: problems and prospects. TIPS 13: 346, 1992.

Greenberg DA et al.: Ethanol and the gamma-aminobutyric acid-benzodiazepine receptor complex. J Neurochem 42: 1068, 1984.

Greenblatt DJ et al.: Influence of magnesium and aluminum hydroxide mixture on chlordiazepoxide absorption. Clin Pharmacol Ther 19: 234, 1976.

Greenblatt DJ et al.: Acute overdosage with benzodiazepine derivatives. Clin Pharmacol Ther 21: 497, 1977.

Greenblatt DJ et al.: Diazepam absorption: effect of antacids and food. Clin Pharmacol Ther 24: 600, 1978.

Greenblatt DJ et al.: Lorazepam kinetics in the elderly. Clin Pharmacol Ther 26: 103, 1979.

Greenblatt DJ et al.: Diazepam disposition determinants. Clin Pharmacol Ther 27: 301, 1980a.

Greenblatt DJ et al.: Oxazepam kinetics: effects of age and sex. J Pharmacol Exp Ther 215: 86, 1980.

Greenblatt DJ et al.: Interaction of cimetidine with oxazepam, lorazepam, and flurazepam. J Clin Pharmacol 24: 187, 1984a.

Greenblatt DJ et al.: Non-interaction of temazepam and cimetidine. J Pharm Sci 73: 399, 1984b.

Greenblatt DJ et al.: Clinical importance of the interaction of diazepam and cimetidine. New Engl J Med 310: 1639, 1984c.

Greenblatt DJ et al.: Absence of interaction of cimetidine and ranitidine with intravenous and oral midazolam. Anesth Analg 65: 176, 1986.

Greenblatt DJ et al.: Fluoxetine impairs clearance of alprazolam but not of clonazepam. Clin Pharmacol Ther 52: 479, 1992.

Gugler R et al: Omeprazole inhibits oxidative drug metabolism—studies with diazepam and phenytoin in vivo and 7- ethoxycoumarin in vitro. Gastroenterology 89: 1235, 1985.

Guven H et al.: Age-related digoxin-alprazolam interaction. Clin Pharmacol Ther 54: 42, 1993.

Hawksworth G et al.: Diazepam beta-adrenergic antagonist interaction. Br J Clin Pharmacol 17: 69, 1984.

Hayes SL et al.: Ethanol and oral diazepam absorption. New Engl J Med 296: 186, 1977.

Henauer SA et al.: Theophylline antagonizes diazepam-induced psychomotor impairment. Eur J Pharmacol 25: 743, 1983.

Hiller A et al.: Unconsciousness associated with midazolam and erythromycin. Br J Anaesth 65: 826, 1990.

Hunter KR et al.: Use of levodopa with other drugs. Lancet 2: 1283, 1970.

Juhl RP et al.: Alprazolam pharmacokinetics in alcoholic liver disease. J Clin Pharmacol 24: 113, 1984.

Klotz U: Lack of effect of nizatidine on drug metabolism. Scand J Gastroenterol 136(suppl): 18, 1987.

Klotz U et al.: The effects of age and liver disease on the disposition and elimination of diazepam in adult man. J Clin Invest 55: 347, 1975.

Klotz V et al.: Delayed clearance of diazepam due to cimetidine. New Engl J Med 302: 1012, 1980.

Klotz V et al.: Pharmacokinetic and pharmacodynamic interaction study of diazepam and metoprolol. Eur J Clin Pharmacol 26: 223, 1984.

Kronbach T et al.: Oxidation of midazolam and triazolam by human liver cytochrome P450IIIA4. Mol Pharmacol 36: 89, 1989.

Lai AA et al.: Time-course of interaction between carbamazepine and clonazepam in normal man. Clin Pharmacol Ther 24: 316, 1978.

Laisi U et al.: Pharmacokinetic and pharmacodynamic interactions of diazepam with different alcoholic beverages. Eur J Clin Pharmacol 16: 263, 1979.

Lasher TA et al.: Pharmacokinetic pharmacodynamic evaluation of the combined administration of alprazolam and fluoxetine. Psychopharmacology (Berlin) 104: 323, 1991.

Lefebvre RA et al.: Influence of lansoprazole treatment on diazepam plasma concentrations. Clin Pharmacol Ther 52: 458, 1992.

Lemberger L et al.: The effect of fluoxetine on the pharmacokinetics and psychomotor responses of diazepam. Clin Pharmacol Ther 43: 412, 1988.

Lemoine A et al.: Major pathway of imipramine metabolism is catalyzed by cytochromes P-450 1A2 and P-450 3A4 in humans. Mol Pharmacol 43: 827, 1993.

Llerena A et al.: Debrisoquine and mephenytoin hydroxylation phenotypes and CPY2D6 genotype in patients treated with neuroleptic and antidepressant agents. Clin Pharmacol Ther 54: 606, 1993.

Linniola M et al.: Effect of adinazolam and diazepam, alone and in combination with ethanol, on psychomotor and cognitive performance and on autonomic nervous system reactivity in healthy volunteers. Eur J Clin Pharmacol 38: 371, 1990.

Locniskar A et al.: Effect of conjugated estrogens or tricyclic antidepressants on the kinetics of diazepam, alprazolam, and lorazepam. Clin Pharmacol Ther 39: 208, 1986a.

Locniskar A et al.: Interaction of diazepam with famotidine and cimetidine, two H2-receptor antagonists. J Clin Pharmacol 26: 299, 1986b.

Loke WH et al.: Caffeine and diazepam: separate and combined effects on mood, memory, and psychomotor performance. Psychopharmacology 87: 344, 1985.

MacLeod SM et al.: Interaction of disulfiram with benzodiazepines. Clin Pharmacol Ther 24: 583, 1978.

Madan BR et al.: Actions of methaminodiazepoxide on cardiac, smooth, and skeletal muscles. Arch Int Pharmacodyn Ther 143: 127, 1963.

Marangos PJ et al.: The benzodiazepines and inosine antagonize caffeine-induced seizures. Psychopharmacology 72: 269, 1981.

Mattila MJ et al.: Oral single doses of erythromycin and roxithromycin may increase the effects of midazolam on human performance. Pharmacol Toxicol 73: 180, 1993.

Merli M et al.: Splanchnic and leg exchange of free fatty acids in patients with liver cirrhosis. J Hepatol 3: 348, 1986.

Murayama T et al.: Flumazenil does not antagonize halothane, thiamylal or propofol anaesthesia in rats. Br J Anaesth 69: 61, 1992.

Naranjo CA et al.: Diurnal variations in plasma diazepam concentrations associated with reciprocal changes in free fraction. Br J Clin Pharmacol 9: 265, 1980a.

Naranjo CA et al.: Fatty acids modulation of meal-induced variations in diazepam free fraction. Br J Clin Pharmacol 10: 308, 1980b.

Naranjo CA et al.: Variability in heparin effect on serum drug binding. Clin Pharmacol Ther 28: 545, 1980c.

Naranjo CA et al.: Nonfatty acid-modulated variations in drug binding due to heparin. Clin Pharmacol Ther 31: 746, 1982.

Nuotto E et al.: Actions and interactions of indomethacin and diazepam on performance in healthy volunteers. Pharmacol Toxicol 62: 293, 1988.

Ochs HR et al.: Diazepam interaction with antituberculosis drugs. Clin Pharmacol Ther 29: 671, 1981.

Ochs HR et al.: Cimetidine impairs nitrazepam clearance. Clin Pharmacol Ther 34: 227, 1983a.

Ochs HR et al.: Differential effect of isoniazid on triazolam oxidation and oxazepam conjugation. Br J Clin Pharmacol 16: 743, 1983b.

Ochs HR et al.: Propranolol interactions with diazepam, lorazepam, and alprazolam. Clin Pharmacol Ther 36: 451, 1984.

Ochs HR et al.: Kinetics of diazepam, midazolam, and lorazepam in cigarette smokers. Chest 87: 223, 1985a.

Ochs HR et al.: Effect of alprazolam on digoxin kinetics and creatinine clearance. Clin Pharmacol Ther 38: 595, 1985b.

Ochs HR et al.: Lack of influence of cigarette smoking on triazolam pharmacokinetics. Br J Clin Pharmacol 23: 759, 1987.

Ochs HR et al.: Influence of propranolol coadministration or cigarette smoking on the kinetics of desmethyldiazepam following intravenous clorazepate. Klin Wochenschr 64: 1217, 1986.

Oetliker H: Action of chlordiazepoxide on contractile mechanism in single fibres of frog muscle. Experientia 26: 682, 1970.

Ohmori S, et al.: Studies on cytochrome P450 responsible for oxidative metabolism of imipramine in human liver microsomes. Biol Pharm Bull 16: 571, 1993.

Olkkola KT et al.: A potentially hazardous interaction between erythromycin and midazolam. Clin Pharmacol Ther 53: 298, 1993.

Olkkola KT et al.: Midazolam should be avoided in patients receiving the systemic antimycotics ketoconazole or itraconazole. Clin Pharmacol Ther 55: 481, 1994.

Patat A et al.: Acute effects of amitriptyline on human performance and interactions with diazepam. Eur J Clin Pharmacol 35: 585, 1988.

Patwardhan RV et al.: Cimetidine spares the glucuronidation of lorazepam and oxazepam. Gastroenterology 79: 912, 1980.

Patwardhan RV et al.: Differential effects of oral contraceptive steroids on the metabolism of benzodiazepines. Hepatology 3: 248, 1983.

Paul SM et al.: Brain-specific benzodiazepine receptors and putative endogenous benzodiazepine-like compounds. Biol Psychiatry 15: 407, 1980.

Perucca E et al.: Inhibition of diazepam metabolism by fluvoxamine: a pharmacokinetic study in normal volunteers. Clin Pharmacol Ther 56: 471, 1994.

Phillips JP et al.: A pharmacokinetic interaction between erythromycin and triazolam. J Clin Psychopharmacol 6: 297, 1986.

Pourbaix S et al.: Pharmacokinetic consequences of long term coadministration of cimetidine and triazolobenzodiazepines, alprazolam and triazolam, in healthy subjects. Int J Clin Pharmacol Ther Toxicol 23: 447, 1985.

Prindle KH et al.: Effect of psychopharmacologic agents on myocardial contractility. J Pharmacol Exp Ther 173: 133, 1970.

Roberts RK et al.: Disposition of chlordiazepoxide: sex differences and effects of oral contraceptives. Clin Pharmacol Ther 25: 826, 1979.

Sanders LD et al.: Interaction of H2-receptor antagonists and benzodiazepine sedation: a double-blind placebo-controlled investigation of the effects of cimetidine and ranitidine on recovery after intravenous midazolam. Anaesthesia 48: 286, 1993.

Sands B et al.: The pharmacology of alcohol abuse. In: Kranzler HR (ed): Handbook of Experimental Pharmacology, Vol. 114. New York, Springer, 1995.

Scavone JM et al.: Alprazolam kinetics in women on low-dose oral contraceptives. J Clin Pharmacol 28:463, 1988a.

Scavone JM et al.: Alprazolam pharmacokinetics in women on low-dose oral contraceptives. J Clin Pharmacol 28: 454, 1988b.

Scavone JM et al.: Lack of effect of influenza vaccine on the pharmacokinetics of antipyrine, alprazolam, paracetamol (acetaminophen) and lorazepam. Clin Pharmacokinet 16: 180, 1989.

Schwleger IM et al.: Anesthetic interactions of midazolam and fentanyl: is their acute tolerance to the opioid? Anesthesiology 70: 667, 1989.

Scott AK et al.: Interaction of metoprolol with lorazepam and bromazepam. Eur J Clin Pharmacol 40: 405, 1991.

Secor JW et al.: Lack of effect of nizatidine on hepatic drug metabolism in man. Br J Clin Pharmacol 20: 710, 1985.

Sellers EM et al.: Inhibition of chlordiazepoxide biotransformation by disulfiram. Clin Res 24: 652A, 1976.

Sellers EM et al.: Intravenous diazepam and oral ethanol interaction. Clin Pharmacol Ther 28: 638, 1980.

Shader RI et al.: Problems with drug interactions in treating brain disorders. Psychiatr Clin North Am 1: 51, 1978.

Shader RI et al.: Steady-state plasma desmethyldiazepam during long-term clorazepate use: effects of antacids. Clin Pharmacol Ther 31: 180, 1982.

Snyder SH et al.: Antischizophrenic drugs and brain cholinergic receptors: affinity for muscarinic sites predicts extrapyramidal effects. Arch Gen Psychiatry 31: 58, 1974.

Sonne J et al.: Single dose pharmacokinetics and pharmacodynamics of oral oxazepam during concomitant administration of propranolol and labetalol. Br J Clin Pharmacol 29: 33, 1990.

Speeg KV et al.: Antagonism of benzodiazepine binding in brain by Antilirium, benzyl alcohol, and physostigmine. J Neurochem 34: 856, 1980.

Suarez E et al.: Effect of halothane anesthesia and trifluoroacetic acid on protein binding of benzodiazepines. Methods Find Exp Clin Pharmacol 13: 693, 1991.

Suzdak PD et al.: Ethanol stimulates gamma-aminobutyric acid receptor-mediated chloride transport in rat brain synaptoneurosomes. Proc Natl Acad Sci, USA 83: 4071, 1986.

Svenson SE, Hamilton RG: A critique of overemphasis on side effects with the psychotropic drugs: an analysis of 18,000 chlordizaepoxide-treated cases. Curr Ther Res Clin Exp 8: 455–464, 1966.

Tassonyi E: Effects of midazolam (Ro 21-3981) on neuromuscular block. Pharmatherapeutica 3: 678, 1984.

Tverskoy M et al.: Midazolam-morphine sedative interactions in patients. Anesth Analg 68: 282, 1989.

Vanderveen RP et al.: Effect of ranitidine on the disposition of orally and intravenously administered triazolam. Clin Pharm 10: 539, 1991.

Viala A et al.: Blood levels of diazepam (Valium) and N-desmethyldiazepam in the epileptic child. Psychiatr Neurol Neurochir 74: 153, 1971.

von Moltke LL et al.: Inhibition of acetaminophen and lorazepam glucuronidation in vitro by probenecid. Biopharm Drug Dispos 14: 119, 1993.

von Moltke LL et al.: Cytochromes in psychopharmacology. J Clin Psychopharmacol 14: 1, 1994a.

von Moltke LL et al.: Inhibitors of alprazolam metabolism in vitro: effect of serotonin reuptake inhibitor antidepressants, ketoconazole, and quinidine. Br J Clin Pharmacol 38: 23, 1994b.

Warot D et al.: Troleandomycin-triazolam interaction in healthy volunteers: pharmacokinetic and psychometric evaluation. Eur J Clin Pharmacol 32: 389, 1987.

Webb SN et al.: Diazepam and neuromuscular blocking agents. Br Med J 3: 690, 1971.

Whiting B et al.: Effect of acute alcohol intoxication on the metabolism and plasma kinetics of chlordiazepoxide. Br J Clin Pharmacol 7: 95, 1979.

Wijnands WJ et al.: Ciprofloxacin does not impair the elimination of diazepam in humans. Drug Metab Dispos 18: 954, 1990.

Wright CE et al.: A pharmacokinetic evaluation of the combined administration of triazolam and fluoxetine. Pharmacotherapy 12: 103, 1992.

Wu D et al.: Inhibition of human cytochrome P450 2D6 (CYP2D6) by methadone. Br J Clin Pharmacol 35: 30, 1993.

Yosselson-Superstine S et al.: Chlordiazepoxide interaction with levodopa. Ann Intern Med 96: 259, 1982.

Yu GCS: Effects of food on hydrodynamically balanced capsule (HBC) of librium. (Personal communication).

6

Anticonvulsants

DOMENIC A. CIRAULO, MICHAEL SLATTERY

The use of anticonvulsants in psychiatry has grown rapidly over the past decade. The general psychiatrist has become as familiar with the prescribing of the mood-stabilizing anticonvulsants as with the prescribing of antipsychotics. In this chapter we review in detail the drug-drug interactions of carbamazepine (Tegretol®), valproate (Depakene®, Depakote®), and phenytoin (Dilantin®). In our practice, these anticonvulsants are the most commonly prescribed. Somewhat less detail is presented regarding interactions of barbiturates (Table 6.1) and primidone.

Carbamazepine is an iminostilbene derivative anticonvulsant that is used in a variety of seizures, impulse-control disorders, sedative-hypnotic withdrawal, and bipolar disorder. It has several characteristics that make it subject to drug-drug interactions (Ketter et al 1991a,b). It is an inducer of the cytochrome P450 system and is subject to autoinduction. Since its metabolism is exclusively hepatic, it may be affected by other drugs that induce or impair hepatic metabolism. Carbamazepine-10-11-epoxide is an active metabolite, and assessment of the clinical impact of drug interactions must consider effects of both the parent compound and the metabolite. Signs and symptoms of toxicity with elevated levels include sedation, nausea, vomiting, vertigo, ataxia, blurred vision, and diplopia.

Valproic acid is a branched-chain fatty acid with antiepileptic activity against a variety of seizures and probable efficacy in bipolar disorder. Most interactions with valproate involve impaired metabolism, although a protein-binding interaction occurs with aspirin.

Table 6.1.
Barbiturate Drug Interactions

Drug	Clinical Effect
Acetaminophen	Barbiturates reduce acetaminophen bioavailability and half-life. With acetaminophen overdoses, chronic phenobarbital treatment increases hepatotoxicity.
Anticoagulants	Barbiturates enhance the metabolism of coumarin anticoagulants. Gastrointestinal absorption of dicumarol, but not warfarin, is decreased. Caution is required when a barbiturate is added or discontinued in patients receiving coumarin anticoagulants.
Antidepressants	Barbiturates induce metabolism of antidepressants resulting in decreased serum levels. In tricyclic overdoses, respiratory depression may occur. (*See* Chapter 2)
Antipyrine	Metabolism of antipyrine is enhanced by barbiturates.
β-Adrenergic blockers	Those β-blockers that are metabolized by the liver (propranolol, metoprolol, alprenolol) will have enhanced elimination during chronic barbiturate therapy. Those β-blockers that are primarily excreted unchanged by the kidneys (atenolol, sotalol, nadolol) will not be affected.
Carbamazepine	Barbiturates stimulate carbamazepine metabolism.
Chloramphenicol	Barbiturates stimulate chloramphenicol metabolism. Chloramphenicol inhibits barbiturate metabolism.
Cimetidine	Chronic phenobarbital treatment induces cimetidine metabolism.
Contraceptives	Barbiturates enhance the metabolism of estrogens, and low dose oral contraceptive agents may be rendered less effective.
Corticosteroids	Barbiturates enhance the metabolism of corticosteroids. Concurrent barbiturate therapy worsens the clinical condition of steroid-dependent asthmatics and decreases renal allograft survival.
Cyclophosphamide	Barbiturates enhance the metabolism of cyclophosphamide to active alkylating metabolites, but also promote elimination of these active agents. Clinical significance not known.
Digitalis glycosides	Barbiturates may lower plasma digitoxin levels and shorten its half-life. Some studies have found no interaction.
Estrogens	Barbiturates induce metabolism of estrogens.
Griseofulvin	Barbiturates impair absorption of griseofulvin.
Lidocaine	Barbiturates reduce oral bioavailability of lidocaine, although this is an uncommon clinical route of administration. They also induce hepatic metabolism of lidocaine. The two drugs given together may cause respiratory depression.
Methoxyflurane	Barbiturates induce metabolism of methoxyflurane to nephrotoxic metabolites, which may also induce renal insufficiency.

(continued)

Barbiturate Drug Interactions

Drug	Clinical Effect
Methyldopa	Findings are contradictory, but barbiturates may reduce methyldopa plasma levels.
Metronidazole	Barbiturates induce metabolism of metronidazole and higher doses may be required.
Monoamine oxidase inhibitors	Tranylcypromine prolongs barbiturate hypnosis in animals. Sedative effects may also be potentiated in humans.
Narcotic analgesics	Barbiturates promote metabolism of meperidine to normeperidine. CNS depression is potentiated.
Phenmetrazine	Concurrent barbiturate therapy reduces weight loss associated with phenmetrazine treatment.
Phenothiazines	Barbiturates induce metabolism (See Chapter 3)
Phenylbutazone	Metabolism induced by barbiturates.
Phenytoin	Therapeutic doses of phenobarbital induce phenytoin metabolism, although large doses may actually inhibit metabolism. Phenytoin may increase plasma levels of phenobarbital. Osteomalacia may be promoted by the combination. (See Phenytoin section)
Primidone	Because primidone is converted to phenobarbital, excessive levels of the latter drug may occur if they are coadministered.
Probenecid	Probenecid may prolong thiopental anesthesia.
Propoxyphene	The addition of propoxyphene to phenobarbital may raise plasma levels of the latter drug.
Pyridoxine	May lower phenobarbital levels.
Quinidine	Barbiturates induce metabolism of quinidine.
Rifampin	Rifampin induces metabolism of hexobarbital.
Sulfonamides	Intravenous sulfisoxazole reduces minimum effective doses of thiopental and shortens wakening time, perhaps via displacement from protein binding sites. Phenobarbital may increase biliary excretion and decrease urinary excretion of sulfasalazine. Acetylation of sulfapyridine is decreased while hydroxylation is increased. Phenobarbital does not affect sulfisoxazole or sulfisomidine.
Tetracycline	Metabolism of doxycycline is induced by barbiturates.
Theophylline	Metabolism is induced by barbiturates.
Valproate	Valproate inhibits phenobarbital metabolism.

Acute toxicity from elevated valproate serum levels is characterized by anorexia, nausea, vomiting, sedation, ataxia, and tremor.

Phenytoin is a hydantoin anticonvulsant that is less widely used as a primary treatment for psychiatric disorders than in years past, although it is still used in some treatment-resistant obsessive compulsive disorders and impulse-control disorders.

Carbamazepine

BARBITURATES (*See* Table 6.1)

β-BLOCKERS (*See* Chapter 7)

CALCIUM CHANNEL BLOCKERS

Evidence of Interaction

Eimer and colleagues (1987) reported a case of carbamazepine (CBZ) neurotoxicity following the addition of diltiazem 30 mg every 6 hours to a patient's medication regimen. Other medications in the regimen included digoxin 0.25 mg/day orally, levothyroxine 0.15 mg daily, nitroglycerin ointment (½ inch every 6 hours), Coumadin® 5 mg alternating with 7.5 mg daily and KCl elixir. One month after the initiation of diltiazem therapy, the patient presented with mental slowing and increased difficulty speaking. The CBZ level was 15.5 μg/liter. Diltiazem was discontinued and a CBZ level on the 4th day of hospitalization was 7.7 μg/ml.

Another case was reported in which three calcium channel blockers—verapamil, diltiazem, and nifedipine—were coadministered at separate times to a 34-year-old man with refractory epilepsy also taking CBZ with levels of 12 to 13 μg/ml (Brodie and MacPhee 1986). Verapamil 120 mg orally 3 times a day produced signs of neurotoxicity during coadministration with CBZ. After 48 hours of coadministration with CBZ, diltiazem 60 mg 3 times a day produced signs of neurotoxicity (dizziness, nausea, ataxia, and diplopia) with a coincident CBZ level of 21 μg/ml. These neurotoxic signs resolved after stopping diltiazem, with a corresponding decrease in CBZ levels. Of interest is that 3 months later nifedipine was given as adjunctive anticonvulsive treatment and a substantial improvement in the control of seizures was noted without signs of neurotoxicity or change in circulating CBZ levels.

In a separate case reported by Macphee and colleagues (1986), verapamil coadministered with CBZ to refractory epileptics resulted in a 94% rise in CBZ levels and coincident neurotoxic signs, which abated with verapamil withdrawal. They also noted a 36% reduction in the CBZE:CBZ ratio during coadministration of these two medications.

Other reports confirm the potential neurotoxicity of the combination of CBZ with diltiazem or verapamil (Ahmad 1990, Bahis et al. 1991, Beattie et al. 1988, Gadde 1990, Price 1988). Felodipine plasma levels were lower on patients taking a variety of anticonvulsants, including CBZ (Capewell et al. 1987).

Mechanism

Inhibition of CBZ metabolism by diltiazem and verapamil is a likely mechanism. Both of these medications have been shown to inhibit hepatic cytochrome P450 monoxygenase activity in mice *in vivo* and *in vitro* (Renton 1985). Brodie and MacPhee (1986) make the point that, although nifedipine does undergo hepatic metabolism, it belongs to a subgroup of calcium channel blockers that are structurally and functionally dissimilar to diltiazem.

Clinical Implications

The combination of CBZ and calcium channel blockers may be used in the treatment of medical conditions, refractory epilepsy, or treatment-resistant psychotic disorders. It appears that there is a substantial risk of CBZ neurotoxicity with the use of either verapamil or diltiazem but not nifedipine. When possible, nifedipine, in contrast to diltiazem or verapamil, should be the drug of choice when considering the coadministration of CBZ with calcium channel blockers.

CIMETIDINE AND H₂-ANTAGONISTS

Evidence of Interaction

Coadministration of a 1,200-mg daily dose of cimetidine with a single dose of CBZ resulted in a 26% increase in the area-under-the-plasma-concentration-time-curve and 18% increase in the elimination half-life of CBZ (Dalton et al. 1985). In a subsequent study by the same authors, CBZ (300 mg orally twice a day) was administered to 8 healthy volunteers for 42 days (days 1–42) and cimetidine was added to the regimen on days 29 to 35. In this study CBZ levels increased by 17% after 2 days of cimetidine treatment but returned to premedication levels by the 7th day of coadministration, indicating a time-dependent interaction (Dalton et al. 1986). Others found no effect of cimetidine 1,200 mg/day on CBZ levels after 7 days of coadministration (Levine et al. 1985). Similarly, Sonne and associates (1983) found no effect of cimetidine 1 g daily for 7 days on CBZ or CBZ-10,11-epoxide levels in 7 epileptic patients.

In another study, cimetidine 400 mg twice a day or placebo was administered to healthy males for 25 days (Macphee et al. 1984). Coadministration with CBZ 200 mg/day for 15 days resulted in a 25 and 33% rise in CBZ concentration during the 1st and 2nd weeks of CBZ administration, respectively.

Webster and associates (1984) studied the pharmacokinetics of a single dose of CBZ 400 mg or VPA 400 mg after 4 weeks of a therapeutic course of either cimetidine (1 g/day, N = 6) or ranitidine (300 mg/day, N = 6). The authors found a decrease in the oral clearance of CBZ of up to 20% after cimetidine treatment (from 20.3 ± 2.2 to 18.0 ± 1.4 ml/hr/kg) with a corresponding prolongation in the elimination half-life from 35.3 (±3.7) to 38.6 (± 1.8) hours. VPA clearance also decreased (10.9 ± 0.8 to 10.0 ± 0.4 ml/hr/kg) with a corresponding prolongation in the elimination half-life. Ranitidine-treated patients failed to show any of the above trends.

Mechanism

Cimetidine inhibits hepatic cytochrome P450.

Clinical Implications

When these medications are coadministered transient increases in CBZ levels may result and clinicians should monitor for CBZ toxicity. Although dosage adjustments are rarely necessary, patients should be advised of the possibility that CBZ side effects may be exacerbated 3 to 5 days after the initiation of cimetidine coadministration. When possible, ranitidine, famotidine, nizatidine, antacid, or sucralfate may be considered as alternate treatment regimens in patients taking CBZ.

CLOZAPINE

Evidence of an Interaction

Raitasuo et al. (1993) described 2 patients in whom an interaction of clozapine and CBZ was suspected. The first patient was a 25-year-old schizophrenic man who had been taking a regimen of clozapine 800 mg/day and CBZ 600 mg/day for several months. After CBZ was discontinued, this patient's clozapine level rose from 1.4 to 2.4 μmol/liter. The second patient was a 36-year-old schizophrenic man with epilepsy taking clozapine 600 mg/day and CBZ 800 mg/day. After CBZ was discontinued in this patient, clozapine levels rose from 1.5 to 3.0 μmol/liter.

Mechanism

CBZ induces the metabolism of clozapine.

Clinical Implications

CBZ and clozapine are sometimes coadministered in patients with seizures and/or complex psychotic disorders. If CBZ is added to clozapine, antipsychotic efficacy may be reduced. When CBZ is stopped, clozapine dosage reduction will be necessary to avoid toxicity. The combined effects of the two drugs on myelopoiesis is unknown (*see* Chapter 3).

CONTRACEPTIVES

Evidence of Interaction

Several reports have documented that the effectiveness of oral contraceptives is reduced in patients on CBZ and phenytoin (Coulam et al. 1979, Janz et al. 1974, Kenyon 1972, Laengner et al. 1974, Rapport 1989). Low plasma norgestrol levels were noted in progestin only formulations in patients taking anticonvulsants. CBZ also alters single-dose pharmacokinetics of ethinylestradiol and levonorgestrel (Crawford et al. 1990).

Mechanism

CBZ (and phenytoin) induce metabolism of contraceptive agents.

Clinical Implications

CBZ and phenytoin should be avoided in patients taking contraceptives. Both the oral contraceptives and Norplant® are affected. Although patients who have breakthrough bleeding are at obvious risk, pregnancy can occur even without this warning.

CORTICOSTEROIDS

Evidence of Interaction

CBZ lowers plasma levels of dexamethasone and invalidates the dexamethasone suppression test (Privatera et al. 1982). Prednisolone and other corticosteroids are probably similarly affected (Olivesi 1986).

Mechanism

CBZ enhances metabolism of corticosteroids.

Clinical Implications

Patients taking CBZ should not receive a dexamethasone suppression test until CBZ has been discontinued for several weeks. Patients on corticosteroid therapy may require dosage adjustments when CBZ is started or discontinued.

CYCLOSPORINE (SANDIMMUNE®)

Evidence of Interaction

CBZ decreases cyclosporine (an immunosuppressive agent) plasma levels (Alvarez 1991, Hillebrand et al. 1987, Lele et al. 1985, Schofield et al. 1990, Yee et al. 1990). The onset of effect is a few days after addition of CBZ, and persists for about 2 to 3 weeks.

Mechanisms

CBZ enhances metabolism of cyclosporine.

Clinical Implications

Some authorities recommend the use of valproate in place of CBZ if possible. If CBZ is used, special attention must be directed to cyclosporine levels after the initiation and termination of CBZ therapy, and appropriate dosage adjustments made.

DANAZOL (DANOCRINE®)

Evidence of Interaction

Danazol, a synthetic androgen used in the treatment of endometriosis, fibrocystic breast disease, and hereditary angioedema may cause increases in CBZ levels. Six epileptic patients with fibrocystic breast disease receiving both CBZ and danazol had CBZ levels increased by almost 2-fold in the presence of danazol (Zielenski et al. 1987).

Mechanism

Using a stable ^{15}N CBZ isotope technique, danazol coadministration increased CBZ elimination half-life (11 to 24.3 hour). CBZ plasma clearance decreased from 57.7 to 23.2 ml/hour/kg. Danazol inhibits the epoxide transdiol pathway of CBZ metabolism (Krämer et al. 1986).

Clinical Implications

Danazol coadministration with CBZ appears to significantly inhibit CBZ metabolism and raise CBZ serum levels. Physicians should monitor patients for the emergence of CBZ side effects or toxicity when these drugs are administered concurrently. CBZ dosage reduction may be necessary.

ERYTHROMYCIN, TROLEANDOMYCIN, AND OTHER MACROLIDE ANTIBIOTICS

Evidence of Interaction

There have been numerous reports of CBZ toxicity precipitated by coadministration with erythromycin. Hedrick and associates (1983) reported 4 cases of epileptic children in which the addition of erythromycin to the medication regimen resulted in an increase in CBZ levels to the toxic range (16–19 μg/ml) and clinical signs of neurotoxicity. Signs of neurotoxicity remitted as CBZ levels decreased after erythromycin was discontinued.

Another case described a 41-year-old woman with epilepsy receiving CBZ 400 mg 3 times daily (level 9.3–13 μg/ml) and phenobarbital (Pb) 100 mg 4 times daily, in whom dizziness, nausea, vomiting, ataxia, and blurred vision developed 3 days after erythromycin stearate was added to her regimen for an infected forehead laceration (Carranco et al. 1985). CBZ level was 28.2 μg/ml and Pb level was 17.2 μg/ml. These symptoms did not reappear within 3 weeks of reinstitution of CBZ and phenobarbital without erythromycin in the regimen.

Another case of erythromycin-induced CBZ toxicity was reported in a 6-year-old epileptic child (Zitelli et al. 1987). Within 5 days of the addition of erythromycin, vomiting, weakness, lethargy, ataxia, nystagmus, and cogwheeling movements developed with a CBZ level of 25.8 μg/ml (CBZ level was 11.9 pre-erythromycin therapy).

Wong and colleagues (1983) performed a controlled two-way crossover study in 8 volunteers with CBZ 400 mg/day alone or with erythromycin 250 mg every 6 hours for 5 days prior to, and 3 days after, concurrent CBZ treatment. They found that the clearance of CBZ was lowered in the presence of erythromycin from 15.0 (±3.0) to 12.1 (±3.1) ml/kg/hr. The mean volume of distribution, elimination rate constant, and absorption rate constant of CBZ were not altered by erythromycin.

Troleandomycin (TAO), like erythromycin, is a macrolide antibiotic that may elevate CBZ serum levels during coadministration. The addition of TAO to the medication regimen of 17 patients with epilepsy led to the development of nausea, vomiting, dizziness, and in 6 patients, a 2- to 4-fold increase in plasma CBZ was also noted, which returned to normal after TAO was withdrawn (Mesdjian et al. 1980). Sixteen of 17 patients were on combination anticonvulsant therapy. Levels of other anticonvulsants were not affected by TAO administration. Another series described symptoms of CBZ toxicity in 8 epileptic patients 24 hours after receiving TAO (Dravet et al. 1977). Of 8 patients, 2 had elevated plasma CBZ levels after TAO was added which decreased after TAO was discontinued. In the other 6, symptoms of toxicity were reported but CBZ plasma levels were not obtained.

Mechanism

CBZ is almost entirely metabolized in the hepatic microsomal system, with only approximately 2% of the dose excreted unchanged in the urine (Bowdle et al. 1979). The primary metabolic pathway is via cytochrome P450, which is also responsible for erythromycin metabolism (Danan et al. 1981, Faigle et al. 1976). TAO may inhibit hepatic metabolism of CBZ, but detailed pharmacokinetic studies have not been published (Mesdjian et al. 1980).

Clinical Implications

Patients taking CBZ who are started on erythromycin antibiotic therapy should be monitored closely for signs and symptoms of CBZ toxicity. The likelihood of the interaction increases with larger doses of erythromycin (Mitsch 1989). Other macrolide antibiotics (e.g. troleandomycin) may also interact with CBZ.

FELBAMATE

Evidence of an Interaction

Coadministration of felbamate, an anticonvulsant, with CBZ results in a decrease in CBZ levels and an increase in the CBZ metabolite CBZ-10,11-epoxide (CBZE). Albani et al. (1991) examined the effect of the administration of felbamate to 22 patients receiving constant CBZ monotherapy in a double-blind controlled study. The authors found that administering felbamate to patients previously receiving CBZ monotherapy resulted in a consistent reduction in the CBZ plasma levels (average of 25% reduction). This effect was evident after 1 week of treatment and reached a plateau after 2 to 4 weeks of coadministration. In addition the authors found a corresponding increase in the CBZE concentration consistently following the reduction in serum CBZ concentrations. Wagner et al. (1993) evaluated the effect of felbamate on the concentrations of carbamazepine and of its metabolites carbamazepine 10,11-epoxide and carbamazepine-trans 10,11-diol (diol) in 26 patients. These authors found that the addition of felbamate increased mean epoxide concentrations from 1.8 μg/ml during placebo or baseline levels to 2.4

μg/ml during felbamate therapy. No significant change in the diol concentration was found.

Mechanism

The likely mechanism of the interaction is an induction of CBZ metabolism after the addition of felbamate.

Clinical Implications

The addition of felbamate to patients already on CBZ may result in a reduction of CBZ levels, but a corresponding increase in the serum concentration of the active CBZ-epoxide metabolite may also occur. Thus, the CBZ-epoxide concentrations as well as CBZ concentrations should be taken into account in patients on this combination before dosage changes are made. Clinical signs of CBZ toxicity may result from increased CBZ-epoxide concentrations if the CBZ dose is increased on the basis of CBZ serum levels alone.

HALOPERIDOL (See CHAPTER 3)

ISONIAZID

Evidence of Interaction

Signs of CBZ toxicity occurred in 10 of 13 patients (disorientation, listlessness, aggression, lethargy, and drowsiness) after isoniazid (INH) 200 mg daily was added to CBZ. Toxic symptoms remitted when CBZ dosage was reduced (Valsalan and Cooper 1982). CBZ levels were monitored in 3 of these patients and were elevated to 26.7, 15.2, and 13.4 μg/ml after the initiation of INH therapy (200 mg every day). The symptoms of CBZ toxicity remitted coincident with decreased levels following CBZ dosage reductions of 2/3, 1/2, and 1/3, respectively.

Another case described a patient who was taking phenytoin 200 mg/day and CBZ 1000 mg/day (with therapeutic levels of both medications). When INH 300 mg/day was added to the patient's regimen, signs of neurotoxicity developed, including ataxia, headaches, vomiting, drowsiness, and confusion (CBZ level = 15 μg/ml) (Block et al. 1982). The phenytoin level was 18 μg/ml at the same time. Her symptoms resolved after INH was discontinued, with anticonvulsant dosages unchanged. CBZ level 1 week later was 6.1 μg/ml; phenytoin was 17.8 μg/ml. A 35-year-old epileptic man on a regimen composed of nitrazepam 10 mg 4 times a day, CBZ 400 mg 4 times a day, and valproic acid 300 mg 4 times a day became drowsy and then stuporous with CBZ levels of 18 to 22 μg/ml 2 days after INH 400 mg/day was started. Prior to INH therapy, CBZ levels were 5 to 8 μg/ml. Valproic acid levels were not altered with INH therapy. Nitrazepam levels were not measured in this study. CBZ clearance was reduced from 6.2 liters/hour before INH to 3.3 liters/hour 3 days after isoniazid treatment was initiated (Wright et al. 1982).

Mechanism

INH decreases clearance of CBZ by inhibiting hepatic microsomal metabolism (Kutt et al. 1970).

Clinical Implications

CBZ metabolism is impaired when INH is coadministered and toxicity may result. CBZ levels should be monitored and signs of CBZ toxicity should be checked in regular clinical assessments.

ISOTRETINOIN (ACCUTANE®)

Summary

Plasma levels of CBZ and CBZE are reduced when CBZ and isotretinoin are coadministered (Marsden 1988).

LAMOTRIGINE

Evidence of an Interaction

Warner et al. (1992) described an interaction between lamotrigine (LTG), an antiepileptic drug, and CBZ. These authors reported that after introduction of LTG to 9 patients already taking CBZ, the mean CBZE concentration increased by 45% and the CBZE:CBZ ratio increased by 19%. There was a variable increase or decrease in concomitant serum CBZ concentration. A mean rise of the CBZ concentration of 16% was noted. In 4 of these patients this change was associated with symptoms of clinical toxicity. Of note is that 3 of the patients in this series were taking other anticonvulsants in addition to CBZ at the time LTG was added. Their respective regimens were as follows: (1) CBZ, VPA; (2) CBZ, PHT (phenytoin); and (3) CBZ, PHT, and clobazam. These, however, were not the patients in whom clinical signs of toxicity developed.

Mechanism

The authors speculate that because these patients showed a marked increase in the CBZE concentration without a consistent reduction in CBZ levels, the likely mechanism of this interaction is an inhibition of the CBZE hydrolase, the enzyme that converts CBZE to CBZ-10,11-dihydroxide.

Clinical Implications

The study described above suggests the potential for toxic symptoms to develop when there is coadministration of LTG and CBZ. Toxic symptoms may occur secondary to the active CBZE metabolite of CBZ. CBZ-epoxide levels should be checked if toxic symptoms develop on this drug combination.

LITHIUM

Evidence of Interaction

Neurotoxicity developed in a series of 5 rapid-cycling manic patients when they were treated with a regimen of CBZ and lithium, despite therapeutic plasma levels of both medications (Shukla 1984). Risk factors for developing neurotoxicity from this combination may include a history of lithium neurotoxicity or the presence of concurrent medical or neurologic illness. Neurotoxic symptoms developed in a 22-year-old woman with bipolar affective disorder when she was treated with a regimen composed of lithium carbonate and CBZ despite therapeutic drug plasma levels (Chaudhry et al. 1983).

Mechanism

The mechanism is unknown.

Clinical Implications

Lithium and CBZ are frequently used in the treatment of rapid-cycling bipolar disorder, and thus there is potential for this interaction to occur in clinical practice. Patients started on this combination should be monitored carefully for signs of neurotoxicity. Patients at high risk may be those with a previous history of lithium neurotoxicity or those with medical or neurologic disorders. In most cases, however, the combination of lithium and CBZ is well tolerated.

MEBENDAZOLE (VERMOX®)

Evidence of Interaction

Plasma levels of mebendazole, a broad spectrum anthelmintic, may be reduced in the presence of CBZ (Luder et al. 1986, Witassek et al. 1983).

Mechanism

CBZ induces hepatic metabolism of mebendazole.

Clinical Implications

The effect of reduced mebendazole plasma levels is probably minimal in the treatment of intestinal organisms such as hookworm or trichuriasis (whipworm). In high-dose applications, such as treatment of hydatid disease, the drug interaction may take on more significance. Valproate does not affect mebendazole metabolism, and may provide an alternative anticonvulsant.

METHADONE

Evidence of Interaction

CBZ may lower methadone plasma levels and lead to opiate withdrawal symptoms (Bell et al. 1988).

Mechanism

CBZ induces methadone metabolism.

Clinical Implications

In patients taking methadone, the addition of CBZ may lower methadone plasma levels and lead to precipitation of opiate withdrawal. Conversely, when CBZ is discontinued, methadone levels may rise. Plasma monitoring of methadone is usually readily available and should be used to guide dosage adjustments under these circumstances.

PHENYTOIN/PHENOBARBITAL/PRIMIDONE

Evidence of Interaction

The plasma levels of CBZ were significantly decreased in patients receiving phenytoin, phenobarbital, or both drugs together compared with CBZ alone (Christiansen and Dam 1973). The average plasma CBZ concentrations in the regimens composed of CBZ alone, CBZ plus phenytoin, CBZ plus phenobarbital, and the combination of CBZ, phenobarbital, and phenytoin were 6.7, 4.4, 5.5, and 3.7 μg/ml, respectively. In a study of 142 epileptic patients, 28 received CBZ alone, while 40, 44, and 30 patients received also phenobarbital (PB), phenytoin, or both drugs, respectively (Johannessen et al. 1975). CBZ levels were significantly decreased in patients receiving co-medication regimens compared with those receiving CBZ alone. The mean serum concentrations of CBZ alone, CBZ + phenytoin, CBZ + PB, and CBZ + PB + phenytoin were 7.2 (±2.5), 5.7 (±2.0), 4.6 (±1.8), and 3.9 (±2.0) μg/ml, respectively.

In a large series of epileptic patients taking CBZ alone or in various combinations with phenytoin, PB, or primidone, there were significantly lower CBZ levels in all patient groups receiving the other anticonvulsants with CBZ than in the group taking CBZ alone (Schneider 1975). A double-blind study of 41 patients given CBZ alone for 3 days and then assigned to one of the following groups: (1) CBZ 1,200 mg + phenytoin 300 mg, (2) CBZ 1,200 mg + PB 300 mg, (3) CBZ 1,200 mg + phenytoin 300 mg + PB 300 mg found that CBZ levels were significantly decreased when CBZ was administered with either phenytoin or phenobarbital or both (Cerenghino et al. 1975)..

Mechanisms and Clinical Implications

CBZ levels are significantly lower in patients who are also taking phenytoin, PB, and/or primidone. Small decreases probably do not affect seizure control, but monitoring serum drug levels may be helpful.

Effect of Carbamazepine on Phenytoin

CBZ coadministration with phenytoin has been noted by various investigators to increase, decrease, and have no effect on phenytoin levels. Zielenski (1983) reported the effect of CBZ-phenytoin coadministration in 24 epileptics. In 50% of the patients, the mean steady-state plasma phenytoin concentration rose from 12.54 (±3.93) to 22.7 (±5.64) μg/ml when phenytoin was given with CBZ, compared with phenytoin alone.

CBZ coadministration has also been reported to decrease phenytoin levels. Hansen et al. (1971) described 5 patients in whom CBZ 600 mg/day was added to phenytoin. The half-life of phenytoin decreased from 10.6 to 6.7 hours with CBZ coadministration after at least 9 days of combined therapy.

Windorfer and Sauer (1977) and Windorfer et al. (1975) found significant decreases in serum phenytoin concentrations when coadministered in long-term therapy with CBZ. Others found serum phenytoin concentrations unaffected by CBZ (Cereghino 1975). The differences among various reports might be accounted for by variations in CBZ and phenytoin doses, duration of therapy, variation in the types and sizes of the study populations, or other factors. Browne and colleagues (1988), studying the combinations in normal volunteers, found that CBZ increased steady-state phenytoin levels by 35%.

Mechanism. The mechanism by which CBZ affects phenytoin levels is unknown.

Effect of Phenytoin on Carbamazepine

Evidence of Interaction. The effect of phenytoin on CBZ levels is well established. Phenytoin reduced CBZ levels in 144 patients, while phenobarbital, methylphenobarbital, primidone, and sulthiame did not (Lander et al. 1975). For each 2 mg/kg/day of phenytoin given, the mean plasma CBZ level fell by 0.9 μg/ml. A study of 60 patients coadministered phenytoin and CBZ also found a reduction in plasma CBZ by phenytoin (Hooper 1974).

Mechanism. Phenytoin may induce CBZ metabolism.

Clinical Implications. When both drugs are coadministered, their plasma levels may be lowered. Effects on phenytoin levels are inconsistent among studies with increases and decreases reported when CBZ is coadministered. Clinical effects on seizure control are possible but not likely. Careful monitoring of serum levels may be required.

PHENOBARBITAL

Evidence of Interaction

Several studies indicate that PB lowers CBZ plasma levels (Cereghino et al. 1975, Christiansen and Dam 1973, Rane et al. 1976).

Mechanism

PB induces hepatic metabolism of CBZ.

Clinical Implications

CBZ levels are significantly lower in patients who are also taking phenytoin, PB, and/or primidone. Small decreases probably do not affect seizure control, but monitoring serum drug levels may be helpful.

PROPOXYPHENE

Evidence of Interaction

Dextropropoxyphene and CBZ are sometimes prescribed in combination for treatment of conditions such as severe herpetic neuralgia. Yu and colleagues (1986) have described 2 cases of CBZ intoxication when used in combination with dextropropoxyphene. Two patients became comatose and another patient became confused when taking this combination for painful acute herpes zoster infection. None were on excessive doses (400, 600, and 400 mg/day) of CBZ yet had toxic CBZ levels.

Dam and colleagues (1977) evaluated the effect of propoxyphene hydrochloride (65 mg 3 times a day) on 7 epileptic outpatients receiving CBZ and found that combined treatment resulted in a marked increase (44–77%) in plasma CBZ levels and a decrease (32–44%) in plasma clearance in 5 patients. Three patients experienced signs of CBZ toxicity. No significant changes in CBZ-10,11-epoxide were noted.

Hansen and associates (1980) evaluated the effects of dextropropoxyphene 65 mg in 6 patients receiving CBZ 600 to 800 mg/day for longer than 6 months. They noted a mean increase of CBZ 66% in serum levels. CBZ-10,11-epoxide levels declined, while CBZ protein binding was unaffected.

Mechanism

Propoxyphene inhibits hepatic metabolism of CBZ.

Clinical Implications

The risk of CBZ toxicity is increased when this combination is used; consider alternate drug regimens for therapy of such conditions as postherpetic neuralgia, or, alternatively, CBZ levels should be monitored closely and the physician should be alert for the signs and symptoms of CBZ toxicity.

THEOPHYLLINE

Evidence of Interaction

An 11-year-old girl with a 2-year history of asthma treated with theophylline 23 mg/kg/day and prednisone 10 mg/day had a generalized seizure. Phenobarbital was started but discontinued because of behavioral problems and she was then started on CBZ therapy (Rosenberry et al. 1983). During coadministration with CBZ, the theophylline elimination half-life fell from 5.25 to 2.75 hours. Theophylline levels, which had been 21 to 23 µg/ml before CBZ initiation, dropped below therapeutic range and the patient had an exacerbation of asthmatic symptoms. CBZ was discontinued and ethotoin was started. The theophylline half-life rose to 6.25 hours within 3 weeks.

Mechanism

CBZ induces metabolism of theophylline.

Clinical Implications

CBZ reduces theophylline half-life and serum concentrations during coadministration. If these medications are coadministered, the physician should be prepared to increase the theophylline dosage. If CBZ is stopped, theophylline doses should be decreased. Careful monitoring of theophylline levels and pulmonary status is necessary.

THYROID HORMONE

Evidence of Interaction

CBZ has a hypothyroid effect, as evidenced by reductions in serum concentrations of total thyroxine, free thyroxine, and triiodothyronine (Cathro et al. 1985, Connell et al. 1984, Roy-Byrne et al. 1984). Requirements for thyroxine replacements increase in hypothyroid patients (Aanderud et al. 1981).

Mechanism

CBZ induces the metabolism of thyroxine and triiodothyronine; it also inhibits compensatory increases in thyrotropin.

Clinical Implications

Thyroid supplementation requirements are altered during CBZ therapy.

VALPROATE (*See* Valproic Acid *section, this chapter*)

VILOXAZINE

Evidence of Interaction

Viloxazine is a "second-generation" antidepressant that has little or no epileptogenic potential (Edwards et al. 1985). It may become an important agent in the treatment of depressed epileptic patients, making coprescription with CBZ increasingly common. Data suggest that CBZ metabolism may be impaired by viloxazine.

Seven epileptic patients on chronic anticonvulsant therapy showed a significant increase in steady-state serum CBZ levels, from 8.1 ($\pm$2.5) to 12.1 ($\pm$2.5) μg/ml (Pisani et al. 1984). Signs of mild CBZ toxicity including dizziness, ataxia, fatigue, and drowsiness were associated with the increased CBZ levels, which remitted when

viloxazine was stopped. CBZ levels returned to baseline after vilox-
azine discontinuation. A later study (Pisani et al. 1986) examined the effect of viloxazine
300 mg/day for 3 weeks on CBZ metabolism in 6 epileptic patients
previously stabilized on CBZ therapy. During viloxazine coadministration, the CBZ concentration increased by 55% compared with
previloxazine levels. The concentration of the active metabolite CBZ-
10,11-epoxide also increased.

Mechanism

The mechanism of the interaction probably involves an inhibition
of the metabolism of both CBZ and its active metabolite CBZ 10,11-
epoxide.

Clinical Implications

Viloxazine has been promoted as having little or no epileptogenic
potential compared with conventional tricyclic antidepressants. Its
use in depressed epileptic patients is substantial in countries where
the antidepressant has been approved. In such circumstances, the
physician prescribing viloxazine to patients on CBZ therapy must
monitor for signs of CBZ toxicity and serum CBZ levels, and should
be prepared to decrease the CBZ dosage.

WARFARIN (COUMADIN®)

Evidence of Interaction

Coadministration of CBZ with warfarin decreased warfarin half-
life and serum levels (Hansen et al. 1971). In a single case study, the
anticoagulant effect of warfarin was neutralized when 400 mg/day
of CBZ was added to the patient's regimen (Kendall and Boivin
1981). This effect was reversed after CBZ had been discontinued for
6 weeks. Reinstitution of CBZ required an 80% increase in warfarin
dose to maintain a therapeutic prothrombin time.

Similarly, CBZ in doses of 300 mg/day coadministered with warfarin required an increase in the daily warfarin dose from 4 to 5.5
mg/day to maintain a therapeutic prothrombin time (Ross and Bee-
ley 1980).

Mechanism

CBZ induces hepatic microsomal enzymes and enhances warfarin
metabolism.

Clinical Implications

When CBZ is administered, the dose of warfarin may need to be increased to maintain a therapeutic prothrombin time. Correspondingly, the dose of warfarin may need to be decreased when CBZ is discontinued.

Phenytoin

ACETAMINOPHEN

Evidence of Interaction

There is some evidence that patients on a combination of antiepileptic agents have reduced acetaminophen bioavailability and half-life (Perucca and Richens 1971). Phenytoin was one of a number of anticonvulsants used in this study. The addition of acetaminophen in oral doses of 1.5 g/day to 9 epileptic patients on phenytoin did not affect serum levels of the latter drug (Neuvonen et al. 1979).

Mechanism

Phenytoin and some other anticonvulsants may increase metabolism or reduce bioavailability of acetaminophen.

Clinical Implications

The clinical significance of this interaction is unknown. There is the potential for decreased effectiveness of acetaminophen in this population and perhaps increased toxicity from its metabolites in circumstances in which clinicians increase the dose or in overdose situations.

ACETAZOLAMIDE

Evidence of Interaction

Case reports have suggested that acetazolamide many accelerate the osteomalacia secondary to anticonvulsants (Mallette 1975, 1977). When acetazolamide was stopped, hyperchloremic acidosis was reversed and urinary calcium excretion decreased.

Mechanism

The mechanism is unknown. It is well recognized that anticonvulsants can induce osteomalacia. Acetazolamide may accelerate this process by increasing calcium and phosphate excretion and causing a systemic acidosis.

Clinical Implications

The evidence supporting the interaction is limited, but caution should be used when prescribing anticonvulsants with carbonic anhydrase inhibitors. Physicians should be aware that osteomalacia may be accelerated in some patients.

ALLOPURINOL (ZYLOPRIM®)

Summary

Allopurinol may inhibit phenytoin metabolism and increase serum phenytoin levels but data are limited (Yokochi et al. 1982).

AMIODARONE

Summary

Phenytoin levels may increase with coadministration of amiodarone, an antiarrhythmic agent (Gore et al. 1984, McGovern et al. 1984).

ANTACIDS

Evidence of Interaction

One multiple-dose and three single-dose studies have examined the interaction of antacids and phenytoin, with conflicting results. Neither aluminum hydroxide 10 ml nor magnesium hydroxide 10 ml every 6 hours administered for 3 days prior to a 100-mg oral dose of phenytoin affected maximum serum concentration, time to maximum concentration, or apparent oral clearance of phenytoin in 6 subjects (O'Brien et al. 1978). Simultaneous administration of an oral dose of 300 mg of phenytoin and antacids (aluminum and magnesium hydroxide 30 ml, aluminum hydroxide/magnesium trisilicate 30 ml, and calcium gluconate 2 g crossover in 2 subjects) showed no effect of the antacids on apparent oral clearance (Chapron et al. 1979). On the other hand, when antacids were given with an oral 600-mg dose of phenytoin and for 6 additional doses following the anticonvulsant, apparent oral clearance was reduced 30.4 and 24.6% with aluminum and magnesium hydroxide 160 mEq, reduced 24.2 and 17.6% with calcium carbonate 160 mEq, but not changed with aluminum hydroxide/magnesium trisilicate as compared with control periods (Garnett et al. 1981). In a multiple-dose study of 12 patients taking 300 to 350 mg of oral phenytoin daily, antacid was added for 7 days. The average serum phenytoin levels were reduced by approximately 12% with aluminum hydroxide/magnesium trisilicate 30 ml but unchanged with calcium carbonate 30 ml (Kulshrestha et al. 1978). Another report describes 3 patients taking phenytoin who had lower serum levels when phenytoin was given alone than with antacids (type unreported, Kutt 1975). When the antacid was given 2 to 3 hours after phenytoin, levels increased. Another clinical report suggests that seizure control was impaired when antacids were ingested with phenytoin (O'Brien et al. 1978).

Mechanism

Several mechanisms have been proposed but none adequately explain the interaction. Decreased gastrointestinal pH, complexation by divalent cations, and antacid-induced diarrhea have been suggested by individual investigators but are not supported by the body of data.

Clinical Implications

The evidence available on the interaction is contradictory. The clinician should be aware that the commonly used antacids may decrease phenytoin bioavailability. Clinical reports suggest that the addition of an antacid to a phenytoin regimen can lower serum levels and impair seizure control. Separating administration by 3 hours or the use of nizatidine, ranitidine, or famotidine, when appropriate, are reasonable alternatives.

ANTICOAGULANTS

Evidence of Interaction

In a study of 6 volunteers given dicumarol (dosed to give prothrombin values of 30%) after 1 week of phenytoin 300 mg/day orally, phenytoin levels increased by 126% over 7 days (Hansen et al. 1966). Radio-labeled intravenous phenytoin was given alone and again after 1 week of dicumarol therapy in 2 volunteers, and elimination half-life of phenytoin was increased in both subjects (from 9 to 36 hours and 9.75 to 44 hours). Another study examined changes in dicumarol level at doses of 40 to 160 mg daily orally and the prothrombin-proconvertin percentage during concurrent phenytoin administration (300 mg/day orally for 1 week). A decreased anticoagulant effect was found and dicumarol levels decreased from a mean 29 µg/ml after 5 days of phenytoin treatment and fell to 21 µg/ml 5 days after phenytoin had been discontinued (Hansen et al.

1971). Other studies (Skovsted et al. 1976) and a case report (Frantzen et al. 1967) support these findings.

The half-life and steady-state serum concentrations of phenytoin do not appear to be affected by coadministration of warfarin (Skovsted et al. 1976), although one case report describes a patient who had been maintained on oral phenytoin 300 mg daily for over a year in whom signs of phenytoin toxicity developed shortly after warfarin was started (Rothermich 1966). Another case report describes an increase in prothrombin time (from 21 to 32 seconds) when phenytoin 300 mg daily orally was added to warfarin (2.5 mg 5 days a week, 5 mg on the other 2 days) (Nappi 1979). Serum levels of phenytoin were increased by about 40%, with an increase in elimination half-life from 9.9 to 14 hours when phenprocoumon was given concurrently (Skovsted et al. 1976), but the anticoagulant does not appear to be affected by phenytoin. Phenytoin levels are unaffected by phenidione (Skovsted et al. 1976).

Mechanism of Interaction

The mechanisms are not fully understood. The hepatic metabolism of phenytoin is probably inhibited by some anticoagulants (dicumarol, phenprocoumon). Phenytoin may displace oral anticoagulants from plasma protein-binding sites, resulting in a transient increase in anticoagulant effect. Phenytoin is known to induce hepatic enzymes and may increase clearance of dicumarol. Phenytoin itself may prolong prothrombin time (Solomon et al. 1972).

Clinical Implications

It would seem advisable to avoid concurrent administration of dicumarol or phenprocoumon with phenytoin when possible. Warfarin may be preferable although initial transient increases in anticoagulant effect may be observed when phenytoin is added to warfarin. Careful clinical and laboratory monitoring should permit appropriate dosage modification to adjust for the interaction.

ANTIHISTAMINES

Evidence of Interaction

There is a single case report describing the development of toxic serum phenytoin levels (60 µg/ml) when a patient was given phenytoin 300 mg/day orally and chlorpheniramine 12 mg/day orally (Pugh 1975).

Mechanism

Unknown.

Clinical Implications

Evidence supporting the interaction is very limited. It may be useful to carefully monitor phenytoin serum levels and observe patients for toxicity when using this drug combination.

ANTINEOPLASTICS

Evidence of Interaction

Intravenous chemotherapy with carmustine, methotrexate, and vinblastine reduced plasma phenytoin levels and increased partial seizures (Bollini et al. 1983). Similar reductions in phenytoin levels with loss of seizure control have been reported in patients receiving bleomycin and cisplatin (Fincham et al. 1979, Sylvester et al. 1984).

Mechanism

Decreased oral bioavailability of phenytoin by antineoplastics is the presumed mechanism of interaction, although altered metabolism is also possible.

Clinical Implications

Phenytoin plasma levels should be monitored during chemotherapy.

BARBITURATES

Evidence of Interaction

The interaction of barbiturates with phenytoin is not straightforward. In most instances barbiturates induce the metabolism of phenytoin; however, it has also been reported that high doses of phenobarbital competitively inhibit the metabolism of phenytoin (Hansten 1974). Five children who were maintained on phenobarbital 5 mg/kg for 28 days were given a single dose of phenytoin 10 mg/kg both before starting and at the completion of drug treatment. Phenytoin levels were 50% lower after 28 days of phenobarbital (Buchanan and Allen 1971). In another study, 12 epileptic patients were given phenytoin (3.7–6.8 mg/kg/day) both with and without phenobarbital (1.4 mg/kg/day). During combined therapy phenytoin levels were depressed; in some patients serum levels dropped as much as 70%. After discontinuation of the phenobarbital, phenytoin levels rose and in some instances led to toxicity (Morselli et al. 1971). Another study of 73 patients found that those receiving combined treatment had lower levels of both drugs than those patients who were taking either alone (Sotaniemi et al. 1970). In one case phenytoin toxicity developed after phenobarbital was discontinued (Morselli et al. 1971). Although some studies have found no interaction (Booker et al. 1971, Kutt et al. 1969, Vapaatola and Lehtinen 1971) most carefully designed studies support the observation that chronic phenobarbital treatment enhances the metabolism of phenytoin, resulting in lower serum levels during combined treatment and increases in phenytoin levels when the phenobarbital is stopped.

Mechanism

Chronic phenobarbital treatment induces the hepatic microsomal enzyme system.

Clinical Implications

Patients receiving phenobarbital (or other barbiturates) with phenytoin should have frequent monitoring of serum levels. With prolonged treatment there is the possibility that serum phenytoin levels will fall below the minimal therapeutic level with loss of seizure control. If the barbiturate is discontinued phenytoin toxicity could result because the enzymes will no longer be induced.

BENZODIAZEPINES (*See* CHAPTER 5)

CALCIUM SULFATE EXCIPIENT

Evidence of Interaction

Phenytoin intoxication occurred in 51 patients when capsules using calcium sulfate as an excipient were replaced by capsules using a lactose excipient (Tyrer et al. 1970). In 3 patients for which serum levels were available before and after the change, there was a 3- to 4-fold increase. In a later study, 13 patients received either phenytoin sodium capsules with lactose or calcium sulfate excipient and then crossed-over (Bochner et al. 1972). Mean serum phenytoin concentrations were 7.7 μg/ml with lactose and 1.7 μg/ml with calcium sulfate.

Mechanism

It has been suggested that a lipid-insoluble complex of phenytoin-calcium sulfate forms which decreases bioavailability.

Clinical Implications

This interaction is primarily of historical interest in the United States, but should serve as a caution to clinicians when different brands of phenytoin are used. Excipients may influence completeness of absorption.

CARBAMAZEPINE

Evidence of Interaction

When administered concurrently, carbamazepine and phenytoin may interact to produce lower steady-state plasma levels. When phenytoin was administered intravenously to 5 patients before and during treatment with carbamazepine 600 mg daily, the elimination half-life of the phenytoin decreased from 10.6 to 6.4 hours after at least 9 days of carbamazepine treatment (Hansen et al. 1971). In the same study, 7 patients on phenytoin treatment received 600 mg of oral carbamazepine daily after steady-state phenytoin levels were achieved. In 3 of the patients the phenytoin level decreased significantly following 4 to 14 days of carbamazepine, from 15 to 7, 18 to 12, and 16 to 10 μg/ml. After the carbamazepine was withdrawn the phenytoin level returned to the original level in 10 days. In 1 subject a transient rise was seen. In general, other reports support the finding that some but not all patients will have lower phenytoin levels on combination therapy (Cereghino et al. 1973, Hooper et al. 1974). Carbamazepine levels have also shown to be reduced by concurrent administration of phenytoin (Cereghino et al. 1975, Christiansen et al. 1973, Rane et al. 1976).

Mechanism

Both phenytoin and carbamazepine induce hepatic metabolism.

Clinical Implications

Although the evidence that plasma levels fall during concurrent therapy is substantial, there is no evidence to suggest that seizure control is compromised with the lower levels. Careful clinical monitoring and the judicious use of serum drug monitoring is recommended when this drug combination is utilized.

CHLORAMPHENICOL

Evidence of Interaction

Chloramphenicol can increase phenytoin serum levels and lead to toxicity. Phenytoin 250 mg/day orally was administered to 2 patients for a 4-day period after which chloramphenicol 2 g/day was also given (Christensen and Skovsted 1969). Both patients showed an increase in serum phenytoin levels, although the data are reported for only one of them. In that patient serum phenytoin rose from 2 μg/ml prior to chloramphenicol to between 7 and 11 μg/ml. In 3 other patients the elimination half-life of phenytoin was increased from 11.75 to 22.75, 16.25 to 38.5, and 9.75 to 25.75 hours when given with chloramphenicol 2 g/day than when administered alone. A single intravenous dose of 3 g of chloramphenicol caused a change in the slope of the β-phase that corresponded to a change in half-life from 10.5 to 22 hours. In another patient a 1.5-g dose caused a change in half-life from 9 to 12.5 hours. A case report describes a patient with a third-ventricle tumor who was taking phenytoin 400 mg/day orally and was given chloramphenicol to treat meningitis (Ballek et al. 1973). Nystagmus on lateral gaze developed in the patient and the serum phenytoin reached 24 μg/ml. When chloramphenicol was stopped the serum phenytoin level dropped to 3 μg/ml on 300 mg daily. A patient with a cavernous hemangioma was being treated with cortisone 2 mg, thyroid extract 3 grains, and phenytoin 300 mg (Rose et al. 1977). Fever developed and the patient was treated with chloramphenicol and other antibiotics. After the 7th day all the antibiotics were discontinued. On the 18th day fever returned and chloramphenicol 1 g every 6 hours was started. The temperature returned to normal but the patient became stuporous. Discontinuation of chloramphenicol led to improved mental status but return of the fever. Reinstitution of the chloramphenicol once again led to the patient being unresponsive to pain, but it was discovered that the serum phenytoin level reached 54 μg/ml. In a review of the serum phenytoin levels during the hospitalization, it was observed that they increased each time chloramphenicol was added.

Mechanism
Chloramphenicol most likely inhibits the hepatic metabolism of phenytoin.

Clinical Implications
Although not a common drug combination, the interaction appears serious and well-documented. Patients who receive the drugs concurrently would be likely to have serious medical illnesses that could be difficult to differentiate from phenytoin toxicity as was the case in the report of Rose and colleagues (1979). Phenytoin serum levels must be monitored if the two drugs are given concurrently.

CIMETIDINE

Evidence of Interaction
Several studies and case reports suggest that cimetidine may impair the metabolism of phenytoin, increasing serum levels of the

anticonvulsant and occasionally leading to phenytoin toxicity (Bartle et al. 1983, Hetzel et al. 1981, Iteogu 1983, Neuvonen et al. 1980, Salem et al. 1983, Watts et al. 1983).

Mechanism

Cimetidine inhibits the hepatic metabolism of phenytoin.

Clinical Implications

Cimetidine, in the usual therapeutic doses, impairs the metabolism of phenytoin and may lead to toxicity. The effect is rapid, beginning within the first 2 days after the addition of cimetidine. After the discontinuation of cimetidine, phenytoin levels will drop within 1 to 2 weeks. Because there appears to be some variability in the magnitude of the effect, frequent serum phenytoin monitoring is recommended. When possible, ranitidine, famotidine, or nizatidine should be used instead of cimetidine.

CIPROFLOXACIN

Summary

Ciprofloxacin inhibits phenytoin metabolism, leading to increased serum concentrations and possible toxicity (Dillard et al. 1992, Hull 1993).

CYCLOSPORINE

Summary

Cyclosporine serum levels are reduced by concomitant phenytoin (Freeman et al. 1984).

DIAZOXIDE

Evidence of Interaction

Low serum phenytoin levels, increased metabolite hydroxyphenyphenylhydantoin (HPPH) formation, and reduced phenytoin half-life have been reported when diazoxide and phenytoin are administered concurrently (Petro et al. 1986, Roe et al. 1975).

Mechanism

Diazoxide appears to induce the metabolism of phenytoin.

Clinical Implications

Serum phenytoin concentrations should be monitored frequently during concomitant therapy.

DIGITALIS GLYCOSIDES

Evidence of Interaction

Serum levels of digoxin and digitoxin are reduced in the presence of phenytoin (Solomon et al. 1971).

Mechanism

Phenytoin is a hepatic enzyme inducer.

Clinical Implications

Serum levels of digitalis glycosides should be monitored frequently whenever phenytoin is added to digoxin or digitoxin, or when it is discontinued after combined therapy.

DISULFIRAM

Evidence of Interaction

Serum phenytoin levels increase with concurrent disulfiram administration (Kiorboe 1966, Olesen 1967). The effect is rapid, within several hours after disulfiram administration, and long lasting, up to 3 weeks following disulfiram discontinuation.

Mechanism

Disulfiram inhibits phenytoin metabolism.

Clinical Implications

Phenytoin serum levels should be closely monitored when disulfiram is added or discontinued. Toxicity has resulted from the administration of disulfiram to patients taking phenytoin when appropriate dosage adjustments were not made.

ENTERAL FEEDING PRODUCTS

Evidence of Interaction

Twenty patients received 1.0-mg loading dose of phenytoin followed by 7 days of 300 mg/day of phenytoin suspension either alone or with 125 ml/hr of Isocal® (Bauer 1982). After the first 7 days, patients were crossed over to the other cell. There was almost a 4-fold increase in levels when phenytoin was given with Isocal®. A case report describes a patient who was receiving phenytoin 400 mg twice daily via nasogastric tube with Osmolite®, resulting in phenytoin serum levels between 2.9 and 4.5 µg/ml (Hatton 1984). Oral phenytoin was discontinued and an intravenous loading dose of 1000 mg was given followed by intravenous doses of 400 mg/day. Over the next month levels ranged from 10 to 20 µg/ml.

Mechanism

The mechanism by which Isocal® and Osmolite® decrease phenytoin bioavailability is unknown.

Clinical Implications

During enteral feedings phenytoin should be administered intravenously if possible. If oral doses must be used, frequent monitoring of serum concentrations is recommended.

ETHANOL

Evidence of Interaction

Abstinent alcoholics metabolize phenytoin more rapidly than non-alcoholics. In a study of 15 alcoholics and 76 control subjects, the mean serum phenytoin level in alcoholics 24 hours after the last dose was half that of control subjects. Mean elimination half-life was 16.3 hours in alcoholics versus 23.5 hours in controls (Kater et al. 1969). Acute ingestion of alcohol in normal volunteers did not affect phenytoin metabolism according to one report (Schmidt 1980).

Mechanism

Chronic ethanol ingestion induces the liver microsomal enzyme system, increasing phenytoin clearance. Acute alcohol usually impairs this system, making it difficult to explain the negative findings of Schmidt (1980).

Clinical Implications

Phenytoin is commonly used for alcoholic patients with a preexisting seizure disorder who require ethanol detoxification. Clinicians should anticipate the need for higher doses in this population.

FLUCONAZOLE (DIFLUCAN®)

Summary

Fluconazole may inhibit phenytoin metabolism and lead to toxicity (Blum et al. 1991, Howitt et al. 1989).

FOLIC ACID

Evidence of Interaction

For many patients, phenytoin treatment leads to folic acid deficiency (Mattson et al. 1973, Norris and Pratt 1974, Reynolds 1973,

Wells 1968). The clinical manifestations of folate deficiency include psychiatric disturbances, neuropathy, and megaloblastic anemia. Some workers have suggested that phenytoin-induced folate deficiency may lead to congenital malformations (Janz 1975, Speidel and Meadow 1974). Replacement of folate may be associated with decreased serum phenytoin, which may lead to lack of seizure control (Baylis et al. 1971, Maxwell et al. 1972, Norris and Pratt 1971, Reynolds 1967, Strauss and Bernstein 1974). Although most patients have relatively small decreases in phenytoin levels and remain in the therapeutic range (Baylis et al. 1971, Furlant et al. 1978, Jensen et al. 1971), reductions of 15 to 25% have been reported.

Mechanism

Folate may increase phenytoin metabolism or reduce its bioavailability. Phenytoin may reduce folate absorption or increase folate utilization as a coenzyme for drug metabolism. Some have suggested that transport of folate from the serum to the central nervous system is impaired by phenytoin. Folic acid when given alone may induce seizures in animals (Hommes and Obbens 1972) and may directly antagonize the action of phenytoin.

Clinical Implications

Phenytoin can reduce folate levels and the addition of folic acid therapy can reduce serum levels of the anticonvulsant. Occasionally, this reduction may lead to impaired seizure control. Serum folate and phenytoin levels should be monitored and patients observed closely for increased seizure activity.

FUROSEMIDE

Evidence of Interaction

Epileptic patients on a variety of anticonvulsants had a slowed onset and a decreased intensity of diuretic effect from furosemide (Ahmad 1974). A study of 5 healthy volunteers found that treatment with phenytoin 300 mg daily for 10 days reduced furosemide oral bioavailability by 50% (Fine et al. 1977).

Mechanism

Phenytoin impairs systemic bioavailability of furosemide probably by reducing gut absorption, although the mechanism is not fully understood. The diuretic response is inhibited, even after intravenous administration, suggesting other mechanisms are also involved.

Clinical Implications

Larger doses of furosemide may be required when phenytoin is administered concurrently.

GLUCAGON

Evidence of Interaction

Patients taking phenytoin may have false-negative glucagon stimulation tests (Kumer et al. 1974). A 44-year-old epileptic man taking phenytoin had the diagnosis of an islet-cell adenoma obscured because no elevation of insulin was observed until phenytoin was discontinued. This observation suggests that phenytoin has the ability to inhibit insulin release (Knopp et al. 1972).

Mechanism

Phenytoin blocks insulin release from the pancreas.

Clinical Implications

Patients treated with phenytoin may have false-negative glucagon stimulation tests.

HALOTHANE AND FLUROXENE (HALOGENATED ANESTHETIC AGENTS)

Evidence of Interaction

Case reports suggest that phenytoin may interact with halogenated anesthetic agents to increase the hepatotoxicity of these agents; this toxicity may in turn cause increased phenytoin levels (Karlin and Kutt 1970, Reynolds et al. 1972). The first case involved a 10-year-old child who had been treated with phenytoin 10 mg/kg/day orally without adverse effects other than gingival hyperplasia and nystagmus. Following anesthesia for 90 minutes, body temperature was elevated for 3 days as was serum glutamic oxaloacetic transaminase (120 units/ml, normal 8–33 units/ml). Serum glutamic pyruvic transaminase level was normal. Intramuscular phenytoin was continued after surgery and the serum phenytoin levels increased to 41 μg/ml. Clinical signs of nystagmus and poor muscle tone and symptoms of lethargy and blurred vision were consistent with phenytoin toxicity. Histologic examination confirmed hepatic necrosis. In the second case, a woman who had been taking phenytoin and phenobarbital died from massive necrosis after fluroxene anesthesia and the authors speculated that phenytoin led to increased hepatotoxicity.

Mechanism

Halothane and fluroxene may cause hepatotoxicity, which may impair phenytoin metabolism. There is no good evidence to suggest that phenytoin increases the likelihood of hepatotoxicity with halogenated anesthetic agents, although it is possible that phenytoin enhances the metabolism of the anesthetic to a hepatotoxic metabolite.

Clinical Implications

The documentation of this interaction is limited, but common sense dictates that caution should be used when halothane or any hepatotoxic drug is administered with phenytoin.

ISONIAZID

Evidence of Interaction

The first indication that phenytoin toxicity could develop with concurrent administration of isoniazid was when the addition of the latter drug to phenytoin and phenobarbital resulted in the onset of drowsiness, ataxia, and incoordination in about 10% of 637 epileptic patients (Murray 1962). In a later study, 6 of 32 patients who were all classified as slow metabolizers of isoniazid showed higher mean serum levels of phenytoin and the typical signs and symptoms of toxicity developed when phenytoin levels increased to above 20 μg/ml (Brennan et al. 1970). In another study, in 6 of 36 patients phenytoin toxicity developed when the received the combination (Kutt et al. 1970). The addition of aminosalicylic acid to the phenytoin-isoniazid combination may increase the risk of phenytoin toxicity (Kutt 1975).

Mechanism

Isoniazid impairs the parahydroxylation of phenytoin. Because this is a dose-related phenomenon, those patients who are the slowest metabolizers of isoniazid are at highest risk.

Clinical Implications

About half of the population are slow metabolizers of isoniazid. Phenytoin toxicity will develop in approximately 10 to 25% of patients taking the phenytoin-isoniazid combination. Those on other antitubercular drugs as well, such as aminosalicylic acid and cycloserine, which inhibit phenytoin metabolism to a lesser degree, may increase the chances of toxicity, although this is controversial. When patients are receiving phenytoin and isoniazid concurrently, frequent serum phenytoin levels and careful observation for signs and symptoms of phenytoin intoxication are necessary. Dosage adjustments must be made when isoniazid is started or discontinued.

LEVODOPA

Evidence of Interaction

In one study phenytoin was successful in the treatment of levodopa-induced dyskinesia but reversed the effect of levodopa on the symptoms of Parkinson's disease (Mendez et al. 1975).

Mechanism

Unknown.

Clinical Implications

There are limited data on this interaction. It would appear wise to avoid the combination if possible, or increase the dose of levodopa when administered with phenytoin.

LIDOCAINE

Evidence of Interaction

The combination of lidocaine and phenytoin is associated with enhanced toxicity, including a case of sinoatrial arrest that was reversed by isoproterenol (Wood 1971). The incidence of less serious side effects (diplopia, nystagmus, nausea, vertigo, hearing disturbance) is also increased (Karlsson et al. 1974).

Mechanism

Drug clearance is not altered to a significant degree during combined therapy. There would appear to be a pharmacodynamic interaction due to enhanced depressant effect on cardiac function.

Clinical Implications

When clinicians use this drug combination, they should be aware of the possibility of toxicity.

METHADONE

Evidence of Interaction

The addition of phenytoin to methadone maintenance therapy may induce withdrawal symptoms (Finelli 1976, Tong 1981).

Mechanism

Phenytoin induces hepatic metabolism of methadone.

Clinical Implications

Enzyme-inducing agents should be avoided in methadone patients. Alternatively, plasma levels of methadone should be followed and appropriate dosage adjustments made.

METHYLPHENIDATE

Evidence of Interaction

Anecdotal reports have suggested that phenytoin toxicity may develop in children who are treated concurrently with phenytoin and methylphenidate (Garrettson et al. 1969) but clinical studies have failed to establish this interaction. A 5-year-old child receiving phenytoin 8.9 mg/kg and primidone 17.7 mg/kg had methylphenidate added to his regimen. Phenytoin levels increased from 8 to 35 μg/ml. Primidone levels increased from 4 to 21 μg/ml and its metabolite phenobarbital increased from 23 to 39 μg/ml. Two other children in the same report did not show elevations of anticonvulsants when methylphenidate was added. One clinical report cites the experience of more than 100 patients taking the combination without adverse consequences (Oettinger 1976). Another report describes an increase in phenytoin concentration during one period of combined administration but not in another (Mirkin and Wright 1971). In two studies there was no interaction noted in 14 patients (Kupferberg et al. 1972, Mirkin and Wright 1971).

Mechanism

In vitro studies indicate that methylphenidate is a competitive inhibitor of hepatic metabolism of phenytoin and other drugs (Hunninghake 1970, Perel and Black 1970). The variability of this effect is substantial.

Clinical Implications

In isolated cases, methylphenidate has been associated with phenytoin toxicity; however, clinical experience and studies suggest the combination usually does not present problems.

PHENYLBUTAZONE

Evidence of Interaction and Mechanism of Interaction

Phenylbutazone and oxyphenbutazone (its major metabolite) impair phenytoin clearance and may lead to phenytoin toxicity (Andreasen et al. 1973, Lunde 1970, Neuvonen et al. 1979, Shoeman et al. 1975).

Clinical Implications

Dosage reduction of phenytoin may be required during concurrent therapy.

PYRIDOXINE

Evidence of Interaction and Mechanism of Interaction

Large doses of pyridoxine 200 mg/day for 4 weeks may enhance phenytoin metabolism and lower serum levels (Hansson et al. 1976).

Clinical Implications

With small doses of pyridoxine, as are found in multivitamin preparations, no special precautions appear necessary. With larger doses, such as daily doses of 200 mg or greater, monitoring of serum phenytoin levels may be necessary.

QUINIDINE

Evidence of Interaction and Mechanism of Interaction

The metabolism of quinidine is enhanced when given with phenytoin (Data et al. 1976, Jaillon et al. 1980).

Clinical Implications

Quinidine levels should be monitored whenever an enzyme-inducing agent such as phenytoin is added or withdrawn from the medication regimen.

SALICYLATES

Evidence of Interaction and Mechanism of Interaction

Salicylates displace phenytoin from plasma protein-binding sites, which could in theory lead to toxicity (Ehrnebo et al. 1977, Fraser et al. 1980, Leonard et al. 1981, Paxton 1980).

Clinical Implications

The clinical importance of this interaction is not documented. Plasma protein-binding interactions usually cause only temporary alterations in free (unbound) drug, so that although total phenytoin concentration may decrease in patients taking high doses of aspirin, free concentration remains relatively constant. Patients at higher therapeutic levels could experience transient toxicity.

STEROIDS

Evidence of Interaction

Phenytoin has been shown to increase the clearance and reduce the elimination half-life of several corticosteroids, including hydrocortisone (Choi et al. 1971), methylprednisolone (Stjernholm et al. 1975), prednisone (Meikle et al. 1975), prednisolone (Petereit et al. 1977, Wassmer et al. 1976), dexamethasone (Brooks et al. 1972, Hague et al. 1972), and metyrapone (Meikle et al. 1969). There are several reports in the literature that document the clinical importance of the interaction. The results of the dexamethasone and metyrapone tests are difficult to interpret in the presence of phenytoin and may yield falsely positive results (Jubiz et al. 1970, Meikle et al. 1969, Werk et al. 1967, 1969). Renal transplant and graft patients taking phenytoin may have a greater rejection rate, presumably due to enhanced clearance of the corticosteroids used as immunosuppressives (Wassner et al. 1976). The effectiveness of dexamethasone in the treatment of cerebral edema may also be reduced in the presence of phenytoin (McClelland and Jack 1978).

Mechanism

Phenytoin induces the hepatic metabolism of corticosteroids.

Clinical Implications

The clinical effectiveness of steroids is reduced when they are given in combination with phenytoin. In these cases the clinician can increase the steroid dose or replace phenytoin with another anticonvulsant that does not induce hepatic metabolism. Some have also suggested that hydrocortisone is affected to a lesser extent than other steroids. This has led to the suggestion that hydrocortisone replace dexamethasone in the suppression test for those patients taking phenytoin (Meikle et al. 1969).

SUCRALFATE

Summary

Sucralfate may reduce phenytoin absorption (Hall et al. 1986, Smart et al. 1985).

SULFONAMIDES

Evidence of Interaction

Phenytoin elimination half-life increased from a mean 11.3 to 20.5 hours following sulfamethizole therapy (4 g/day taken orally) (Lumholtz et al. 1975, Siersbaek-Nielsen et al. 1973). Sulfaphenazole may also inhibit phenytoin metabolism, but sulfisoxazole, sulfadimethoxine, and sulfamethoxypyridazine do not.

Mechanism

Some sulfonamides inhibit hepatic metabolism of phenytoin.

Clinical Implications

Serum phenytoin monitoring and reduced dosage may be required in the presence of some sulfonamides (Hansen et al. 1966, 1975, 1979, Lumholtz et al. 1975, Siersbaek-Nielsen et al. 1973).

SULTHIAME

Evidence of Interaction

Several studies have documented an increase in plasma phenytoin when sulthiame is coadministered, and toxicity may develop (Frantzen 1967, Hansen et al. 1968, Houghton et al. 1974a,b, 1975, Olesen et al. 1969, Richens et al. 1973).

Mechanism

Sulthiame inhibits hepatic metabolism of phenytoin.

Clinical Implications

Clinicians should be aware that the addition of sulthiame to phenytoin can raise serum levels of the latter drug by 75%. Sulthiame is an anticonvulsant that is not marketed in the United States.

TETRACYCLINES

Evidence of Interaction

The elimination half-life of doxycycline was approximately 50% shorter in patients taking phenytoin than control subjects (7.1 vs. 15.1 hours) (Alestig 1974, Penttila et al. 1974, Neuvonen et al. 1974, 1975, 1979). Chlortetracycline, demeclocycline, methacycline, oxytetracycline are not affected by phenytoin.

Mechanism

Phenytoin enhances metabolism of doxycycline.

Clinical Implications

Phenytoin may lower doxycycline levels below minimum therapeutic concentrations. Alternative antibiotics or appropriate dosage adjustments should be made.

THEOPHYLLINE

Evidence of Interaction

Theophylline clearance is higher, and elimination half-life and clinical effect are reduced by concomitant phenytoin administration (Marquis et al. 1982, Taylor et al. 1980).

Mechanism

Phenytoin stimulates hepatic metabolism of theophylline.

Clinical Implications

Theophylline dosage adjustment and plasma level monitoring may be necessary when phenytoin is added to or withdrawn from treatment (Marquis et al. 1982, Taylor et al. 1980).

THYROID HORMONES

Evidence of Interaction

Phenytoin may increase the metabolism of thyroid hormone, requiring changes in dosage of replacement therapy (Blackshear et al. 1983). One case report cites the occurrence of supraventricular tachycardia in a patient with hypothyroidism who was treated with replacement therapy when phenytoin was administered intravenously for atrial flutter (Fulop et al. 1966).

Mechanism

Phenytoin enhances the metabolism of thyroid hormones.

Clinical Implications

Phenytoin administration may alter required dosage of thyroid replacement hormone.

VALPROATE

Evidence of Interaction

Clinical studies suggest that phenytoin may in some but not all cases increase the metabolism of valproate when the two drugs are given in combination. In addition, phenytoin levels may transiently decrease when valproate is added, although the literature is contradictory. Four adult patients with intractable seizures were stabilized on phenytoin (between 4.1 and 5.5 mg/kg/day); 1 patient was also taking phenobarbital 90 to 120 mg/day (Bruni et al. 1980a). The patients were then given valproate in doses determined by their clinicians (plasma concentrations ranged from 36.8 to 56.2 µg/ml, dosages not reported) and were observed for 22 to 32 weeks. Within 2 weeks of starting the valproate, the patients had total phenytoin plasma concentrations that decreased transiently and returned to baseline in 3 of the 4 patients by about 5 weeks. In all 4 patients, the percentage of unbound phenytoin increased 2 weeks after valproate was started. It remained elevated in 3 patients over a 22-week follow-up period. Urinary concentration of the metabolite of phenytoin, HPPH, increased during weeks 2 to 5, but decreased over 5 to 22 weeks. Elimination half-life was nonsignificantly reduced during 2 to 5 weeks and significantly increased during weeks 5 to 22. This study confirmed an earlier animal study and in vitro study of human plasma, which suggested that valproate displaced phenytoin from its protein-binding sites (Patsalos et al. 1977). This is of dubious clinical importance because the excess phenytoin is metabolized (as indicated by increased HPPH). Although total plasma phenytoin may decrease, seizure control is generally not jeopardized. In another study, 23 patients with uncontrolled seizures of a generalized or partial type were given an open clinical trial of valproate in addition to phenytoin (Mattson et al. 1978). During initiation of valproate there was a decline in total serum phenytoin concentration (16.5–10.2 µg/ml), while the percentage of free phenytoin increased (10.9 to 20%). In another study of the interactions of valproate and other anticonvulsant drugs, 10 of 15 patients had a decrease in phenytoin concentrations during valproate therapy (Wilder et al. 1978).

Decreases ranged from slight to greater than 50% in those patients. In a 1-year follow-up of 8 patients, the phenytoin levels were similar to the prevalproate levels in 7, suggesting that any effect is merely temporary (Bruni et al. 1980b). A study of 5 children reported that after the addition of valproate to phenytoin there was an increase in the serum levels of the latter drug for the first few days followed by return to prevalproate levels or lower (Windorfer et al. 1975). Another study found that the administration of a single 800-mg valproate dose to patients who had been taking phenytoin for 3 months resulted in both a decrease in total serum phenytoin concentration and percentage of protein found (Monks et al. 1980). Phenytoin may also induce the metabolism of valproate. In a study of 7 patients taking valproate alone (mean dose 14.8 mg/kg) and 12 patients taking the combination, the serum concentration of valproate was lower in the combined group than in the former group (205 vs. 333 μmol/liter, Reunanen et al. 1980).

The case of a 31-year-old man taking valproate in whom delirium and increased seizure frequency developed after phenytoin (1.0 g oral loading dose followed by maintenance) was added was described (Hansten 1982).

Mechanism

Phenytoin enhances the metabolism of valproate while the latter drug may displace phenytoin from its protein-binding sites.

Clinical Implications

In most cases this will not be a clinically significant interaction. Theoretically the displacement of phenytoin from its binding sites could lead to toxicity if a patient has a particularly high level to begin with. When valproate is added to phenytoin, it is possible that there will be a transient increase in the unbound phenytoin level with a temporary decrease in total plasma phenytoin level for a few weeks, with return to prevalproate levels in about 5 weeks. Reports of the interaction affecting seizure control are not common; however, the clinican should monitor such patients carefully.

Primidone

ACETAZOLAMIDE

Evidence of Interaction

Syversen and associates (1976) studied the effects of acetazolamide on primidone plasma levels in 3 epileptic patients. They coadministered acetazolamide 250 mg 12 hours before and concurrently with the primidone dose 500 mg. Serum and urine levels of primidone were measured under both conditions. Each patient participated in two studies with a time interval of 2 to 17 days between studies. In one patient, primidone was not detected in the plasma when given with acetazolamide. In another patient, the peak serum primidone concentration was delayed, with corresponding delays in the urinary excretion of primidone and metabolites (phenylethylmalonamide and phenobarbital). The third patient had a higher peak concentration in the primidone alone experiment, but had no difference in the urinary excretion of drug or metabolites.

Mechanism

The investigators suggest that acetazolamide interferes with primidone absorption.

Clinical Implications

After the addition of acetazolamide to a medication regimen containing primidone, serum primidone levels should be checked and appropriate dosage changes made.

PHENYTOIN

Evidence of Interaction

Fincham and colleagues (1974) studied the effect of phenytoin on the phenobarbital (a primidone metabolite)/primidone ratio in epileptic patients. Fifteen patients taking primidone alone had a low ratio (1.05 ± 0.2). The ratio in 44 patients taking both phenytoin and primidone was notably higher (4.35 ± 0.5). Another case study supports these findings. Porro and associates (1982) reported a case in which an interaction was found between primidone and phenytoin in an epileptic patient treated with the combination for 3 months. The addition of phenytoin (level 20.7 μg/ml ± 0.5) to the medication regimen increased steady-state levels of primidone metabolites phenobarbital and phenylethylmalonamide (pema). Serum levels of primidone decreased (9.5 μg/ml (± 0.08) to 7.8 μg/ml (± 0.9) as did serum levels of p-hydroxyphenobarbital, a metabolite of phenobarbital. The urinary excretion of primidone and its metabolites paralleled the changes observed in their plasma levels after the addition of phenytoin. The urinary excretion of unchanged primidone significantly decreased 271 (± 21.2 mg/24 hours) to 114.7 (± 21.8 mg/24 hours) and the urinary output of pema and unchanged phenobarbital significantly increased. The percentage of unconjugated p-hydroxyphenobarbital in the urine remained unchanged throughout the course of study. After withdrawal of phenytoin, plasma phenobarbital and primidone levels slowly returned to previous steady-state levels.

Mechanism

Phenytoin induces the biotransformation of primidone to pema and phenobarbital.

Clinical Implications

When phenytoin is coadministered with primidone the physician should be aware of a potential interaction, which may require frequent plasma anticonvulsant monitoring.

ISONIAZID

Evidence of Interaction

A single case report describes a 46-year-old epileptic woman with miliary tuberculosis who was treated with a combination of isoniazid (INH) 300 mg/day and primidone 250 mg every 6 hours (Sutton et al. 1975). As a result, the steady-state serum level of primidone rose from 14.7 to 26.9 µg/ml and the serum levels of primidone metabolites, Pb and pema, fell (Pb 36.4–32 µg/ml, pema 12.4–8.8 µg/ml). The elimination half-life of primidone increased from 8.7 to 14.0 hours and the steady-state primidone levels rose by 83%. Pb and pema levels fell by 12 and 29%, respectively.

Mechanism

INH inhibits hepatic metabolism of primidone.

Clinical Implications

Primidone toxicity may occur during administration with INH. Monitoring of primidone levels and dosage adjustments may be required.

PHENOBARBITAL

Evidence of Interaction

Serum levels of phenobarbital may be elevated in patients receiving primidone plus phenobarbital therapy (Griffin et al. 1976).

Mechanism

Since a portion of primidone is converted to phenobarbital in the body, coadministration of these medications may lead to phenobarbital toxicity via progressive accumulation.

Clinical Implications

Because primidone is metabolized to phenobarbital, coprescription of these agents is unwarranted.

NICOTINAMIDE

Evidence of Interaction

Nicotinamide is a water-soluble vitamin used in the treatment of pellagra. It also has been used in conjunction with primidone in cases of refractory epilepsy. A significant interaction between primidone and nicotinamide was reported in mice and 3 epileptic patients (Bourgeois et al. 1982). In mice, 200 mg/kg of nicotinamide increased the elimination half-life of primidone by 47.6%. The conversion of primidone to its metabolites Pb and pema was decreased in mice by 32.4 and 14.5%, respectively. Nicotinamide was also found to decrease the conversion of primidone to phenobarbital in 3 epileptic patients when added to their regimen. Nicotinamide at doses of 41 to 178 mg/kg/day increased the primidone/phenobarbital ratio and decreased the primidone clearance. The dose of nicotinamide correlated directly with the primidone/phenobarbital ratio for all patients.

Mechanism

Nicotinamide may inhibit the hepatic cytochrome P450 enzymes involved in primidone metabolism.

Clinical Implications

Nicotinamide may be used in conjunction with primidone to improve seizure control or reduce toxicity by lowering levels of phenobarbital. In addition, nicotinamide may be useful in patients with psychiatric symptoms of pellagra (acute psychosis, violence, hallucinations, and delusions of persecution). When using the combination, the physician should be aware of the potential shifts in the primidone:Pb ratio. One group suggests that in epilepsy the primidone:Pb ratio should be maintained at or above 1 to avoid phenobarbital neurotoxicity (Bourgeois et al. 1982).

VALPROIC ACID

Evidence of Interaction

The steady-state levels of the primidone metabolite, phenobarbital, may increase with the addition of valproate (Adams et al. 1978). The addition of valproate to a regimen containing primidone caused an initial increase and then a decrease in plasma primidone levels in 7 epileptic children (Windorfer et al. 1975).

Mechanism
Valproate initially impairs phenobarbital metabolism, but after long-term therapy (1–3 months) metabolism may normalize.

Clinical Implications
Primidone levels should be monitored closely and dosage adjustments made as necessary during coadministration with valproate.

Valproic Acid

ANTACIDS

Evidence of Interaction
A small study involving 7 healthy volunteers given an aluminum hydroxide-magnesium antacid and a single 500-mg dose of valproic acid (VPA) had 12% higher area-under-the-curve with the combination than with VPA alone (May et al. 1982).

Mechanism
Unknown.

Clinical Implications
Antacids are commonly given for the gastrointestinal side effects of VPA. Although this does not appear to be a significant interaction, it can easily be avoided by separating the dose of antacid and VPA by an hour or more.

AMITRIPTYLINE

Evidence of Interaction
Pisani et al. (1986) evaluated 6 patients during coadministration of amitriptyline (AT) and VPA. The authors found that during AT treatment, a slight but significant increase in both the apparent volume of distribution and elimination half-life of VPA occurred.

Mechanism
The mechanism of the interaction is unknown.

Clinical Significance

VPA and AT are sometimes used together in the treatment of postherpetic neuralgia and rarely in the treatment of bipolar disorder. This combination could also potentially be used in the treatment of epilepsy patients with chronic pain or headaches. VPA toxicity may occur if AT is administered concurrently.

ASPIRIN

Evidence of Interaction

Orr and associates (1982) found that in 5 of 6 epileptic children who were taking 18 to 49 mg/kg/day of VPA, the steady-state free fraction of VPA rose from 12 to 43% during coadministration of antipyretic doses of aspirin. Some evidence suggests valproate toxicity may result from the combination (Goulden et al. 1987).

Mechanism

VPA is highly protein bound at therapeutic concentrations and has a small volume of distribution (Rotne et al. 1980). In vitro, salicylate has been reported to displace VPA from its plasma protein-binding sites (Fleitman et al. 1980, Schobben et al. 1978). In addition, salicylates have been shown to inhibit β-oxidation of VPA. Abbott and associates (1986) noted that all metabolites of VPA β-oxidation (2-ene-VPA, 3-OH-VPA, and 3-keto-VPA) were significantly decreased in the urine during ASA-VPA coadministration. There was also significant increase in the urinary VPA glucuronide conjugates as well as the 4-ene-VPA metabolites. 4-ene-VPA itself may be a potent inhibitor of the hepatic fatty acid β-oxidation sequence by sequestering acetylcoenzyme A.

Clinical Implications

The above evidence suggests that the potential for VPA toxicity may be increased during coadministration of salicylates and VPA.

BENZODIAZEPINES

Evidence of Interaction

Dhillon et al. (1982) found that when 10 mg of diazepam was administered intravenously to healthy young volunteers, each receiving 1,500 mg of valproate daily, the concentration of unbound diazepam in serum increased by approximately 2-fold compared with diazepam administered alone. The intrinsic clearance and volume of distribution of unbound diazepam were significantly reduced during coadministration. In addition, mean serum levels of the diazepam metabolite *N*-desmethyldiazepam were significantly lower during valproate coadministration. Absence seizures have been reported with the combination of clonazepam and valproate, but causality has not been established (Browne 1979, Watson 1979).

Mechanism
Valproate displaces diazepam from plasma protein-binding sites and inhibits its metabolism.

Clinical Implications
Coadministration of diazepam and valproic acid may result in increased effects of diazepam.

CIMETIDINE

Evidence of Interaction
VPA clearance was decreased and elimination half-life was increased when VPA was coadministered with cimetidine, but not ranitidine (Webster et al. 1984).

Mechanism
Cimetidine inhibits the metabolism of sodium valproate.

Clinical Implications
Dosage adjustments in sodium valproate will be necessary when the clinician is initiating or discontinuing cimetidine therapy. Alternatively, ranitidine, famotidine, or nizatidine may be used.

CARBAMAZEPINE

Evidence of Interaction and Mechanism of Interaction
The combination of VPA and carbamazepine (CBZ) resulted in higher plasma levels of the CBZ active metabolite, carbamazepine-10,11-epoxide (CBZE), while CBZ levels were not significantly affected (McKauge et al. 1982). Another study found that VPA reduced the binding of CBZ to plasma protein *in vitro* (Mattson et al. 1982). Levy and associates (1984) administered VPA (1 g twice a day for 1 week) to 7 epileptic patients receiving CBZ therapy and found that CBZ serum levels were reduced by 3 to 59% in 6 of 7 patients and were unchanged in 1 patient. The plasma concentration ratio of CBZE:CBZ increased in all patients by 11 to 500%. In the

plasma protein-binding portion of the study, the mean CBZ free fraction was increased in 3 subjects, decreased in 1 subject, and remained unchanged in 2 subjects with VPA-CBZ coadministration. The same authors also found that the coadministration of CBZ with 24-hour infusions of VPA at 75 and 150 mg/hour in rhesus monkeys resulted in a decrease in the mean clearance of free CBZ from 7.96 (± 1.75) to 4.84 (± 1.26) liter/hour/kg ($P < 0.01$) and 4.12 (± 1.75) liter/hour/kg ($P < 0.01$), respectively. These results suggest that VPA inhibits CBZ metabolism. Pisani and associates (1986) evaluated the comparative effects of VPA and valpromide (VPM), a prodrug of VPA, on plasma levels and protein binding of CBZ and CBZE in 12 epileptic patients. The authors found that CBZ levels were not affected by either treatment. In the VPA-treated group, CBZE levels increased by 101% (range 29–238%) within 1 week of combined therapy and returned to baseline after VPA was stopped. In the VPM-treated group, levels of CBZE increased by an average of 330%. The plasma protein binding of CBZ and CBZE was not significantly affected by either VPM or VPA. The authors suggest that VPA and VPM inhibit the epoxide hydroxylase enzyme in CBZE metabolism.

Clinical Implications

CBZ and VPA are frequently used in combination for the treatment of epilepsy. In addition, both of these drugs have been used for treatment-resistant schizophrenic and bipolar patients, making the interaction of possible clinical importance for psychiatrists. Since VPA appears to increase the level of CBZE, an active metabolite of CBZ, and may cause protein-binding displacement of CBZ, there is the possibility that CBZ toxicity may develop when using these medications in combination.

ETHOSUXIMIDE

Evidence of Interaction

Pisani and associates (1984) found that, when 500 mg of ethosuximide (ESM) was administered during the course of VPA therapy (800–1,600 mg/day titrated to therapeutic levels), there was a significant increase in ESM serum elimination half-life (from 44 to 54 hours). Also ESM total body clearance was significantly decreased (from 11.2 to 9.5 ml/min on average) during coadministration with VPA. The ESM renal clearance was unchanged during coadministration.

Mechanism

The authors suggest that VPA increases ESM's half-life and decreases total body clearance of ESM via an inhibition of hepatic metabolism.

Clinical Implications

VPA, when coadministered with ESM, increases the risk of ESM toxicity. A different anticonvulsant combination should be chosen or ESM doses decreased to minimize the risk of toxicity.

FELBAMATE

Evidence of an Interaction

Wagner et al. (1994) in a random crossover study administered felbamate 600 mg and 1,200 mg twice daily to 10 patients already maintained on VPA 9.5 to 26.2 mg/kg/day. These authors found that the addition of felbamate to VPA resulted in increased serum concentrations of VPA. Coadministration of felbamate increased average VPA steady-state concentrations and decreased VPA clearance.

Mechanism

Felbamate may inhibit metabolism of VPA.

Clinical Implications

Coadministration of felbamate and VPA may result in increased levels of VPA and toxicity. Thus, if this combination is prescribed, VPA levels should be monitored closely and dosage reductions of VPA should be made when appropriate.

LAMOTRIGINE

Evidence of Interaction

Yuen et al. (1992) examined the effect of VPA on lamotrigine (LTG) metabolism in 6 male subjects. Each subject received 100 mg of LTG orally on two occasions at a minimum of 14 days apart. One of these doses was given alone and the other concomitantly with VPA at a dose of 200 mg every 8 hours, the first dose of which was given 1 hour before LTG was initiated. The authors found that coadministration of LTG and VPA resulted in the slower elimination of

LTG and a 21% reduction in LTG clearance, with a corresponding increase in LTG elimination half-life. Reduced elimination occurred within the first hour after administration. Reutens et al. (1993) reported that disabling tremor developed when LTG and VPA were coadministered. The first case was a patient with complex partial seizures. On a regimen of LTG, 200 mg/day and VPA 2,000 mg/day, a severe tremor developed in the patient. The corresponding random serum concentration of LTG was 628 μmol/liter and that of VPA was 53 μmol/liter. This patient's tremor resolved after the LTG dose was reduced to 100 mg/day. The second case was a patient with multiple seizure types including myoclonus, generalized tonic clinic seizures, and absence seizures. Titubation and a disabling postural and action tremor developed while this patient was taking a regimen of LTG 150 mg/day and VPA 2,500 mg/day. The VPA concentration was 1,030 μmol/liter. This patient's tremor resolved when the VPA dose was reduced to 2,000 mg/day. A third more complicated case was also described. In a patient taking a combination of phenytoin 425 mg/day, VPA 2,500 mg/day, and LTG 200 mg/day, ataxia and upper extremity action tremor developed only after phenytoin was discontinued from the regimen. Random plasma levels of LTG and VPA were 55 and 868 μmol/liter, respectively. These symptoms resolved after LTG was decreased to 100 mg/day. Thus the authors speculated that the withdrawal of phenytoin from this regimen induced toxic symptoms, presumably by unmasking the VPA/LTG interaction since phenytoin induces the hepatic enzymes responsible for the metabolism of LTG and VPA (Peck 1991). Finally, Pisani et al. (1993) described 7 patients with refractory partial seizures whom, when taking the combination of VPA and LTG, had high concentrations of LTG that at times resulted in toxic symptoms of sedation, ataxia, and fatigue that resolved after the LTG dosage was reduced.

Mechanism

Yuen et al. (1992) postulate that VPA impairs the hepatic glucuronidation of LTG via competitive inhibition of enzymes.

Clinical Implications

The coadministration of VPA and LTG may result in clinical signs of toxicity; thus, with this combination, serum levels of both drugs need to be monitored carefully and dose adjustments made if necessary.

PHENOBARBITAL

Evidence of Interaction

VPA appears to impair the metabolism of phenobarbital (PB) and increase plasma PB levels (Bruni et al. 1980a, Wilder et al. 1978). Patel and colleagues (1980) performed a randomized crossover study of 6 normal subjects and found that when steady-state VPA concentrations of 20 to 30 μg/ml were achieved, mean PB elimination half-life was prolonged from 96 to 142 hours. In addition, mean PB clearance was reduced from 4.2 to 3.0 ml/hr/kg. The renal clearance of PB, urine pH, and PB volume of distribution did not change significantly.

Mechanism

Metabolic studies in 4 patients coadministered PB and VPA found a decrease in the hepatic conversion of phenobarbital to hydroxyphenylphenobarbital and decreased the urinary hydroxyphenylphenobarbital:PB ratio (Bruni et al. 1980a). These data imply an inhibition of the hepatic microsomal enzymes. The VPA-mediated inhibition of PB hepatic metabolism may be secondary to VPA's short-chain fatty acid structures; fatty acids have been shown to nonspecifically inhibit hepatic oxidative and/or conjugative metabolic processes (Lang 1976, Patel et al. 1980).

PHENYTOIN (*See* PHENYTOIN *section in this chapter.*)

NAPROXEN

Evidence of Interaction

A single study in healthy volunteers suggested that naproxen may displace valproic acid from its protein-binding sites (Grimaldi et al. 1984).

Mechanism

Naproxen displaces valproic acid from its protein-binding sites.

Clinical Implications

This is probably not a clinically significant interaction, although if a patient had high serum levels of VPA, a temporary increase in unbound levels could lead to transient adverse effects.

NEUROLEPTICS (CHLORPROMAZINE AND HALOPERIDOL)

Evidence of Interaction

Ishizaka and colleagues (1984) administered VPA 400 mg/day to 6 schizophrenic patients, measured the minimum trough levels of VPA (C_{min}), and compared these values to C_{min} of VPA after a single 400-mg dose of chlorpromazine was coadministered. The mean C_{min} of VPA when coadministered with chlorpromazine (33.2 ± 1.7 μg/ml) was significantly greater ($P < 0.01$) than when VPA was administered alone (27 ± 1.4 μg/ml). With discontinuation of the chlorpromazine (after a 2-week washout period) the mean VPA elimination half-life was shortened from 15.4 (±1.4) to 13.5 (±1.2) hours ($P < 0.05$), with a corresponding increase in VPA clearance from 7.18 (±0.38) to 8.32 (±0.34) ml/hr/kg ($P < 0.01$). Of note is that this study was nonblind and no placebo was used. The same investigators found that haloperidol (6–10 mg/day) had no significant effect on the C_{min}, half-life, or clearance of VPA.

Mechanism

Chlorpromazine may competitively inhibit the metabolism of VPA. VPA and chlorpromazine share common metabolic pathways, while haloperidol is metabolized primarily via oxidative dealkylation.

Clinical Implications

VPA increases endogenous brain γ-aminobutyric acid levels (Pinder et al. 1977) and may improve psychotic symptoms (Linnoila et al. 1980). Given the possible effectiveness in schizophrenia and mania, there is the potential for valproate and chlorpromazine to be used in combination. Chlorpromazine has been shown to increase the C_{min} and elimination half-life and to decrease the clearance of VPA, which may lead to VPA toxicity. Thus, the physician should monitor VPA serum concentrations closely and make VPA dosage adjustments as necessary.

THIOPENTAL

Evidence of Interaction

There is an increase in the unbound fraction of the anesthetic agent thiopental in rabbits also receiving valproate (Aguilera et al. 1986). In the absence of VPA, the unbound fraction of thiopental was 15.2% (±0.64%) but with the concentration of VPA above the therapeutic range, the unbound fraction of thiopental was increased to 22.42% (±1.65%). In addition, the recovery time from the hypnotic effects of thiopental was increased in the presence of VPA.

Mechanism

It would appear from the above study that VPA, which is extensively protein bound, causes protein displacement of thiopental, increasing the unbound fraction.

Clinical Implications

Because unbound thiopental would be more accessible to the central nervous system, leading to prolonged hypnotic anesthetic effects, doses of thiopental in the anesthesia of epileptic or psychiatric patients taking VPA may require downward adjustments.

ZIDOVUDINE (AZT)

Evidence of Interaction

In vitro studies in human liver microsomes suggest that valproic acid may impair zidovudine metabolism (Rajaonarison et al. 1992). Coadministration of zidovudine and valproic acid increased plasma area-under-the-curve for zidovudine 2-fold (Lertora et al. 1994).

Mechanism

Valproic acid impairs glucuronidation of zidovudine.

Clinical Implications

Unknown.

REFERENCES

Aanderud S et al.: The influence of carbamazepine on thyroid hormones and thyroxine-binding globulin in hypothyroid patients substituted with thyroxine. Clin Endocrinol 15: 247, 1981.
Abbott FS et al.: The effects of aspirin on valproic acid metabolism. Clin Pharmacol Ther 40: 94, 1986.
Adams DJ et al.: Sodium valproate in the treatment of intractable seizure disorders, a clinical and electroencephalographic study. Neurology 28: 152, 1978.
Aguilera L et al.: Interaction between thiopentone and sodium valproate. Br J Anaesth 58: 1380, 1986.
Ahmad S.: Diltiazem-carbamazepine interaction. Am Heart J 120: 1485, 1990.
Ahmad S et al.: Renal sensitivity to frusemide caused by chronic anticonvulsant therapy. Br Med J 3: 657, 1974.
Alestig K et al.: Studies on the intestinal excretion of doxycycline. Scand J Infect Dis 6: 265, 1974.

Alvarez JS et al.: Effect of carbamazepine on cyclosporine blood level. Nephron 58: 235, 1991.

Andreasen PB et al.: Diphenylhydantoin half-life in man and its inhibition by phenylbutazone: the role of genetic factors. Acta Med Scand 193: 561, 1973.

Bahls F et al.: Interactions between calcium channel blockers and the anticonvulsants carbamazepine and phenytoin. Neurology 41: 740, 1991.

Ballek RE et al.: Inhibition of diphenylhydantoin metabolism by chloramphenicol (letter). Lancet 1: 150, 1973.

Bartle WR et al.: Dose-dependent effect of cimetidine on phenytoin kinetics. Clin Pharmacol Ther 33: 649, 1983.

Bauer LA: Interference of oral phenytoin absorption by continuous nasogastric feedings. Neurology 32: 570-572, 1982.

Baylis EM et al.: Influence of folic acid on blood phenytoin levels. Lancet 1: 62, 1971.

Beattie F et al.: Verapamil induced carbamazepine neurotoxicity. Eur Neurol 28: 104, 1988.

Bell J et al.: The use of serum methadone levels in patients receiving methadone maintenance. Clin Pharmacol Ther 43: 623, 1988.

Blackshear JL et al.: Thyroxine replacement requirements in hypothyroid patients receiving phenytoin. Ann Intern Med 99: 341, 1983.

Block SH et al.: Carbamazepine-isoniazid interaction. Pediatrics 69: 494, 1982.

Blum RA et al.: Effect of fluconazole on the disposition of phenytoin. Clin Pharmacol Ther 49: 420, 1991.

Bochner F et al.: Factors involved in an outbreak of phenytoin intoxication. J Neurol Scand 16: 481, 1972

Bollini P et al.: Decreased phenytoin level during antineoplastic therapy: a case report. Epilepsia 24: 75, 1983.

Booker HE et al.: Concurrent administration of phenobarbital and diphenylhydantoin: lack of interference effect. Neurology 21: 383, 1971.

Bourgeois BFD et al.: Interactions between carbamazepine and nicotinamide. Neurology 32: 1122, 1982.

Bowdle TA et al.: Effects of carbamazepine on valproic acid kinetics in normal subjects. Clin Pharmacol Ther 26: 629, 1979.

Brennan RW et al.: Diphenylhydantoin intoxication attendant to slow intoxication of isoniazid. Neurology 20: 687, 1970.

Brodie MJ, Macphee GJ: Carbamazepine neurotoxicity precipitated by diltiazem. Br Med J 292: 1170, 1986.

Brooks SM et al.: Adverse effects of phenobarbital on corticosteroid metabolism in patients with bronchial asthma. N Engl J Med 86: 1125, 1972.

Browne TR: Interaction between clonazepam and sodium valproate (reply). N Engl J Med 300: 678, 1979.

Browne TR et al.: Carbamazepine increases phenytoin serum concentrations and reduces phenytoin clearance. Neurology 38: 1146, 1988.

Bruni J et al.: Valproic acid and plasma levels of phenobarbital. Neurology 30: 94, 1980a.

Bruni J et al.: Interactions of valproic acid with phenytoin. Neurology 30: 1233, 1980b.

Buchanan RA, Allen RJ: Diphenylhydantoin and phenobarbital blood levels of epileptic children. Neurology 21: 866, 1971.

Capewell S et al.: Gross reduction in felodipine bioavailability in patients taking anticonvulsants. Br J Clin Pharmacol 24: 243, 1987.

Carranco E et al.: Carbamazepine toxicity induced by concurrent erythromycin therapy. Arch Neurol 42: 187, 1985.

Cathro DM et al.: Case report: sub-normal serum thyroxine levels associated with carbamazepine and valproic acid treatment. Nebr Med J 70: 235, 1985.

Cereghino JJ: Preliminary observations on serum carbamazepine concentrations in epileptic patients. Neurology 23: 357, 1973.

Cereghino JJ et al.: The efficacy of carbamazepine combinations in epilepsy. Clin Pharmacol Ther 18: 733, 1975.

Chapron DJ et al.: Effect of calcium and antacids on phenytoin bioavailability. Arch Neurol 36: 439, 1979.

Chaudhry RP et al.: Lithium and carbamazepine interaction: possible neurotoxicity. J Clin Psychiatry 44: 1, 1983.

Christiansen J, Dam M: Influence of phenobarbital and diphenylhydantoin on plasma carbamazepine levels in patients with epilepsy. Acta Neurol Scand 49: 453, 1973.

Christiansen LK, Skovsted L: Inhibition of drug metabolism by chloramphenicol. Lancet 2: 1397, 1969.

Choi Y et al.: Effect of diphenylhydantoin on cortisol kinetics in humans. J Pharmacol Exp Ther 176: 27, 1971.

Connell JMC et al.: Changes in circulating thyroid hormones during short-term hepatic enzyme induction with carbamazepine. Eur J Clin Pharmacol 26: 453, 1984.

Coulam CB et al.: Do anticonvulsants reduce the efficacy of oral contraceptives? Epilepsia 20: 519, 1979.

Crawford P et al.: The interaction of phenytoin and carbamazepine with combined oral contraceptive steroids. Br J Clin Pharmacol. 30: 892, 1990.

Dalton MJ et al.: The influence of cimetidine on a single dose carbamazepine pharmacokinetics. Epilepsia 26: 127, 1985.

Dalton MJ et al.: Cimetidine and carbamazepine: a complex drug interaction. Epilepsia 27: 553, 1986.

Dam M et al.: Interaction between carbamazepine and propoxyphene in man. Acta Neurol Scand 566: 603, 1977.

Danan G et al.: Self induction by erythromycin of its own transformation into a metabolite forming an inactive complex with cytochrome P450. J Pharmacol Exp Ther 218: 509, 1981.

Data JL et al.: Interaction of quinidine with anticonvulsant drugs. N Engl J Med 294: 699, 1976.

Dhillon SA et al.: Valproic acid and diazepam interactions in vivo. Br J Clin Pharmacol 13: 353, 1982.

Dillard ML et al.: Ciprofloxacin-phenytoin interaction (letter). Ann Pharmacother 26: 263, 1992.

Dravet C et al.: Interaction between carbamazepine and triacetyloleandomycin. Lancet 1: 810, 1977.

Edwards JG et al.: Antidepressants and seizures: epidemiological and clinical aspects. In: Trimble MR (ed.): The Psychopharmacology of Epilepsy, Chichester, John Wiley, 1985, p. 119.

Ehrnebo M et al.: Distribution of phenobarbital and diphenylhydantoin between plasma and cells in blood: effect of salicylic acid, temperature and total drug concentration. Eur J Clin Pharmacol 11: 37, 1977.

Eimer M et al.: Elevated serum carbamazepine concentrations following diltiazem initiation. Drug Intell Clin Pharm 21: 340, 1987.

Faigle JW et al.: The biotransformation of carbamazepine. In: Birkmayer W (ed.): Epileptic Seizures Behavior and Pain, Baltimore, University Park Press, 1976.

Fincham RW et al.: The influence of diphenylhydantoin on primidone metabolism. Arch Neurol 30: 259, 1974.

Fincham RW et al.: Decreased phenytoin levels in antineoplastic therapy. Ther Drug Monit 1: 277, 1979.

Fine A et al.: Malabsorption of frusemide caused by phenytoin. Br Med J 3: 1061, 1977.

Finelli PF: Phenytoin and methadone tolerance. N Engl J Med 294: 227, 1976.

Fleitman JS et al.: Albumin binding interaction of sodium valproate. J Clin Pharmacol 20: 514, 1980.

Frantzen E et al.: Phenytoin (Dilantin) intoxication. Acta Neurol Scand 43: 440, 1967.

Fraser DG et al.: Displacement of phenytoin from plasma binding sites by salicylate. Clin Pharmacol Ther 27: 165, 1980.

Freeman DJ et al.: Evaluation of cyclosporin-phenytoin interaction with observations of cyclosporin metabolites. Br J Clin Pharmacol 18: 887, 1984.

Fulop M et al.: Possible diphenylhydantoin induced arrhythmia in hypothyroidism. JAMA 196: 454, 1966.

Furlant M et al.: Effects of folic acid on phenytoin kinetics in healthy subjects. Clin Pharmacol Ther 24: 294, 1978.

Gadde K et al.: Diltiazem effect on carbamazepine levels in manic depression. J Clin Psych 10: 378, 1990.

Garnett WR et al.: Bioavailability of phenytoin administered with antacids. Ther Drug Monit 1: 435, 1979.

Garrettson LK et al.: Methylphenidate interaction with both anticonvulsants and ethyl biscoumacetate: a new action of methylphenidate. JAMA 207: 2053, 1969.

Gore JM et al.: Interaction of amiodarone and diphenylhydantoin. Am J Cardiol 54: 1145, 1984.

Goulden KJ et al.: Clinical valproate toxicity induced by acetylsalicylic acid. Neurology 37:1392, 1987.

Griffin GD et al.: Primidone-phenobarbital intoxication. Drug Ther 60: 76, 1976.

Grimaldi R et al.: In vivo plasma protein binding interaction between valproic acid and naproxen. Eur J Drug Metab Pharmacokinet 9: 359, 1984.

Hague N et al.: Studies on dexamethasone metabolism in man: effect of diphenylhydantoin. J Clin Endocrinol Metab 34: 44, 1972.

Hall TG et al.: Effect of sucralfate on phenytoin bioavailability. Drug Intell Clin Pharm 20: 607, 1986.

Hansen BS et al.: Influence of dextropropoxyphene on steady-state serum level and protein binding of three anti-epileptic drugs in man. Acta Neurol Scand 61: 357, 1980.

Hansen JM et al.: Dicoumarol-induced diphenylhydantoin intoxication. Lancet 2: 265, 1966.

Hansen JM et al.: Sulthiame (Ospolot [R]) as an inhibitor of diphenylhydantoin metabolism. Epilepsia 9: 17, 1968.

Hansen JM et al.: Carbamazepine induced acceleration of diphenylhydantoin and warfarin metabolism in man. Clin Pharmacol Ther 12: 539, 1971.

Hansen JM et al.: Potentiation of warfarin by co-trimoxazole. Br Med J 1: 684, 1975.

Hansen JM et al.: The effect of different sulfonamides on phenytoin metabolism in man. Acta Med Scand Suppl 624: 106, 1979.

Hansson O et al.: Pyridoxine and serum concentrations of phenytoin and phenobarbitone. Lancet 1: 256, 1976.

Hansten PD: Interactions between anticonvulsant drugs: primidone, diphenylhydantoin and phenobarbital. Northwest Med 1: 17, 1974.

Hansten P: Drug Interactions Newsletter 2:43-44, 1982.

Hatton RC: Dietary interaction with phenytoin (letter). Clin Pharmacol 3: 110, 1984.

Hedrick R et al.: Carbamazepine-erythromycin interaction leading to carbamazepine toxicity in four epileptic children. Ther Drug Monit 5: 405, 1983.

Hetzel DJ et al.: Cimetidine interaction with phenytoin. Br Med J 282: 1512, 1981.

Hillebrand G et al.: Valproate for epilepsy in renal transplant recipients receiving cyclosporine. Transplantation 43: 915, 1987.

Hommes OR and Obbens EA. The epileptogenic action of Na-folate in the rat. J Neurol Sci 16: 271–281, 1972.

Hooper WD et al.: Preliminary observations on the clinical pharmacology of carbamazepine. Proc Aus Assoc Neurol 11: 189, 1974.

Houghton GW et al.: Inhibition of phenytoin metabolism by sulthiame in epileptic patients. Br J Clin Pharm 1: 59, 1974a.

Houghton GW et al.: Phenytoin intoxication induced by sulthiame in epileptic patients. J Neurol Neurosurg Psychiatry 37: 275, 1974b.

Houghton GW et al.: Inhibition of phenytoin metabolism by other drugs during epilepsy. Int J Clin Pharmacol 12: 210, 1975.

Howitt KM et al.: Phenytoin toxicity induced by fluconazole (letter). Med J Aust 151: 603, 1989.

Hull RL.: Possible phenytoin-ciprofloxacin interaction (letter). Ann Pharmacother 27: 1283, 1993.

Hunninghake DB: Drug interactions. Postgrad Med 47: 71, 1970.

Ishizaka T et al.: The effects of neuroleptics (haloperidol and chlorpromazine) on the pharmacokinetics of valproic acid in schizophrenic patients. J Clin Psychopharmacol 4: 254, 1984.

Iteogu MD et al.: Effect of cimetidine on single-dose phenytoin kinetics. Clin Pharm 2: 302, 1983.

Jaillon P et al.: Phenytoin induced changes in quinidine and 3-hydroxyquinidine pharmacokinetics in conscious dogs. J Pharmacol Exp Ther 213: 33, 1980.

Janz D: The teratogenic risk of antiepileptic drugs. Epilepsia 16: 159, 1975.

Janz D et al.: Anti-epileptic drugs and failure of oral contraceptives (letter). Lancet 1: 1113, 1974.

Jensen ON et al.: Subnormal serum folate due to anticonvulsive therapy: a double-blind study of the effect of folic acid treatment in patients with drug-induced subnormal serum folates. Arch Neurology 22: 181, 1971.

Johannessen SI et al.: The influence of phenobarbital and phenytoin on carbamazepine serum levels. In Schneider H, Janz D, Garoner-Thorpe C et al. (eds.): Clinical Pharmacology of Anti-epileptic Drugs, New York, Springer, 1975, p. 201.

Jubiz W et al.: Effect of diphenylhydantoin on the metabolism of dexamethasone. Mechanism of the abnormal dexamethasone suppression in humans. N Engl J Med 283: 11, 1970.

Karlin JM, Kutt H: Acute diphenylhydantoin intoxication following halothane anesthesia. J Pediatr 76: 941, 1970.

Karlsson E et al.: Plasma levels of lidocaine during combined treatment with phenytoin and procainamide. Eur J Clin Pharm 7:455, 1974.

Kater RMH et al.: Increased rate of clearance of drugs from the circulation of alcoholics. Am J Med Sci 258: 35, 1969.

Kendall AG, Boivin M: Warfarin-carbamazepine interaction (letter). Ann Intern Med 94: 280, 1981.

Kenyon IE: Unplanned pregnancy in an epileptic. Br Med J 1: 686, 1972.

Ketter TA et al.: Principles of clinically important drug interactions with carbamazepine, part I. J Clin Psychopharm 11: 198, 1991a.

Ketter TA et al.: Principles of clinically important drug interactions with carbamazepine, part II. J Clin Psychopharm 11: 306, 1991b.

Kiorboe E.: Phenytoin intoxication during treatment with Antabuse (disulfiram). Epilepsia 7: 246, 1966.

Knopp RH et al.: Diphenylhydantoin and an insulin-secreting islet adenoma. Arch Intern Med 130: 904, 1972.

Krämer G et al.: Carbamazepine-danazol drug interaction: its mechanism examined by a stable isotope technique. Ther Drug Monit 8: 387, 1986.

Kulshrestha VK et al.: Interaction between phenytoin and antacids. Br J Clin Pharmacol 6: 177, 1978.

Kumer D et al.: Diagnostic use of glucagon-induced insulin response: studies of patients with insulinoma or other hypoglycemic conditions. Ann Intern Med 80: 697, 1974.

Kupferberg HJ et al.: Effect of methylphenidate on plasma anticonvulsant levels. Clin Pharmacol Ther 13: 201, 1972.

Kutt H et al.: Depression of parahydroxylation of diphenylhydantoin by antituberculosis chemotherapy. Neurology 16: 594, 1966.

Kutt H et al.: The effect of phenobarbital on plasma diphenylhydantoin level and metabolism in man and in rat liver microsomes. Neurology 19: 611, 1969.

Kutt H et al.: Diphenylhydantoin intoxication: a complication of isoniazid therapy. Am Rev Respir Dis 101: 377, 1970.

Kutt H: Interaction of antiepileptic drugs. Epilepsia 16: 393, 1975.

Laengner H et al.: Antiepileptic drugs and failure of oral contraceptives (letter). Lancet 2: 600, 1974.

Lander CM et al.: Interactions between anticonvulsants. Proc Aust Assoc Neurol 12: 111, 1975.

Lang M et al.: Depression of drug metabolism in liver microsomes after treating rats with unsaturated fatty acids. Gen Pharmacol 415, 1976.

Lele P et al.: Cyclosporine and tegretol—another drug interaction. Kidney Int 27: 344, 1985.

Leonard RF et al.: Phenytoin-salicylate interaction. Clin Pharmacol Ther 29: 56, 1981.

Lertora JJ et al.: Pharmacokinetic interaction between zidovudine and valproic acid in patients infected with human immunodeficiency virus. Clin Pharmacol Ther 56: 272, 1994.

Levine M et al.: Differential effect of cimetidine on serum concentrators of carbamazepine and phenytoin. Neurology 35: 562, 1985.

Levy RH et al.: Carbamazepine-valproic acid interaction in man and rhesus monkey. Epilepsia 25: 338, 1984.

Linnoila M et al.: Effects of sodium valproate on tardive dyskinesia. Br J Psychiatry 137: 240, 1980.

Luder PJ et al.: Treatment of hydatid disease with high oral doses of mebendazole: long-term follow-up of plasma mebendazole levels and drug interactions. Eur J Clin Pharmacol 31: 443, 1986.

Lumholtz B et al.: Sulfamethizole-induced inhibition of diphenylhydantoin, tolbutamide and warfarin metabolism. Clin Pharmacol Ther 17: 731, 1975.

Lunde PKM: Plasma protein binding of diphenylhydantoin in man: interaction with other drugs and the effect of temperature and plasma dilution. Clin Pharmacol Ther 11: 846, 1970.

Macphee GJ et al.: Effects of cimetidine on carbamazepine auto and heteroinduction in man. Br J Clin Pharmacol 18: 411, 1984.

Macphee GJ et al.: Verapamil potentiates carbamazepine neurotoxicity: a clinically important interaction. Lancet 1: 700, 1986.

Mallette LE: Anticonvulsants, acetazolamide, and osteomalacia (letter). N Engl J Med 293: 668, 1975.

Mallette LE: Acetazolamide-accelerated anticonvulsant osteomalacia. Arch Intern Med 137: 1013, 1977.

Marquis SF et al.: Phenytoin-theophylline interaction. N Engl J Med 307: 1189, 1982.

Marsden JR: Effect of isotretinoin on carbamazepine pharmacokinetics. Br J Derm 119: 403, 1988.

Mattson RH et al.: Folate therapy in epilepsy: clinical and pharmacological effects. Arch Neurol 29: 79, 1973.

Mattson RH et al.: Valproic acid in epilepsy: clinical and pharmacological effects. Ann Neurol 3: 20, 1978.

Mattson GF et al.: Interaction between valproic acid and carbamazepine in an in vitro study of protein binding. Ther Drug Monit 4: 181, 1982.

Maxwell JD et al.: Folate deficiency after anticonvulsant drugs: an effect of hepatic enzyme induction? Br Med J 1: 297, 1972.

May CA et al.: Effects of three antacids on the bioavailability of valproic acid. Clin Pharm 1: 244, 1982.

McGovern B et al.: Possible interaction between amiodarone and phenytoin. Ann Intern Med 101: 650, 1984.

McKauge L et al.: Factors influencing simultaneous concentrations of carbamazepine and its epoxide in plasma. Ther Drug Monit 4: 181, 1982.

McLelland J, Jack W: Phenytoin-dexamethasone interactions: a clinical problem. Lancet i: 1096, 1978.

Meikle AW et al.: Effect of diphenylhydantoin on the metabolism of metyrapone and the release of ACTH in man. J Clin Endocrinol Metab 29: 1553, 1969.

Meikle AW et al.: Kinetics and interconversion of prednisolone and prednisone studied with new radioimmunoassays. J Clin Endocrinol Metab 41: 717, 1975.

Mendez JS et al.: Diphenylhydantoin blocking of levodopa effects. Arch Neurol 32: 44, 1975.

Mesdjian E et al.: Carbamazepine intoxication due to triacetyloleandomycin administration in epileptic patients. Epilepsia 21: 489, 1980.

Mirkin BL, Wright F: Drug interactions: effect of methylphenidate on the disposition of diphenylhydantoin in man. Neurology 21: 1123, 1971.

Mitsch RA.: Carbamazepine toxicity precipitated by intravenous erythromycin. Drug Intell Clin Phar 23: 878, 1989.

Monks A et al.: Effect of single doses of sodium valproate on serum levels and protein binding in epileptic patients. Clin Pharmacol Ther 27: 89, 1980.

Morselli PL et al.: Interaction between phenobarbital and diphenylhydantoin in animals and in epileptic patients. Ann NY Acad Sci 179: 88, 1971.

Murray FJ: Outbreak of unexpected reactions among epileptics taking isoniazid. Am Rev Respir Dis 86: 729, 1962.

Nappi JM: Warfarin and phenytoin interaction. Ann Intern Med 90: 852, 1979.

Neuvonen PJ et al.: Interaction between doxycycline and barbiturates. Br Med J 1: 535, 1974.

Neuvonen PJ et al.: Effect of antiepileptic drugs on the elimination of various tetracycline derivatives. Eur J Clin Pharmacol 9: 147, 1975.

Neuvonen PJ et al.: Antipyretic analgesics in patients on antiepileptic drug therapy. Eur J Clin Pharmacol 15: 263, 1979.

Neuvonen PJ et al.: Cimetidine-phenytoin interaction: effect on serum phenytoin concentration and antipyrine test in man. Naunyn-Schmied Arch Pharmacol 313(suppl): R60, 1980.

Norris JW, Pratt RF: A controlled study of folic acid in epilepsy. Neurology 21: 659, 1971.

Norris JW, Pratt RF: Folic acid deficiency and epilepsy. Drugs 8: 366, 1974.

O'Brien WM et al.: Failure of antacids to alter the pharmacokinetics of phenytoin. Br J Clin Pharmacol 6: 276, 1978.

Oettinger L.: Interaction of methylphenidate and diphenylhydantoin. Drug Ther 5: 107, 1976.

Olesen OV et al.: The influence of disulfiram and calcium carbamide on the serum diphenylhydantoin. Arch Neurol 16: 642, 1967.

Olesen OV et al.: Drug-interaction between sulthiame (Ospolot [R]) and phenytoin in the treatment of epilepsy. Dan Med Bull 16: 154, 1969.

Olivesi A.: Modified elimination of prednisolone in epileptic patients on carbamazepine monotherapy, and in women using low-dose oral contraceptives. Biomed Pharmacother 40: 301, 1986.

Orr J et al.: Interaction between valproic acid and aspirin in epileptic children: serum protein binding and metabolic effects. Clin Pharmacol Ther 31: 642, 1982.

Patel IH et al.: Phenobarbital-valproic acid interaction. Clin Pharmacol Ther 27: 515, 1980.

Patsalos PN et al.: Effect of sodium valproate on plasma protein binding of diphenylhydantoin. J Neurol Neurosurg Psychiatry 40: 570, 1977.

Paxton JW: Effects of aspirin on salivary and serum phenytoin kinetics in healthy subjects. Clin Pharmacol Ther 27: 170, 1980.

Peck AW: Clinical pharmacology of lamotrigine. Epilepsia 32(S): S9, 1991.

Penttila O et al.: Interaction between doxycycline and some antiepileptic drugs. Br Med J 2: 470, 1974.

Perel JM, Black N: In vitro metabolism studies with methylphenidate. Fed Proc 29: 315, 1970.

Perucca E and Richens A: Paracetamol disposition in normal subjects and in patients treated with antiepileptic drugs. Br J Clin Pharmacol 7: 201, 1971.

Petereit LB et al.: Effectiveness of prednisolone during phenytoin therapy. Clin Pharmacol Ther 22: 912, 1977.

Petro DJ et al.: Diazoxide-diphenylhydantoin interaction. J Pediatr 89: 331, 1975.

Pinder PM et al.: Sodium valproate: a review of its pharmacological properties and therapeutic efficacy. Drugs 13: 81, 1977.

Pisani F et al.: Valproic acid-ethosuximide interaction: a pharmacokinetic study. Epilepsy 25: 229, 1984.

Pisani F et al.: Carbamazepine-viloxazine interaction in patients with epilepsy. J Neurol Neurosurg Psychiatry 49: 1142, 1986.

Pisani F et al.: Interaction of lamotrigine with sodium valproate. Lancet 341: 445, 1993.

Porro M et al.: Phenytoin: an inhibitor and inducer of primidone metabolism in an epileptic patient. Br J Clin Pharmacol 14: 294, 1982.

Price WA. Verapamil-carbamazepine neurotoxicity. J Clin Psych 49: 80, 1988.

Privitera M et al.: Interference by carbamazepine with the dexamethasone suppression test. Biol Psychiatry 17: 611, 1982.

Pugh RNH et al.: Interaction of phenytoin with chlorpheniramine (letter). Br J Clin Pharmacol 2: 174, 1975.

Raitaxuo V et al.: Carbamazepine and plasma levels of clozapine (letter). Am J Psychiatry 150: 169, 1993.

Rajaonarison JF et al.: 3'-azido-3'-deoxythymidine drug interactions: screening for inhibitors in human liver microsomes. Drug Metab Dispos 20: 578, 1992.

Rane A et al.: Kinetics of carbamazepine and its 10,11-epoxide metabolite in children. Clin Pharmacol Ther 19: 276, 1976.

Rapport DJ et al.: Interactions between carbamazepine and birth control pills (letter). Psychosomatics 30: 462, 1989.

Renton KW: Inhibition of hepatic microsomal drug metabolism by calcium channel blockers diltiazem and verapamil. Biochem Pharmacol 34: 2549, 1985.

Reunanen MI et al.: Low serum valproic acid concentrations in epileptic patients on combination therapy. Curr Ther Res 28: 456, 1980.

Reutens DC et al.: Disabling tremor after lamotrigine with sodium valproate. Lancet 342: 185, 1993.

Reynolds EH: Effects of folic acid on the mental state and fit-frequency of drug-treated epileptic patients. Lancet 1: 1086, 1967.

Reynolds EH: Anticonvulsants, folic acid, and epilepsy. Lancet 1: 376, 1973.

Reynolds ES et al.: Massive hepatic necrosis after fluroxene anesthesia—a case of drug interaction? N Engl J Med 286: 530, 1972.

Richens A et al.: Phenytoin intoxication caused by sulthiame. Lancet 2: 1442, 1973.

Roe TF et al.: Drug interaction, diazoxide and diphenylhydantoin. J Pediatr 89: 331, 1975.

Rose JQ et al.: Intoxication caused by interaction of chloramphenicol and phenytoin. JAMA 237: 2630, 1977.

Rose JQ et al.: Prednisolone pharmacokinetics in relation to dose (letter). J Pediatr 94: 1014, 1979.

Rosenberry KR et al.: Reduced theophylline half-life induced by carbamazepine therapy. J Pediatr 102: 472, 1983.

Ross JR and Belley L: Interaction between carbamazepine and warfarin. Br Med J 2: 1415, 1980.

Rothermich NO: Diphenylhydantoin intoxication. Lancet 2: 640, 1966.

Rotne H et al.: Pharmacokinetics of 2-propylaleric acid (Depakene) in epileptic children. In: Johannessen S (ed.): *Antiepileptic Therapy: Advances in Drug Monitoring*, New York, Raven, 1980, p. 57.

Roy-Byrne PP et al.: Carbamazepine and thyroid function in affectively ill patients: clinical and theoretical implications. Arch Gen Psychiatry 41: 1150, 1984.

Salem RB et al.: Effect of cimetidine on phenytoin serum levels. Epilepsia 24: 284, 1983.

Schmidt D: Effects of ethanol intake on phenytoin metabolism in volunteers. Experientia 31: 1313, 1980.

Schneider H: Carbamazepine: the influence of other antiepileptic drugs on its serum level. In: Schneider H, Janz D, Gardner-Thorpe C et al. (eds.): *Clinical Pharmacology of Antiepileptic Drugs*, New York, Springer, 1975, p. 189.

Schobben F et al.: Pharmacokinetics, metabolism and distribution of 2-propylpentanoate (sodium valproate) and the influence of salicylate co-medication. In: Meinardi H, Rowan AJ (eds.): *Advances in Epileptology*, Amsterdam, Swet and Zeiftinger, 1978, p. 271.

Schofield OMV et al.: Cyclosporin A in psoriasis: interaction with carbamazepine (letter). Br J Dermatol 122: 425, 1190.

Shoeman DM et al.: Diphenylhydantoin potency and plasma protein binding. J Pharmacol Exp Ther 195: 84, 1975.

Shukla S et al.: Lithium-carbamazepine neurotoxicity and risk factors. Am J Psychiatry 141: 1604, 1984.

Siersbaek-Nielsen K et al.: Sulphamethizole-induced inhibition of diphenylhydantoin and tolbutamide metabolism in man. Clin Pharmacol Ther 14: 148, 1973.

Skovsted L et al.: The effect of different oral anticoagulants on diphenylhydantoin (DPH) and tolbutamide metabolism (abstract). Acta Med Scand 199: 513, 1976.

Smart HL et al.: The effects of sucralfate upon phenytoin absorption in man. Br J Clin Pharmacol 20: 238, 1985.

Solomon GE et al.: Coagulation defects caused by diphenylhydantoin. Neurology 22: 1165, 1972.

Solomon HM et al.: Interactions between digitoxin and other drugs *in vitro* and *in vivo*. Ann NY Acad Sci 179: 362, 1971.

Sonne J et al.: Lack of interaction between cimetidine and carbamazepine. Acta Neurol Scan 68: 253, 1983.

Soyaniemi E et al.: The clinical significance of microsomal enzyme induction in the therapy of epileptic patients. Ann Clin Res 2: 223, 1970.

Speidel BD, Meadow SR: Epilepsy, anticonvulsants and congenital malformations. Drugs 8: 354, 1974.

Stjernholm MR et al.: Effects of diphenylhydantoin, phenobarbital, and diazepam on the metabolism of methylprednisolone and its sodium succinate. J Clin Endocrinol Metab 41: 887, 1975.

Strauss RG, Bernstein R: Folic acid and dilantin antagonism in pregnancy. Obstet Gynecol 44: 345, 1974.

Sutton G et al.: Isoniazid as an inhibitor of primidone metabolism. Neurology 25: 1179, 1975.

Sylvester RK et al.: Impaired phenytoin bioavailability secondary to cisplatin, vinblastine, and bleomycin. Ther Drug Monit 6: 302, 1984.

Syversen GB et al.: Acetazolamide-induced interference with primidone absorption. Arch Neurol 34: 80, 1977.

Taylor JW et al.: The interaction of phenytoin and theophylline. Drug Intell Clin Pharm 14: 638, 1980.

Tong TG: Phenytoin induced methadone withdrawal. Ann Intern Med 94: 349, 1981.

Tyrer JH et al.: Outbreak of anticonvulsant intoxication in an Australian city. Br Med J 4: 271, 1970.

Valsalan VC, Cooper GL: Carbamazepine intoxication caused by interaction with isoniazid. Br Med J 285: 261, 1982.

Vapaatalo H, Lehtinen L: Variations of serum diphenylhydantoin concentrations in epileptic out-patients. Eur Neurol 5: 303–310, 1971.

Wagner ML et al.: Effect of felbamate on carbamazepine and its major metabolite. Clin Pharmacol Ther 53: 536, 1993.

Wagner ML et al.: The effect of felbamate on valproic acid disposition. Clin Pharmacol Ther 56: 494, 1994.

Warner T et al.: Lamotrigine-induced carbamazepine toxicity: an interaction with carbamazepine-10,11-epoxide. Epilepsy Res 11: 147, 1992.

Wassner SJ et al.: The adverse effect of anticonvulsant therapy on renal allograft survival. J Pediatr 88: 134, 1976.

Watson WA.: Interaction between clonazepam and sodium valproate. N Engl J Med 300: 678, 1979.

Watts RW et al.: Lack of interaction between ranitidine and phenytoin (letter). Br J Clin Pharmacol 15: 499, 1983.

Webster LK et al.: Effect of cimetidine and ranitidine on carbamazepine and sodium valproate pharmacokinetics. Eur J Clin Pharmacol 27: 341, 1984.

Wells DG: Folic acid and neuropathy in epilepsy. Lancet 2: 543, 1968.

Werk EE Jr. et al.: Failure of metyrapone to inhibit 11-hydroxylation of 11-deoxycortisol during drug therapy. J Clin Endocrinol Metab 27: 1358, 1967.

Werk EE Jr et al.: Interference in the effect of dexamethasone by diphenylhydantoin. N Engl J Med 281: 32, 1969.

Wilder BJ et al.: Valproic acid: interaction with other anticonvulsant drugs. Neurology 28: 892, 1978.

Windorfer A, Sauer W: Drug interactions during anticonvulsant therapy in childhood; diphenylhydantoin, primidone phenobarbitone, clonazepam, nitrazepam, carbamazepine, and dipropylacetate. Neuropediatrics 8: 29, 1977.

Windorfer A et al.: Elevation of diphenylhydantoin and primidone serum concentration by addition of dipropylacetate, a new anticonvulsant drug. Acta Paediatr Scand 64: 771, 1975.

Witassek F et al.: Chemotherapy of larval echinococcosis with mebendazole: microsomal liver function and cholestasis as determinants of plasma drug level. Eur J Clin Pharmacol 25: 85, 1983.

Wong YY et al.: Effect of erythromycin on carbamazepine pharmacokinetics. Clin Pharmacol Ther 33: 460, 1983.

Wood RA: Sinoatrial arrest: an interaction between phenytoin and lignocaine. Br Med J 1: 645, 1971.

Wright JM et al.: Isoniazid-induced carbamazepine toxicity and vice versa. Med Intell 307: 1325, 1982.

Yee GC et al.: Pharmacokinetic drug interactions with cyclosporine, part 1. Clin Pharmacokinet 19: 319, 1190.

Yokochi K et al.: Phenytoin-allopurinol interaction: Michaelis Menten kinetic parameters of phenytoin with and without allopurinol in a child with Lesch Nyhan syndrome. Ther Drug Monit 4: 353, 1982.

Yu Y et al.: Interaction between carbamazepine and dextropropoxyphene. Postgrad Med J 62: 231, 1986.

Yuen AW et al.: Sodium valproate acutely inhibits lamotrigine metabolism. Br J Clin Pharmacol 33: 511, 1992.

Zielenski JJ et al.: Carbamazepine-phenytoin interactions: elevation of plasma phenytoin concentrations due to carbamazepine co-medication. Ther Drug Monit 7: 51, 1983.

Zielenski JJ et al.: Clinically significant danazol carbamazepine interaction. Ther Drug Monit 9: 24, 1987.

Zitelli BJ et al.: Erythromycin induced drug interactions. Clin Pediatr 26: 117, 1987.

7

β-Blockers

JOHN J. RATEY and KATHLEEN L. MACNAUGHTON

β-Adrenergic blockers made their debut in the medical community in the 1960s as a treatment for hypertension and angina pectoris (Goodman and Gilman 1986). Researchers studying the effects of β-blockers on heart rate, cardiac output, blood pressure, and blood flow in patients with hypertension noticed that some patients reported an increased tolerance to psychological stressors. β-Blockers are beginning to be recognized for their therapeutic value in treating anxiety disorders, tremor, aggression and violent behavior, social phobias, and as adjuncts in the treatment of alcohol withdrawal, mania, and schizophrenia.

Currently there are 14 β-blockers available in the United States. Half-life, metabolism, membrane stabilization, and liposolubility are the most important properties to be considered in β-blocker selection. See Table 7.1 for pharmacologic characteristics to consider when prescribing β-blockers in a psychiatric population. Before initiating treatment with β-blockers, a patient's history should be thoroughly reviewed for contraindicators including the following (Williams et al. 1982, Yudofsky et al. 1981):

- History of allergy to β-adrenergic blocking agents
- History of chronic obstructive pulmonary disease
- History of bronchial asthma
- History of allergic or nonallergic bronchospasm—for example, emphysema
- History of congestive heart failure
- History of severe sinus bradycardia
- History of ventricular failure or cardiac shock
- History of insulin-treated diabetes mellitus

Table 7.1.
Pharmacologic Properties of β-Blockers

Compound	Trade Name	Half-life (hr)	Elimination	Selectivity	Liposolubility
Acebutol	Sectral	3–4	60% Hepatic, 40% Intestinal	β_1, β_2	Medium
Atenolol	Tenormin	6–9	Renal	β_1	Low
Betaxolol	Kerlone	14–22	80% Hepatic	β_1	Low
Bisoprolol	Zebeta	9–12	50% Renal, 50% Hepatic	β_1	Low
Carteolol	Cartrol	5–6	50–70% Renal	$\beta_1, \beta_2, \alpha_1$	Low
Esmolol	Brevibloc	0.15	Esterases	β_1	Low
Labetalol	Trandate	6–8	95% Hepatic, 5% Renal	β_2	Medium
Metoprolol	Lopressor	3–7	Hepatic	β_1	Medium
Nadolol	Corgard	20–24	Renal	β_1, β_2	Low
Penbutolol	Levatol	5	Hepatic and renal	β_2	High
Pindolol	Visken	3–4	60% Hepatic, 40% Renal	β_1, β_2	Medium
Propranolol	Inderal	4–6	Hepatic	β_2	High
Sotalol	Befapace	12	Renal	β_1, β_2	Low
Timolol	Blocadren	4–5	80% Hepatic, 20% Renal	β_1, β_2	Medium

- History of hypoglycemia
- Current or recent (<2 weeks) administration of adrenergic-augmenting psychotropic drugs

Medical screening should include liver and kidney functioning information and measurement of general blood chemistry. When there is indication of hyperthyroidism, hypothyroidism, or liver or renal dysfunction, medications should be reviewed and β-blockers should not be initiated until these levels are within normal limits. A current electrocardiogram (ECG) should be conducted to eliminate patients with a history of pathologic cardiac conduction, including arteriovenous block greater than first-degree, cardiogenic shock, sinus bradycardia with greater than first-degree block, and congestive heart failure.

The dose of β-blockers used is of importance; however, the length of drug administration is also an important variable which can not be overemphasized. Hypotensive side effects often limit the amount of drug tolerated; thus dosage ought to be tailored to the individual patient. Even at low doses, positive effects on behavior can be noted, especially if they are viewed longitudinally. Our experience suggests that behavioral changes can occur in the first month of treatment but may take as long as 6 months before the maximum effect can be noted.

Patients should be withdrawn slowly from β-blockers. Gradual withdrawal is an option due to the nontoxicity of β-blockers. Reduction of total daily dose by one-fourth to one-third every month is standard. In the advent of a negative response—for example, bronchospasm, marked hypotension, or bradycardia—the β-blocker should be discontinued immediately while the heart rate and blood pressure are monitored simultaneously. β-Blockers with the longest half-lives—for example, nadolol—are the safest to discontinue immediately.

The side-effect profile for propranolol includes hypotension, dizziness, nausea, sleep disturbances, and depression. Hypotension is the side effect most likely to occur. Should unfavorable symptoms occur, a moderate decrease in dosage will normally alleviate unfavorable symptoms. β-Blockers with low lipid solubility have fewer CNS side effects and may be a viable alternative to propranolol. Work done with propranolol supports its use in psychiatric disorders, and evidence is accumulating for the use of other β-blockers as well.

α-Adrenoreceptor Antagonists

CLONIDINE

Evidence of Interaction

Numerous case reports and studies have reported that combined therapy with β-blockers enhances the hypertensive response following clonidine withdrawal (Bailey et al. 1991, Bruce 1979, Cairns and Marshall 1976, Harris et al. 1976, Lilja et al. 1980, Rosenthal et al. 1981, Saarimaa 1976, Strauss 1977, Vernon and Sakula 1979, Warren et al. 1979, Yudkin 1977). This interaction possibly caused a fatal cerebellar hemorrhage in 1 patient (Vernon and Sakula 1979). Gradual withdrawal of clonidine in patients who are β-blocked has also been reported to cause hypertensive reactions (Cairns and Marshall 1976, Strauss 1977). Additionally, a paradoxical hypertensive response was reported in patients on continued clonidine therapy who were concomitantly receiving propranolol (Warren et al. 1979) and sotalol (Saarimaa 1976). In one study of 12 patients treated with clonidine, addition of propranolol or sotalol failed to increase blood pressure (Lilja et al. 1980). The hypertensive effect of continued clonidine therapy with the addition of β-blockade has not been established.

Mechanism

During rapid clonidine withdrawal, hypertension is most likely the result of increased circulating catecholamine levels. When patients are receiving a β-blocker and are concurrently undergoing clonidine withdrawal, the vasodilating β response of epinephrine would be blocked, which would subsequently result in an exaggerated vasoconstricting α-response, thus producing hypertension.

Clinical Implications

Discontinuing the β-blocker prior to withdrawing clonidine may reduce the risk of rebound hypertension. Labetalol, which has both α- and β-blocking activity, may be useful in preventing rebound hypertension following the discontinuation of clonidine (Rosenthal et al. 1981). Patients who are maintained on a β-blocker during clonidine withdrawal should be carefully monitored in case of a hypertensive response.

DIHYDROERGOTAMINE

Evidence of Interaction

A case was reported where a 26-year-old normotensive woman taking propranolol prophylactically for migraine headaches was administered oxygen, compazine 5 mg, and dihydroergotamine 0.75 mg intravenously for an acute migraine headache (Gandy et al. 1990). The patient immediately became hypertensive with complaints of crushing substernal chest pain and blood pressure of 180/120 mm Hg. She was hospitalized and was discovered to be hyperthyroid. Although Raskin reported good results in treating presumably euthyroid patients with dihydroergotamine and propranolol (Raskin 1986), others have observed severe peripheral vasoconstriction and ischemia when these drugs were used simultaneously (Baumrucker 1973, Gandy et al. 1990, Venter 1984).

Mechanism

Not established. In this particular patient, the hypermetabolic state associated with hyperthyroidism may have played an instrumental part in causing the observed reaction.

Clinical Implications

Physicians should exercise caution in administering dihydroergotamine to hyperthyroid patients who are receiving therapy with a β-blocker.

Anesthetics

Evidence of Interaction

In a case report of a 68-year-old woman treated concomitantly with digoxin 1 mg/day and metoprolol 50 mg/day for hypertension, a low dose of bupivacaine for intercostal nerve block (ICB) resulted in cardiotoxicity (Roitman et al. 1993). The patient received an uneventful ICB with 94 mg of bupivacaine on the 2d postoperative day. On the 3d postoperative day the patient requested an ICB due to discomfort. Shortly (about 12 minutes) after the ICB the patient experienced abrupt slowing of the heart rate and the ECG depicted bradycardia. The patient experienced cardiac arrest and regained responsiveness within 48 hours. Both metoprolol and digoxin have high depressive potential on the cardiac conduction system; thus it is highly probably that all three drugs interacted to slow impulse propagation through the heart.

The effects of bupivacaine were studied in 26 patients receiving long-term β-receptor blocking therapy (Ponten et al. 1982a). The patients were being treated with β-blockers for hypertension and/or ischemic heart disease, and all were scheduled for gall bladder surgery. Thirteen patients underwent a gradual preoperative withdrawal of the β-receptor blockers, while the remaining 13 were continued on the β-blockers until surgery. Bupivacaine did not produce cardiovascular changes in patients receiving long-term β-receptor blocking therapy. However, 1 patient with cardiac failure showed signs of transient cardiodepression. The authors concluded that bupivacaine did not negatively affect the cardiovascular stability in patients receiving β-blocker therapy. Similar results were obtained in a study of 43 men treated with β-blockers for hypertension and/ or ischemic heart disease (Ponten et al. 1982b). The patients were scheduled for transurethral resections under spinal anesthesia with tetracaine. All patients were randomly subjected to either continuation of or gradual preoperative withdrawal of the β-blocker. In those patients who underwent β-receptor blocker withdrawal, elevated heart rates, arrhythmias, angina pectoris, and postoperative ST-T changes were consistently seen. These changes were not exhibited in the patients who continued their β-receptor blocker therapy during and after spinal anesthesia.

A study of bupivacaine and cardiovascular drugs in closed-chest dogs demonstrated that propranolol increased conduction time and lengthened QRS duration (Timour et al. 1990). An animal study examining the effects of various anesthetic agents (urethane, pentobarbitone, halothane, amobarbitone, ketamine, or chloralose) on propranolol and atenolol demonstrated that anesthetic agents differentially affect the mean arterial pressure response to a β-blocker (Abdelraham et al. 1992). A study of the pulmonary reactivity to methacholine during β-blockade by propranolol and esmolol in rats demonstrated that both esmolol and propranolol significantly decreased heart rate and mean arterial pressure. Propranolol significantly shifted the methacholine dose-response curve so that methacholine increased pulmonary resistance; esmolol did not have this effect (Tobias et al. 1990).

Mechanism

Severe hypertensive reactions may be due to a propranolol-induced blockade of the β-adrenergic stimulatory effect of epinephrine (Foster and Aston 1983).

Clinical Implications

Results from these studies suggest that β-blockers do not need to be discontinued prior to bupivacaine or tetracaine treatment; however, clinicians should watch for evidence of cardiodepression. Additionally, esmolol, which appears to be relatively cardioselective, may be a better choice than a nonselective β-blocker in situations where β-blockers must be used in patients with reactive airway disease (Tobias et al. 1990).

Antacids

Evidence of Interaction

Dobbs and colleagues (1977) conducted a study on 5 normal subjects to determine the interaction between 30 ml of aluminum hydroxide gel and 80 mg of propranolol. Concomitant administration resulted in a mean decrease in maximum plasma concentration of 57% compared with propranolol alone in the same 5 subjects. This indicates that the absorption of propranolol is at least delayed by aluminum hydroxide administration. The total bioavailability also demonstrated a decrease, as evidenced by the 58% reduction in the area-under-the-plasma-concentration-time-curve (AUC).

Hong and colleagues (cited in Gugler 1990) found contrasting results in a study of the plasma concentration of propranolol 40 mg and exercise-induced heart rate when administered concomitantly with 30 ml of aluminum hydroxide gel. The antacid did not alter the bioavailability or the β-adrenoceptor-blocking activity of propranolol. The effects of an aluminum-magnesium hydroxide antacid on the bioavailability of metoprolol and atenolol were studied in 6 healthy volunteers (Regardh et al. 1981). The subjects received (in random order) metoprolol 100 mg, or atenolol 100 mg alone or together with 30 ml of an antacid suspension with an *in vitro* binding capacity of

52.5 mmol HCl by 10 ml of the antacid. Results demonstrated that concomitant administration of the antacid increased the C_{max} of metoprolol by 25% and the AUC by 11%. Both the t_{max} and elimination half-life of metoprolol remained unchanged. The C_{max} of atenolol was significantly reduced by 37% and the AUC by 33% during concomitant administration with the antacid. In a study of 6 healthy subjects receiving atenolol 100 mg in combination with furosemide 40 mg, calcium 500 mg, or with aluminum hydroxide 5.6 g, the aluminum hydroxide produced an insignificant reduction of mean peak plasma levels (about 20%) (Kirch et al. 1981). Combination therapy with calcium had a significant effect on atenolol. The mean peak plasma levels of atenolol decreased by 51% and the elimination half-life increased to a mean of 11.0 hours (compared with 6.2 hours with atenolol alone). The effect of the reduced atenolol bioavailability seems to be somewhat offset by the increased elimination half-life. The prolonged elimination half-life led to atenolol accumulation. Twelve hours after atenolol 100 mg and calcium 500 mg were coadministered, exercise tachycardia was lower than with atenolol alone.

It appears that the gastrointestinal absorption of atenolol and propranolol may be reduced by combined administration with aluminum or magnesium antacids. However, the absorption of metoprolol does not appear to be altered.

Mechanism

Antacids may inhibit the gastrointestinal absorption of some β-adrenoceptor blockers.

Clinical Significance

One should separate doses of β-blockers and antacids by at least 1 hour. Clinicians should be alert for evidence of altered response to β-blockers if antacids are initiated or discontinued. If a change in clinical status occurs, β-blocker dose adjustment may be necessary due to possible accumulation of atenolol or decreased absorption of propranolol.

Antiinflammatory Agents

Evidence of Interaction

In a well-controlled study of 26 obese hypertensive patients, indomethacin, when administered concurrently with labetalol, produced minor increases in diastolic blood pressure and weight (Abate et al. 1991). Concomitant treatment of sulindac, indomethacin and labetalol resulted in significantly increased sitting and standing systolic blood pressure. The effects of sulindac and indomethacin on systolic blood pressure, diastolic blood pressure, and weight did not differ significantly. However, sulindac in combination with labetalol did not increase diastolic blood pressure or weight. In a study of 17 patients with hypertension and osteoarthritis, concomitant treatment of propranolol and sulindac or naproxen did not produce significant differences in mean sitting or standing blood pressure (Schuna et al. 1989). Indomethacin was found to partially antagonize the hypotensive effects of propranolol in a study of 15 patients with essential hypertension (Watkins et al. 1980). Similar results were obtained in a study of 7 hypertensive patients where inhibition of prostaglandin synthesis by indomethacin significantly suppressed or abolished the antihypertensive effect of pindolol and propranolol (Durao et al. 1977). In another study the antihypertensive response to oxprenolol was reduced by about 50% when administered concomitantly with indomethacin (Salvetti et al. 1982).

Mechanism

Not established. These studies with indomethacin suggest that the antihypertensive effect of β-blockers is antagonized (Durao et al. 1977). If the hypotensive effect of propranolol is partly due to increased production of a vasodilator, such as prostacyclin, then it is possible that indomethacin reversed the hypotensive effect of propranolol (Watkins et al. 1980), or perhaps the interaction is due to the mild sodium retention that accompanies indomethacin (Watkins et al. 1980).

Clinical Implications

When administering combination therapy with β-blockers and an antiinflammatory agent, clinicians should monitor patients for altered β-blocker response.

ANTIBIOTICS

Clinical Implications

In a study of 8 healthy subjects nadolol was investigated to determine whether it undergoes enterohepatic circulation and whether activated charcoal or antibiotics affect its metabolism (Souich et al. 1983). For 2 days the mean peak plasma nadolol concentration more than doubled following a single oral dose of nadolol (80 mg) and oral erythromycin 0.5 g 4 times daily and oral neomycin 0.5 g 4 times daily.

It was determined that there is enterohepatic circulation for nadolol. In addition the results suggested that activated charcoal decreases nadolol bioavailability and that erythromycin may increase the nadolol effect. Interactions between atenolol with aspirin, allopurinol, and ampicillin were studied in 6 healthy subjects (Schafer-Korting 1983). Both allopurinol and aspirin did not alter the kinetics of atenolol. Following long-term treatment with atenolol and ampicillin, the bioavailability of atenolol decreased. Ampicillin reduced atenolol-induced inhibition of exercise tachycardia, suggesting that the plasma concentration of atenolol was reduced.

Mechanism

Erythromycin increases the effect of nadolol by increasing the rate of nadolol absorption while simultaneously increasing the extrarenal elimination of nadolol (Souich et al. 1983).

Clinical Implications

Clinicians should be aware of possible altered β-blocker effects when concomitant antibiotics are administered. With regard to the antihypertensive effect of atenolol, it may be necessary to double the atenolol dose during combination therapy with ampicillin in order to achieve the desired antihypertensive effect (Schafer-Korting et al. 1983).

ANTICHOLINERGICS

Evidence of Interaction

Regardh and colleagues (1981) found that propantheline slowed the absorption rate of atenolol, but bioavailability of atenolol increased by 36%. The study was conducted on 6 healthy subjects who each received atenolol 100 mg with and without propantheline 30 mg. One would expect that under conditions of multiple dosing the atenolol response would be enhanced; however, this has not been examined.

Mechanism

Anticholinergics may increase the bioavailability of atenolol, possibly by slowing gut motility.

Clinical Implications

During concomitant treatment with anticholinergics and β-blockers, one should be alert for altered response to either drug.

Antidepressants

IMIPRAMINE

Evidence of Interaction

In a study of 12 healthy males, concomitant treatment with labetalol and imipramine resulted in an increase in relative bioavailability of imipramine. Additionally, the oral clearance of imipramine was decreased (Hermann et al. 1992).

Mechanism

Labetalol decreases oral clearance of imipramine as it inhibits the hydroxylation of imipramine and desipramine to their respective 2-hydroxy metabolites. It appears that labetalol inhibits the P450-IID6 isozyme, which is responsible for the hydroxylation of imipramine and desipramine (Hermann et al. 1992).

Clinical Implications

One should monitor patients taking imipramine and β-blockers for signs and symptoms of toxicity.

PHENELZINE

Evidence of Interaction

Propranolol has been reported to be well tolerated in combination with phenelzine (Davidson et al. 1984). However, Risch and colleagues (1982) have found combination therapy with monoamine oxidase inhibitors (MAOIs) and propranolol to result in severe hypertensive crises.

Two cases have been reported of the development significant bradycardia developing in elderly patients during concomitant treatment with phenelzine and a β-blocker (Reggev and Vollhardt 1989). This first case involves a 75-year-old man with diet-controlled, adult-onset diabetes, hypertension, and angina. The patient was receiving nadolol 40 mg daily for blood pressure and angina, when phenelzine (started 30 mg daily, increased to 60 mg daily) was added for recurrent major depression. Over the course of 8 days, the patient's pulse decreased from 62 to 80 to 46 to 50 beats/minute. Nadolol was reduced to 20 mg daily, and the patient's pulse returned to 70 to 80 beats/minute.

In the second case, a 63-year-old hypertensive woman was taking metoprolol 150 mg daily. Following a course of electroconvulsive treatment, phenelzine 60 mg daily was added to her treatment regimen. The patient remained asymptomatic after her pulse fell below 60 beats/minute. Metoprolol was discontinued, and the patient's pulse rate returned to 70 to 80 beats/minute.

Mechanism

Chronic administration of MAOIs is associated with a reduction of peripheral adrenergic activity. The hypertensive response resulting from the interaction of β-blockers and phenelzine is apparently due to β-receptor blockade in the presence of unopposed α-adrenergic activity. This interaction may involve a number of pharmacodynamic mechanisms at different sites. The possibilities include altered β-receptor activity at the sinoatrial node, a central nervous system effect of chronic MAOI therapy, or it may involve both reduced peripheral adrenergic activity of norepinephrine by phenelzine and blockade of peripheral receptors by the β-blockers.

Clinical Implications

During concomitant administration of MAOIs and β-blockers, the doses of both drugs should be reduced and blood pressure and pulse monitored. Since aging further alters β-receptor function, we advise close monitoring of the cardiac functioning of geriatric patients.

ANTIDIABETIC AGENTS

Evidence of Interaction (Hansten and Horn 1993)

1. Delayed Rate of Glucose Recovery during Hypoglycemia. Following insulin-induced hypoglycemia, propranolol appears to inhibit glucose recovery (Hansten 1980). Propranolol may increase the potential for hypoglycemia in predisposed patients who are not receiving insulin. Predisposing factors include the following: liver dysfunction, hemodialysis, prolonged exercise, fasting, large propranolol doses, and, possibly, youth (Grajower et al. 1980, Hansten 1980, Hesse and Pedersen 1973, Holm et al. 1981, Kallen et al. 1980, Pelsor et al. 1981, Wray and Sutcliffe 1972). Metoprolol may slightly prolong insulin-induced hypoglycemia (Newman et al. 1976). Practolol, penbutolol, and atenolol have not demonstrated an affect on the magnitude or duration of insulin-induced hypoglycemia (Deacon et al. 1977, Newman 1976). In 1 case, timolol eye drops may have contributed to a hypoglycemic episode (Angelo-Nelsen et al. 1980).

2. Hypertension during Hypoglycemia. Numerous clinical studies and case reports have documented increased blood pressure and bradycardia during hypoglycemia in the presence of propranolol treatment (Hansten 1980, Ryan et al. 1982). It has been proposed that other nonselective β-blockers such as alprenolol, nadolol, oxprenolol, sotalol, and timolol would have a similar effect (Ostman et al. 1982). Metoprolol and atenolol are less likely to produce hypertension during hypoglycemia as they have a decreased inhibitory effect on vasodilatory β-2 receptors (Hansten 1980, Ostman et al. 1982). Although large doses of metoprolol produce more β-2-blockade and can therefore be expected to increase blood pressure during hypoglycemia (Hansten and Horn 1993). One patient receiving metoprolol 100 mg twice daily experienced hypoglycemia-induced hypertension; however, serum metoprolol levels may have been increased due to concurrent drug therapy (Shepherd et al. 1981).

3. Inhibition of the Symptoms of Hypoglycemia. The tachycardia which normally accompanies hypoglycemia is inhibited by propranolol (Hansten 1980). Reflex bradycardia may occur due to increased blood pressure when hypoglycemia occurs in the presence of propranolol. Metoprolol has also been reported to inhibit the tachycardia occurring during hypoglycemia, although metoprolol is less likely to produce reflex bradycardia as blood pressure does not change to a significant degree (Lager et al. 1979). Additionally atenolol (Deacon and Barnett 1976), acebutolol (Deacon et al. 1977, Newman 1976), penbutolol (Sharma et al. 1979), and alprenolol (Ostman et al. 1982) have been documented as inhibiting hypoglycemia-induced tachycardia. Sweating due to hypoglycemia is not inhibited by β-blockers; in fact it may actually be prolonged (Hansten 1980, Waal-Manning 1979).

4. Inhibition of Insulin Secretion. Propranolol inhibits the insulin response to glucose (Meyers and Hope-Gill 1979) and tolbutamide (Scandellari et al. 1978). Some patients with insulinoma have used propranolol to inhibit insulin secretion (Blum et al. 1975, 1978). Furthermore, long-term propranolol therapy has been associated with a decrease in glucose tolerance (Groop et al. 1982, Hansten 1980, Mohler et al. 1979, Nardone and Bouma 1979). Metoprolol, which is less likely to inhibit insulin secretions, appears to be less likely than propranolol to impair glucose tolerance (Ekberg and Hansson 1977, Groop et al. 1982, Reeves et al. 1982, Waal-Manning 1976). Cardioselective β-blockers may not have as great of an inhibitory effect on insulin secretion when compared with nonselective β-blockers, as stimulation of β-2 receptors in the pancreas tends to stimulate insulin secretion (Hansten and Horn 1993, Wood 1983).

5. Impaired Peripheral Circulation. Propranolol may be associated with reduced circulation to the extremities, leading to gangrene in some extreme cases (Hansten 1980). This may pose a serious problem to a diabetic who may already have impaired peripheral circulation (Hansten and Horn 1993). Cardioselective β-blockers, which have less effect on β-2 receptors in peripheral arterioles, theoretically should be less likely to negatively affect peripheral circulation.

Mechanism (Hansten and Horn 1993)

1. The delayed glucose recovery from insulin-induced hypoglycemia during β-blockade is most likely related to inhibition of the hyperglycemic effect of the epinephrine released in response to hypoglycemia (Popp et al. 1982, Santiago et al. 1980).
2. Hypertension induced by β-blockers during hypoglycemia is related to blockade of the β-2 effects of epinephrine released in response to hypoglycemia. This leaves unopposed α-(vasoconstrictor) effects which increase the blood pressure.
3. β-Blocker induced inhibition of tachycardia during hypoglycemia is related to inhibition of the cardiac stimulatory effect of the epinephrine released in response to hypoglycemia.
4. Under certain conditions β-blockers may inhibit insulin secretion, which may lead to a hyperglycemic effect.
5. β-Blockers may impair peripheral circulation.

Clinical Implications

When treating diabetic patients, the clinician is advised to use the cardioselective β-blockers (metoprolol, atenolol) because they are less likely to produce the unwanted effects described above. However, if any β-blocker is used in diabetic patients adequate warning should be given. Patients should understand that they are not likely to have the same warning symptoms of hypoglycemia (tachycardia). Cardioselective β-blockers are only relatively effective in avoiding β-2 effects; thus, when using large doses of cardioselective β-blockers, both β1 and β2 blockade will be achieved eliminating any advantage.

Antihypertensives and Miscellaneous Cardiovascular Agents

PROPAFENONE

Evidence of Interaction

Steady-state plasma concentrations of both metoprolol and propafenone alone and in combination were analyzed in two studies:

one with 8 patients treated for cardiovascular disease, and the second using 6 healthy volunteers (Wagner et al. 1987). Metoprolol concentrations increased 7-fold in all 4 cardiovascular patients treated with metoprolol and propafenone. The increased concentration corresponded to a decrease in oral clearance of metoprolol in these 4 patients. In the 4 patients treated originally with the drug combination followed by discontinuation of metoprolol, the concentration of propafenone was not affected by concomitant administration with metoprolol. Two patients experienced major side effects during concomitant treatment. One suffered from nightmares and the other experienced acute left ventricular failure with pulmonary edema and hemoptysis. Both of these side effects disappeared after reduction or discontinuation of metoprolol treatment. In the study of the healthy volunteers, all but 1 subject exhibited higher concentrations of metoprolol following the addition of propafenone to the treatment regimen. The β-adrenergic blocking effect of metoprolol is more pronounced following combination therapy as evidenced by the more than 20% reduction in exercise-induced tachycardia.

A case report depicts a 41-year-old man who experienced nightmares and became severely disoriented after beginning metoprolol treatment. The physician initiated propafenone while beginning to gradually withdraw metoprolol. On the 8th day the patient was brought to a clinic and diagnosed with acute metoprolol-induced brain syndrome. It appeared that the syndrome was aggravated by the concomitant administration of propafenone. Within 24 hours of withdrawal of both metoprolol and propafenone the delirium disappeared.

A study of 12 healthy men evaluated the effects of propafenone on propranolol during concomitant therapy (Kowey et al. 1989). Following combined administration of propafenone and propranolol, plasma propranolol concentrations increased and plasma 4-hydroxypropranolol concentrations decreased in all 12 subjects. Exercise tachycardia was reduced by 19.4% during propranolol treatment. A modest enhancement of β-adrenergic blocking effect is evidenced by a 25.1% reduction in exercise tachycardia following combination therapy with propranolol and propafenone. Prior abnormalities of the conduction system or of ventricular function may exaggerate the interaction; thus these results apply only to healthy subjects.

Mechanism

It is speculated that increased metoprolol plasma levels are due to a reduced first-pass metabolism and reduced systemic clearance of metoprolol in the presence of propafenone.

Clinical Implications

During combined treatment with propafenone and metoprolol it may be necessary to reduce the dosage of metoprolol. One should watch for nightmares, evidence of cardiac failure or any evidence of toxic delirium, in which case the clinician should consider discontinuing either propafenone or the β-blocker.

PRAZOSIN

Evidence of Interaction

Acute postural hypotension and tachycardia often result as a first-dose response following the initiation of prazosin therapy. A study of 8 healthy men evaluated the effects of propranolol 80 mg and primidolol 100 mg in response to oral prazosin (1 mg) (Elliott et al. 1981). Both the severity and duration of the orthostatic fall in blood pressure (and the occurrence of hypotensive symptoms) were increased by concomitant β-blocker therapy. Similar results were obtained in hypertensive patients taking propranolol when prazosin (2 mg) was added to their treatment regimen (Graham et al. 1976). In these patients it was observed that the acute postural hypotension following the first dose of prazosin was enhanced. In a study of hypertensive patients taking alprenolol, a similar increase in the first-dose hypotensive response to prazosin was observed (Seideman et al. 1982). A study using animal paradigms found concomitant administration of propranolol and prazosin caused the mean arterial pressure to increase 20% above the control mean arterial pressure prior to the administration of drugs (Tabrizchi and Pang 1989).

Mechanism

The cardiovascular response that would normally follow prazosin-induced hypotension may be inhibited by β-blockade.

Clinical Implications

Caution should be taken when initiating prazosin therapy to patients who are being treated with β-blockers. Conservative doses should be used.

METHYLDOPA

Evidence of Interaction

A case report has been presented discussing a 36-year-old hypertensive man treated with methyldopa and hydralazine (Nies et al. 1973). Propranolol (5 mg by slow intravenous injection) was administered following a cerebrovascular accident. Following the initiation of propranolol the patient's blood pressure rose from 240/130 to 290/175. The same investigators administered α-methyl-norepinephrine to 6 mongrel dogs who were all pretreated with propranolol. The combination resulted in a pressor response similar to that of norepinephrine. They proposed that propranolol allows unopposed alpha adrenergic vasoconstriction, thus shifting the dose-response curve and changing its slope so that the pressor response to α-methyl-norepinephrine resembles the response to norepinephrine.

In a similarly described case, a patient receiving methyldopa, atropine, and practolol was administered neostigmine, which was followed by a hypertensive reaction (260/140 mm Hg) (Palmer 1975). The authors proposed that stimulation of nicotine receptors in the ganglia by neostigmine resulted in release of α-methyl-norepinephrine and/or norepinephrine from nerve endings and possibly some epinephrine from the adrenals. The β-blockade that remained in the patient would result in an overbalance of α-vasoconstrictor activity.

Mechanism

Nies and colleagues (1973) have proposed that methyldopa results in accumulation of α-methyl-norepinephrine in storage sites of the adrenergic neuron. When propranolol is administered, the β-adrenergic stimulation of α-methyl-norepinephrine is inhibited and this results in unopposed α-adrenergic stimulation, thus increasing pressor response.

Clinical Implications

Patients receiving β-blockers and methyldopa should be monitored for hypertensive episodes. If a hypertensive crisis occurs, phentolamine (Regitine®) should be administered (Nies et al. 1973).

QUINIDINE

Evidence of Interaction

Six healthy males were studied to determine whether an interaction occurs during concomitant treatment with quinidine (50 mg) and propranolol, both of which bind to the cytochrome P450 responsible for the oxidation of desbrisoquin (Zhou et al. 1990). The area under the plasma concentration time curve for propranolol doubled and there was a reduction in the clearance of propranolol during concomitant administration of quinidine. This increased concentration of propranolol resulted in increased β-blockade which was measured by a reduction in exercise heart rate and prolongation of the QTc and PR interval.

Mechanism

The authors proposed that quinidine stereoselectively inhibits the metabolism of propranolol through inhibition of the desbrisoquin isozyme.

Clinical Implications

Lower doses of β-blockers should be used during concomitant administration with quinidine.

Barbiturates

Evidence of Interaction

The effect of pentobarbital on plasma levels of alprenolol, its metabolite 4-hydroxy-alprenolol, and the inhibition of exercise tachycardia were studied in 6 healthy subjects (Collste et al. 1979). For 10 days, at bedtime, the subjects were given placebo and a single oral dose of alprenolol 0.2 g before and after pentobarbital 0.1 g. Seven hours later the plasma concentrations and the inhibition of exercise tachycardia were studied. Both alprenolol and 4-hydroxy-alprenolol plasma levels decreased by about 40% following pentobarbital; however plasma half-lives remained the same. The degree of induction differed markedly between subjects. There did not appear to be an association between the change of alprenolol and 4-hydroxy-alprenolol plasma levels and pentobarbital plasma levels. Inhibition of exercise tachycardia was reduced from 14.0% to 10.7%; this was proportional to the decreased drug plasma levels.

Similar results were obtained in a study of 8 healthy subjects pretreated with pentobarbital 0.1 g for 10 days (Haglund et al. 1979). When these subjects were concomitantly administered metoprolol 0.1 g orally, the area-under-the-plasma-concentration-time-curve for metoprolol was reduced by 32%. Comparable results were attained in a study of 5 healthy subjects who were administered orally (200 mg) and intravenously (5.0 mg) alprenolol following pentobarbital 0.1 g (Alvan et al. 1977). After the oral dose of alprenolol, the area-under-the-alprenolol-plasma-concentration-time-curve decreased; however, elimination rate was not significantly changed. Disposition of the intravenous dose of alprenolol did not change significantly after pentobarbital treatment.

Sontaniemi and colleagues (1979) examined plasma clearance of propranolol, sotalol, and hepatic drug-metabolizing enzyme activity in 68 patients. Three patients who were taking enzyme inducers (2 patients taking phenytoin, 1 taking pentobarbital) had a higher plasma clearance of propranolol than those not on enzyme inducers. Plasma clearance of sotalol did not seem to be affected by the enzyme inducers.

Mechanism

The metabolism of extensively metabolized β-blockers (propranolol, metoprolol, alprenolol) appears to be stimulated by barbiturates.

Clinical Significance

When patients are receiving concomitant treatment with β-blockers that are metabolized by the liver (e.g. propranolol, metoprolol, alprenolol) and barbiturates, clinicians should watch for evidence of diminished response to the β-blocker due to increased metabolism. It may be necessary to increase the β-blocker dosage. β-blockers that are excreted primarily unchanged by the kidneys (e.g. atenolol, nadolol, sotalol) are not likely to interact with barbiturates and thus could be used to avoid this interaction.

Caffeine

Evidence of Interaction

Caffeine did not affect plasma binding of propranolol in 16 healthy subjects who took caffeine 250 mg orally (Patwardhan et al. 1980). In spite of a rise in free fatty acids, there was no change in plasma binding of propranolol. The effect of coffee on blood pressure and forearm blood flow was not altered by treatment with propranolol or metoprolol in a study of 12 normotensive subjects (Smits et al. 1983). However, coffee-induced decrease in heart rate was somewhat greater during pretreatment with propranolol.

Mechanism

None.

Clinical Implications

No special precautions appear to be necessary.

Calcium Channel Blockers

DILTIAZEM

Evidence of Interaction

A study was conducted to evaluate hemodynamic tolerability and safety of high-dose intravenous diltiazem in 9 patients receiving long-term metoprolol treatment for coronary artery disease (Wiesfeld et al. 1992). The results from this study indicate that in patients with normal ventricular function taking chronic β-blocking therapy, high dosages of intravenous diltiazem have no negative effects on cardiac pump function and do not result in negative chronotropic properties or conduction disturbances. The authors concluded that patients receiving long-term β blocking therapy will tolerate high-dose intravenous diltiazem.

Combined administration of diltiazem and β-blockers can cause bradycardia, the life-threatening nature of which has been reported. The charts of 10 patients concomitantly treated with oral diltiazem and a β-blocker who were all admitted to the intensive coronary care unit with symptomatic bradycardia were studied (Sagie et al. 1991). The chart review revealed that the drug interaction was not dose dependent and even occurred in very low doses of each drug (diltiazem 90 mg/day, propranolol 30 mg/day). The mean age of the patients involved was 70 years; thus it appeared in mainly elderly patients. The interaction occurred anywhere from within a few hours of onset of concomitant treatment to after up to 2 years of concomitant therapy. In almost all of the reported cases bradyarrhythmias resolved spontaneously within 24 hours of discontinuing both drugs. Electophysiologic abnormalities in all 10 patients were localized to the sinus node and the primary rhythm disorders were junctional escape rhythm, sinus bradycardia and sinus pause.

Yust and colleagues (1992) reported 4 cases in which the combined administration of diltiazem and a β-blocker caused bradycardia due to sinus node dysfunction or atrioventricular block. All four cases were severe and produced life-threatening circumstances. The first case involved an 86-year-old woman receiving metoprolol 100 mg daily and diltiazem 60 mg 3 times daily. She was admitted due to complaints of weakness. An electrocardiogram (ECG) revealed right bundle branch block, sinoatrial arrest, and extremely slow junctional bradycardia. The second was a 66-year-old man receiving atenolol 100 mg daily and diltiazem 30 mg 3 times a day. He experienced severe dizziness and had two near-syncopal episodes. The ECG demonstrated atrial fibrillation with very slow ventricular response and intermittent prolonged RR pauses. The third case involved a 75-year-old man who was administered atenolol 25 mg in addition to his diltiazem 30 mg 3 times a day regimen. Two days later an ECG revealed junctional bradycardia. The fourth case involved a 74-year-old woman who was admitted for dizziness. One week previously she had begun therapy with propranolol 20 mg 4 times daily, diltiazem 60 mg 3 times daily, and isosorbide mononitrate 20 mg 3 times daily. The ECG showed sinoatrial arrest with a slow junctional escape rhythm.

Combined treatment with β-blockers and calcium channel blockers may either enhance or unmask intrinsic drug properties that may result in either increased therapeutic efficacy or harmful adverse effects (Sagie et al. 1991). Patients with normal left ventricular function and no evidence of conduction system disease usually benefit from increased antianginal potency. Combined treatment in patients with antecedent sinoatrial or atrioventricular (AV) nodal conduction abnormality or in patients with clinically significant left ventricle (LV) dysfunction may be associated with adverse drug interaction effect. Verapamil is the most likely to produce negative inotropic, chronotropic, and dromotropic effects when used alone or in combination with β-blockers.

Mechanism

In the presence of β-blockers the reflex increase in heart rate resulting from peripheral vasodilation produced by diltiazem is reduced, thus allowing the negative inotropic effect of diltiazem to remain unopposed.

Clinical Implications

Although diltiazem-β-blocker combination therapy is of great therapeutic value in ischemic syndromes, caution should be advised when using this combination especially in the elderly or patients with left ventricular dysfunction or antecedent sinoatrial or atrioventricular conduction abnormality.

VERAPAMIL

Evidence of Interaction

Murthy and colleagues (1991) investigated the effect of concomitant administration of verapamil and metoprolol in dogs. The results of this study demonstrate that verapamil 3 mg/kg inhibits the plasma metoprolol clearance after both intravenous 0.51 mg/kg and oral administration 1.37 mg/kg of metoprolol in dogs. The authors noted that the magnitude of inhibition in oral clearance observed in the dogs is comparable to that reported in angina patients.

Bailey and colleagues (1991) conducted three randomized, double-blind, crossover trials to evaluate submaximal exercise hemodynamics in 8 healthy men following treatment with oral verapamil 120 mg alone and in combination with a β-blocker. The β-blockers administered in this study were propranolol 80 mg, metoprolol 100 mg, and pindolol 5 mg. Combined administration with verapamil and β-blockers produced greater decreases in heart rate and prolongation of PR interval than did either drug administered alone. Increased reduction of systolic blood pressure and prolongation of rate-adjusted PR interval was only demonstrated during combined therapy with verapamil and propranolol. Exercise fatigue and resting first-degree heart block were frequent adverse events seen in all verapamil and β-blocker combinations. The authors concluded that combination therapy results in enhanced negative chronotropic effects in healthy volunteers during submaximal exercise testing. They noted that verapamil and propranolol produce additional negative inotropic and dromotropic effects. This suggests that β-blockers with β1 selectivity or intrinsic stimulatory activity may result in decreased hemodynamic depression when combined with verapamil.

The effects of combination treatment with verapamil and propranolol was studied in a double-blind, randomized, balanced, crossover study with 6 healthy males (Murdoch et al. 1991). The first study looked at the effect of repeated propranolol therapy on verapamil after a single oral or intravenous dose. The second study examined the pharmacodynamics and pharmacokinetics of verapamil and propranolol alone and in combination after single and repeated oral doses. The authors concluded that although they are unable to exclude a clinically relevant drug interaction between verapamil and propranolol, they thought their findings represented hemodynamic responses due to the summation of the drugs' individual influences.

There has been an accumulation of evidence that supports the prior conclusion that the combination of verapamil and β-blockade results in additive cardiodepressant effects (Kieval et al 1982, Packer et al. 1982a,b, Winniford et al. 1982, 1983). A few cases have been reported in which marked bradycardia, cardiac failure, and severe hypotension have developed in patients as a result of the concomitant administration of both drugs (Packer 1982a, Wayne et al. 1982).

Mechanism

Verapamil's intrinsic depressant effect on myocardial contractility is offset by a reflex increase in heart rate as a result of peripheral vasodilation which is also produced by verapamil (Hansten 1985). When β-blockers are concomitantly administered, the reflex increase in heart rate is reduced, thus allowing the negative inotropic effect of verapamil to remain unopposed. Intrinsic cardiodepressant effect of β-blockers may be additive with that of verapamil.

Clinical Implications

Combined treatment with verapamil and β-blockers may be advantageous in cases of refractory angina pectoris. Clinicians should watch for evidence of additive cardiodepressant effects in patients receiving concomitant therapy.

NIFEDIPINE

Evidence of Interaction

As with the other calcium channel blockers, numerous studies have documented the positive clinical response in patients with angina pectoris or hypertension to combination therapy with nifedipine and a β-blocker (Christensen et al. 1982, Daly et al. 1982, Dargie et al. 1981, Dean and Kendall 1981, DePonti et al. 1981, Eggertsen and Hannson 1982, Husted et al. 1982, Krikler et al. 1982, Pfisterer et al. 1982, Young and MacDonald 1982). Several case reports have described cardiac failure or severe hypotension associated with concomitant therapy between nifedipine and β-blockers (Anastassiades 1980, 1982, Robson and Vishwanath 1982, Staffurth and Emery 1981). In a study of 12 patients treated with nifedipine 10 mg sublingually during β-blockade with atenolol 100 mg 4 times daily, a negative inotropic response to nifedipine was observed (Joshi et al. 1981). Another study examining the effect of nifedipine on propranolol found that nifedipine increased propranolol concentrations during the absorption phase (Bauer et al. 1989). They concluded that nifedipine does not alter propranolol metabolism since no change was found in propranolol total AUC, half-life ($t\frac{1}{2}$) or oral clearance.

Mechanism

In the presence of β-blockers the reflex increase in heart rate resulting from peripheral vasodilation produced by nifedipine is reduced, thus allowing the negative inotropic effect of nifedipine to remain unopposed (Hansten 1985).

Clinical Implications

When prescribing combination therapy of nifedipine and a β-blocker, clinicians should watch for excessive cardiodepressant effects and hypotension.

LACIDIPINE

Evidence of Interaction

A study of 24 healthy men examined the pharmacokinetic and pharmacodynamic effects of concomitant administration of lacidipine 4 mg and propranolol 160 mg (Hall et al. 1991). Propranolol significantly decreased the maximum plasma concentration (38%) and area-under-the-plasma-concentration-time curve (42%) for lacidipine. Lacidipine significantly increased the maximum plasma concentration (35%) and area-under-the-plasma-concentration-time curve (26%) of propranolol. An increased reduction in supine systolic blood pressure, diastolic blood pressure, and pulse rate compared with the reduction produced by lacidipine alone was observed during concomitant therapy. A significant reduction in supine systolic blood pressure compared with the reduction produced by propranolol was observed, but there was no marked difference in supine diastolic blood pressure and pulse rate. The authors concluded that a modest pharmacokinetic and pharmacodynamic interaction is evident and should be evaluated further.

Mechanism

The authors propose that because both drugs undergo extensive first-pass metabolism after oral dosing, increased concentrations as a consequence of competition for cytochrome P450 may have been expected. However, as propranolol decreases hepatic blood flow, this may result in an increased first-pass loss of highly extracted drugs. This effect on blood flow of the presystemic clearance of lacidipine may have been significantly greater than any effect on cytochrome P450; thus this is a possible explanation of the observed decrease in systemic availability of lacidipine. Because lacidipine is a vasodilator and causes cardiac output to be increased, hepatic blood flow may have been affected. Any increase in this parameter may cause presystemic clearance of propranolol to be decreased, thus resulting in elevated drug concentrations.

Clinical Implications

The effects of combined treatment with lacidipine and β-blockers needs to be further evaluated to ascertain whether these pharmacodynamic changes are clinically relevant.

NISOLDIPINE

Evidence of Interaction

A study of the interaction between nisoldipine and atenolol and propranolol was conducted in two groups of healthy volunteers (Elliott et al. 1991). Nisoldipine significantly increased the peak plasma concentrations of both atenolol and propranolol; additionally the AUC of propranolol was increased. Exercise tests produced no evidence that would suggest that β-blockade was compromised with the addition of nisoldipine. The results from this study are consistent with the known advantageous therapeutic effects of combined treatment with calcium channel blockers and β-blockers in patients suffering from angina and/or hypertension.

Mechanism

In the presence of β-blockers the reflex increase in heart rate resulting from peripheral vasodilation produced by nisoldipine is reduced, thus allowing the negative inotropic effect of nisoldipine to remain unopposed.

Clinical Implications

As with the other calcium channel blockers, clinicians should be alert for signs of excessive cardiodepression and hypotension.

Carbamazepine

Evidence of Interaction

The interaction between carbamazepine and β-blockers is largely theoretical. In a study of 17 patients receiving carbamazepine, the serum levels of α1-acid glycoprotein were 23% higher when compared with 21 control subjects (Tiula and Neuvonen 1982). Propranolol binding was not determined in this study. It is possible that carbamazepine increases the metabolism of β-blockers metabolized by the liver.

Mechanism

Carbamazepine therapy increases serum levels of α_1-acid glycoprotein, a protein that propranolol is bound to in the serum. Carbamazepine stimulates hepatic drug-metabolizing enzymes, which may increase propranolol metabolism.

Clinical Implications

The clinical significance has not been established; thus one should observe patients for altered propranolol response during combined therapy with carbamazepine.

Diuretics

Evidence of Interaction

A study of 10 healthy subjects examined the effect of furosemide 25 mg orally on the plasma concentration and β-blockade by propranolol 40 mg orally (Chiariello et al. 1979). Results demonstrated increased blood levels of propranolol after concomitant administration of propranolol and furosemide. In a study aimed at measuring β-blocking action of propranolol alone and with furosemide, results indicated that furosemide-induced increases in propranolol blood concentrations accompanied a simultaneous increase in β-adreno-ceptor blockade (Chiariello et al. 1977). During combined administration of furosemide, practolol showed reduced renal clearance (Tilstone et al. 1977). Atenolol, however, was unaffected by concurrent furosemide treatment (Kirch et al. 1981).

Mechanism

Not established.

Clinical Implications

One should be aware of the possibility of altered effect of β-blockade if furosemide is administered concomitantly with propranolol.

Epinephrine

Evidence of Interaction

A number of studies with hypertensive patients suffering from angina and in healthy subjects have demonstrated that propranolol enhances the pressor response to epinephrine, usually with accompanying bradycardia (Gandy 1989, Houben et al. 1979, 1982, Kram et al. 1974, Varma et al. 1976, VanHerwaarden et al. 1977a,b, Yasue et al. 1976). In 1 patient, an intracerebral hemorrhage developed due to a marked hypertensive response (Hansbrough and Near 1980). The marked bradycardia may be associated with AV block or other cardiac arrhythmias (Kram et al. 1974, Lampman et al. 1981).

Patients who were receiving chronic propranolol therapy experienced severe hypertensive reactions following infiltration of lidocaine with epinephrine (Foster and Aston 1983). It has been demonstrated that labetalol increased diastolic pressure and slowed the heart rate during epinephrine infusions (Richards et al. 1979). Metoprolol, however, has a minimal effect on the pressor response to epinephrine (Houben et al. 1979, 1982, VanHerwaarden et al. 1977a,b). Propranolol has been shown to inhibit the pressor and bronchodilation response of epinephrine patients with anaphylaxis (Jacobs et al. 1981, Newman and Schultz 1981).

Mechanism

Epinephrine has both α- and β-adrenergic effects. Using the β-blockers, by definition, blocks the β-adrenergic effects; thus, in the presence of a β-blocker epinephrine will have its α-adrenergic effects (vasoconstriction) with a diminution of its β-adrenergic (vasodilation, bronchodilation, and cardiac stimulation) effects. This can result in hypertension with a reflex increase in vagal tone resulting in bradycardia.

Clinical Implications

When possible, epinephrine should not be used by patients receiving β-blocker therapy (Gandy 1989). If necessary, epinephrine should be administered with extreme caution. Blood pressure should be monitored carefully, and continuous cardiac monitoring is advised. Pharmacologic treatment of rapid blood pressure increases is aimed at relieving α-vasoconstriction. Hydralazine, given as an IV infusion of 20 mg in 250 mL saline at 40 to 45 drops/min, has been recommended (Brummett 1984) and used effectively in 2 patients (Foster and Aston 1983). Droperidol, which has mild alpha-blocking effects, appeared to be helpful in 1 patient (Foster and Aston 1983). Chlorpromazine also has alpha-blocking effects and has been recommended (Foster and Aston 1983). This is given by diluting 1 mL (25 mg) with 24 mL saline and administering it in 1-mg increments, generally to a maximum of 5 mg. Sodium nitroprusside infusion also is effective in reducing afterload and would be suitable in this setting. Phentolamine, a short-acting alpha-blocker (half-life, 19 minutes), offers the advantages of ease of administration and rapid onset of action. It is given in a dose of 5 mg IV over one minute. Maximal effects should be present within two minutes of injection (Gandy 1989). When using epinephrine to treat anaphylaxis, one should be aware that the response to epinephrine may be poor in the presence of β-blockade and vigorous supportive care may be needed. Selective β1 blockers may be less likely than nonselective β-blockers to result in hypertension with bradycardia and to decrease broncho-dilation during concurrent administration of epinephrine or endogenous epinephrine release. This is the main reason why β-blockers should not be used in patients with a history of asthma. If a β-blocker is used in a patient with a history of asthma or chronic obstructive pulmonary disease (COPD), then a cardioselective β-blocker is indicated. However, cardioselective β-blockers are only relatively effective in preventing β2 effects; thus, when using large doses of cardioselective β-blockers, both β1 and β2 blockade will be achieved, eliminating any advantage of the cardioselective β-blocker.

Ethanol

Evidence of Interaction

Sotaniemi and colleagues (1981) conducted a study to investigate the effects of alcohol on the metabolism of both propranolol and sotalol. The subjects were 14 healthy students, none of whom took medication, smoked, or drank alcohol regularly. The subjects were given either propranolol (two 40-mg tablets), sotalol (two 80-mg tablets), or placebo. After a full dinner, alcohol was ingested between 7 p.m. and 2 a.m. The following morning, 6 hours after the last drink, the patients were given the drugs again and food was taken 2 hours after alcohol. The results from the study indicated that alcohol increased the clearance rate and bioavailability of propranolol, but reduced the clearance rate of sotalol. These changes in metabolism were reflected in a diminished and increased ability of propranolol and sotalol, respectively, to decrease blood pressure. Both drugs reduced the heart rate following alcohol administration; however, they were not able to entirely counteract the alcohol-induced rise in heart rate. Additionally, the antiarrhythmic action of atenolol was studied in rats that were either dependent or nondependent on ethanol (Filipek et al. 1989). Joint administration of atenolol and ethanol produced a weaker antiarrhythmic effect than atenolol alone in adrenaline-induced arrhythmia. However, no significant effect of atenolol on ethanol blood concentration was discovered.

Mechanism

The exact mechanism has not been established. Effects are possibly due to ethanol-induced increases in hepatic blood flow, thus increasing the clearance of β-blockers from the system.

Clinical Implications

Patients should be advised that ingesting alcohol may reduce the effect of propranolol and increase the effect of sotalol.

Food

Evidence of Interaction

Food enhanced the bioavailability of both metoprolol and propranolol in 13 healthy volunteers (Melander et al. 1977). This was demonstrated by an increased peak serum concentration and a larger area-under-the-curve when metoprolol and propranolol were administered with food compared with during a fasting state. Another study found that when the drug was taken with food, the absorption of propranolol was delayed (Shand et al. 1970). However, this occurred without change in the peak concentration of the drug.

Mechanism

The gastrointestinal absorption of metoprolol and propranolol appears to be complete. The enhanced bioavailability may be due to changes in metabolism of the drug during first pass through the liver (Melander et al. 1977).

Clinical Implications

With regard to meals, β-blockers should be taken in a consistent manner to minimize variation in absorption.

H$_2$-Receptor Antagonists

CIMETIDINE AND RANITIDINE

Evidence of Interaction

A number of studies have demonstrated that cimetidine substantially increases plasma propranolol levels. Heagerty and colleagues (1981) studied whole-blood propranolol concentrations in 6 patients receiving cimetidine for peptic ulcerations for at least 2 weeks prior to the onset of the study. The patients were given a single 80-mg oral dose of propranolol after an overnight fast. Two weeks after the patients had terminated cimetidine treatment the study was repeated using the same dose of propranolol. Results demonstrated that mean blood propranolol levels were higher during the period when the patients were concomitantly taking cimetidine than when they were not. Additionally the mean relative bioavailability of propranolol was significantly higher when the patients were taking cimetidine. Bioavailability had a mean increase of 58%, and results were consistent in each subject.

Resting pulse rates are significantly lower in patients receiving cimetidine in combination with propranolol than in those taking propranolol alone (Feely et al. 1981), although in one study cimetidine failed to alter exercise-induced tachycardia in patients receiving concomitant administration with metoprolol or propranolol (Kirch et al. 1982). In the same study the plasma levels of both metoprolol and propranolol were increased. The plasma levels of atenolol, which is extensively excreted by the kidneys, were minimally affected by cimetidine therapy. Similar results for atenolol were documented in a single-dose study (Houtzagers et al. 1982). This same study reported that metoprolol 100 mg did not affect cimetidine. A preliminary report demonstrated that cimetidine increases the bioavailability of labetalol by about 80% (Daneshmend et al. 1981).

The influence of ranitidine and cimetidine on propranolol was studied in 5 healthy subjects (Reimann et al. 1982). β-Blocker effect was measured by a bicycle ergometer exercise test. The propranolol plasma levels were also measured. During the 3 hours of dynamic tests the propranolol plasma levels increased from 25% to 67% in subjects receiving concomitant treatment with cimetidine. Propranolol plasma levels of subjects receiving ranitidine remained unchanged. Propranolol-induced heart rate and blood pressure changes during exercise or during the isoproterenol sensitivity test did not reflect changes induced by concomitant treatment with either cimetidine or ranitidine.

A further report indicated that ranitidine 150 mg twice daily failed to affect the pharmacokinetics of propranolol 80 mg after concomitant administration in 6 healthy volunteers (Heagerty et al. 1982). Ranitidine differs from cimetidine in that it does not appear to affect the hepatic metabolism of certain drugs. Thus, Spahn and colleagues (1983) undertook a preliminary study to examine the effect of ranitidine on metoprolol, a β-blocker that is primarily metabolized in the liver. Atenolol, a renally excreted β-blocker, was used as a control. Six healthy subjects were administered combined treatment with ranitidine 150 mg twice daily, metoprolol 100 mg twice daily, and atenolol 100 mg twice daily. The results indicated that atenolol was not significantly altered by ranitidine. However, the plasma concentration time curve for metoprolol increased by about 50% during concomitant administration of ranitidine. This effect does not appear to be consistent with ranitidine's reported lack of effect on propranolol.

Mechanism

Cimetidine reduces the activity of the hepatic microsomal enzymes that metabolize propranolol. It appears that cimetidine decreases propranolol metabolism by reducing blood flow.

Clinical Implications

When patients are receiving combined treatment of cimetidine and propranolol, labetalol and possible other β-blockers, clinicians should watch for evidence of increased β-blocker response. If clinical status changes, the clinicians should consider lowering the dose of the β-blocker. Ranitidine, famotidine, and nizatidine may be alternatives to cimetidine in patients taking propranolol requiring concomitant treatment.

HMG-CoA Reductase Inhibitors

Evidence of Interaction

In a randomized, 4-way crossover study, 16 healthy males were given pravastatin and lovastatin either with or without concomitant propranolol. Coadministration of propranolol reduced the mean area-under-the-serum-concentration-time-curve of both pravastatin and lovastatin (Pan et al. 1991).

Mechanism

Propranolol may have decreased the oral bioavailability of pravastatin and lovastatin by lowering hepatic blood flow, thus increasing first-pass extraction (Pan et al. 1991).

Clinical Implications

Unknown, but likely to be small.

β-Adrenergic Bronchodilators

ISOPROTERENOL

Evidence of Interaction

It has been demonstrated that asthmatic patients who are pretreated with propranolol are resistant to the bronchodilating effects of isoproterenol as measured by the forced expiratory volume in 1 second (FEV1) (Johnson et al. 1975, Thringer and Svedmyr 1976). In the same studies, selective β1-receptor blockers (metoprolol and practolol) did not appear to inhibit isoproterenol increased in FEV1. In normal subjects, it has been demonstrated that β-blockers inhibit isoproterenol-induced increases in pulse rate, decreases in diastolic blood pressure, and increases in plasma cyclic adenosine amino-phosphate (cAMP) (Messerli et al. 1976, Perruca et al. 1981).

Mechanism

β-Adrenergic blockers inhibit the actions of isoproterenol, which is a β-adrenergic stimulant.

Clinical Implications

Concomitant use with β-blockers and isoproterenol is not recommended due to their antagonistic effects. Therapy with β-blockers should be avoided in asthmatic patients treated with isoproterenol. If β-blocker therapy is unavoidable, cardioselective β-blockers (e.g. metoprolol) may be preferable to propranolol in asthmatic patients, since bronchodilation from isoproterenol is less likely to be reduced.

TERBUTALINE

Evidence of Interaction

Formgren and Eriksson (1975) administered practolol to 29 asthmatic patients who used the bronchodilator terbutaline. Practolol did not appear to impair the bronchodilator activity of terbutaline.

Mechanism

Cardioselective β-adrenergic blockers are expected to have little effect on bronchoselective β agonists such as terbutaline.

Clinical Implications

β-Blockers should always be administered with extreme caution in asthmatic patients; however, the combination of practolol and terbutaline appears to be relatively safe.

Levodopa

Evidence of Interaction

In a study of 25 parkinsonian patients with tremor as a dominant clinical feature, concomitant treatment of propranolol (not less than 60 mg daily), and levodopa produced better results than either drug given alone (Kissel et al. 1974). Tremor was either rapidly reduced or abolished in all except 2 patients who had undergone thalamotomy. Improvement was maintained during 6-month to 2-year followup periods. A study conducted by Lotti and colleagues (1974) confirmed the potentiating effect of propranolol on normal and obese subjects. They also demonstrated an increase in plasma-growth hormone following concomitant levodopa and practolol treatment. Sandler and colleagues (1975) failed to find additional improvement in 4 parkinsonian patients when oxprenolol was added to levodopa therapy. After levodopa, propranolol enhances the elevated plasma growth hormone levels. These increased levels of growth hormone were reportedly close to those seen in acromegaly (Camanni and Massara 1974).

Mechanism

The β-blockers antagonize the β-adrenergic properties of levodopa. The β-blockers treat the tremor of Parkinson's disease, thus enhancing the therapeutic effect of levodopa. In addition, β-blockers increase the stimulation of growth hormone secretion by levodopa.

Clinical Implications

In all cases, combined therapy with levodopa and β-blockers appears to enhance the therapeutic effects of levodopa. This appears to be a favorable interaction; however, until the magnitude and clinical significance of elevated growth hormone levels is well determined, those patients receiving combined therapy for prolonged periods should be monitored closely.

Marijuana

Evidence of Interaction

Sulkowski and colleagues (1977) administered propranolol 120 mg to 6 healthy, experienced marijuana smokers. Propranolol inhibited the increase in heart rate and systolic blood pressure that normally follows smoking 10 mg of marijuana. Propranolol may have also prevented marijuana-induced reddening of the eyes, and impairment on learning task.

Mechanism

It has been proposed that propranolol blocks β-adrenergic stimulation produced by marijuana.

Clinical Implications

None.

Neuroleptics/Antipsychotics

CHLORPROMAZINE

Evidence of Interaction

In a study involving two 7-week treatment phases, chronic schizophrenic inpatients (9 male, 1 female) were treated with a fixed dose
of chlorpromazine individually determined on the basis of past medication history (Peet et al. 1980). During one of the 7-week periods
the subjects received concomitant doses of propranolol and chlorpromazine. Propranolol was titrated during the first 4 weeks to a
maximum of 10 mg/kg daily. If the pulse rate fell below 50/min or
the systolic blood pressure fell below 90 mm Hg the dose was not
increased further and/or was reduced. Four subjects did not complete
the study. Concomitant treatment with chlorpromazine and propranolol results in elevated plasma levels of both chlorpromazine
and propranolol. Vestal and colleagues (1979) examined the effects
of chlorpromazine on the disposition and effectiveness of propranolol
in 5 male subjects (4 normal, 1 hypertensive). They demonstrated
that chlorpromazine increased steady-state blood levels and lowered
oral clearance of propranolol. Plasma binding remained unchanged,
which the authors believed indicated that chlorpromazine inhibits
propranolol metabolism. In one case report a woman with chronic
schizophrenia experienced delirium, grand mal seizure, and photo-
sensitivity after propranolol was added to her neuroleptic regimen
(Miller and Rampling 1982). The author cites augmented plasma
neuroleptic levels induced by propranolol as the precursor to the
seizures.

Mechanism

Chlorpromazine increases the steady-state blood levels and lowers the oral clearance of propranolol, which is consistent with metabolic inhibition (Vestal et al. 1979). At high doses propranolol may
have an antipsychotic effect, which may be due to a synergistic or
additive effect on receptor sites. Neuroleptics are α-adrenergic blocking agents; thus, like β-blockers, they lower blood pressure.

Clinical Implications

These studies illustrate the potential for toxic complications during concomitant treatment with β-blockers and chlorpromazine.
Schizophrenic patients who are unresponsive to standard antipsychotic therapy may respond in selected cases to combined treatment
with propranolol and an antipsychotic agent. Propranolol as a treat-

ment for schizophrenia remains experimental and controversial. Clinicians should undertake this combination with great caution. The antipsychotic drugs produce varying degrees of α-adrenergic blockade. Chlorpromazine, thioridazine, and mesoridazine administered singularly are the antipsychotics that have the greatest potential to produce hypotensive reactions. When antipsychotics are combined with β-blockers the risk of hypotension increases dramatically. Of the antipsychotics, haloperidol, trifluoperazine, and fluphenazine have the least α-adrenergic blocking action, and consequently are least likely to produce hypotensive reactions. During concomitant administration of β-blockers and antipsychotics, blood pressure and pulse should be regularly monitored. If blood pressure goes below 90/60 mm Hg or if pulse rate falls below 55 beats/min, administration of β-blockers should be delayed until blood pressure and pulse normalize.

THIORIDAZINE

Evidence of Interaction

Greendyke and Kanter (1987) conducted a study to determine the effect of long-acting propranolol on plasma levels of thioridazine and haloperidol in five patients with organic brain disease. Concomitant administration of propranolol increased blood levels of thioridazine and its major metabolites. The magnitude of the increase in thioridazine/sulforidazine/mesoridazine plasma levels significantly correlated with increases in plasma propranolol level. The blood plasma levels of haloperidol were not affected by joint treatment with propranolol.

Prior to conducting a study aimed at assessing the efficacy of propranolol in the treatment of aggression in psychiatric patients, Silver and colleagues (1986) conducted a pilot study to assess the drug interactions between propranolol and thioridazine. The first patient was a 34-year-old man diagnosed with schizophrenia. Over a period of 40 days, propranolol was added to a total dose of 800 mg/day to his pharmacologic regimen, which previously consisted of thioridazine 400 mg twice daily. The second patient, a 27-year-old schizophrenic woman with generalized seizure disorder, was taking thioridazine 300 mg twice daily, and phenytoin 100 mg three times daily at the onset of the study. Propranolol was introduced and increased over a period of 26 days to a total dose of 800 mg/day. The addition of propranolol produced a 3-fold and 5-fold increase in plasma thioridazine levels. This increase placed both patients in a potentially toxic range; however, neither patient exhibited signs or symptoms of thioridazine toxicity.

In a study of 26 male patients with intermittent explosive disorder secondary to organic brain disease, the effects of pindolol on the serum levels of thioridazine, haloperidol, phenytoin, and phenobarbital were examined (Greendyke and Gulya 1988). No significant increases in haloperidol, phenytoin, or phenobarbital were discovered during concomitant administration of pindolol. Both pindolol and thioridazine levels were elevated when the drugs were coadministered. Pindolol's effect on the serum blood levels of thioridazine was less pronounced than the effects demonstrated in previous studies with propranolol.

Mechanism

Competitive interference with hepatic metabolism is suggested by the mutual elevation of pindolol and thioridazine levels (Greendyke and Gulya 1988). At high doses propranolol may have an antipsychotic effect, which suggests a synergistic or additive effect on receptor sites. Neuroleptics are α-adrenergic blocking agents; thus, like β-blockers, they lower blood pressure.

Clinical Implications

These studies demonstrate the potential for toxic complications in patients receiving thioridazine and β-blockers. (See Clinical Implications for Chlorpromazine.)

HALOPERIDOL

Evidence of Interaction

Hypotension and cardiopulmonary arrest are reported in a 48-year-old schizophrenic woman treated with haloperidol and propranolol (Alexander et al. 1984). The patient tolerated haloperidol 20 mg daily with trichlormethiazide 4 mg daily; however, during a subsequent hospitalization she was treated with an 80 mg dose of propranolol 80 mg, followed 10 hours later with oral haloperidol 10 mg. Ninety minutes later the patient fell to the floor and became unresponsive. Her breathing became shallow and she became cyanotic. The patient's blood pressure fell to 80/0 mm Hg. She responded to respiratory assistance and was eventually discharged on haloperidol and trichlormethiazide. Ten months later she was once again given 10 mg of haloperidol and 40 mg of propranolol. Once more she became unresponsive and cyanotic, and stopped breathing. She was revived and discharged on loxapine, propranolol, and trichlormethiazide. The patient had an identical response 5 months later when again she received haloperidol 10 mg and propranolol 80 mg.

In a study of 14 hospitalized chronic schizophrenics, propranolol (400–500 mg) was added to the previous neuroleptic regimen (Yorkston et al. 1977). When compared with the placebo group, the propranolol group showed a greater improvement on the Brief Psychiatric Rating Scale, the psychiatrists' global assessment and nursing ratings. On the physicians' ratings, improvement was seen by week 8, and by week 19 florid psychotic symptoms had diminished in all 7 propranolol patients.

Mechanism

It is possible that propranolol increased the plasma level of haloperidol and the total level of active metabolites. At high doses propranolol may have an antipsychotic effect, which suggests a synergistic or additive effect on receptor sites. Neuroleptics are α-adrenergic blocking agents; thus, like β-blockers, they lower blood pressure.

Clinical Implications

(*See* Clinical Implications for Chlorpromazine)

Opioid Analgesics

Evidence of Interaction

Pretreatment with propranolol in chronically instrumented dogs receiving sufentanil alone or in combination with the nondepolarizing neuromuscular-blocking agent vecuronium resulted in a decreased left ventricular +dP/dt without other hemodynamic alterations. Sufentanil produced statistically significant, dose-dependent decreases in heart rate and +dP/dt after pretreatment with propranolol. Mean and diastolic coronary vascular resistance was also increased. The combined pretreatment of diltiazem and propranolol resulted in significantly greater bradycardia than did no pretreatment or pretreatment with propranolol alone. The concomitant administration of sufentanil and vecuronium after combined pretreatment of propranolol and diltiazem produced bradyarrhythmias and two episodes of asystole. The authors concluded that the appearance of cardiac conduction disturbances in dogs treated with sufentanil and vecuronium are more likely to occur after pretreatment with diltiazem and propranolol (Schmeling et al. 1989). In a study of first-pass uptake of fentanyl in human and rat lungs, propranolol was found to alter the pulmonary accumulation of fentanyl. First-pass uptake of fentanyl was decreased, representing a potential drug interaction (Roerig et al. 1989).

Mechanism
Not established.

Clinical Implications
Not established.

Oral Contraceptives

Evidence of Interaction
Kendall and colleagues (1982) administered a 100-mg single oral dose of metoprolol to 23 healthy women. Twelve of these women were also receiving a low-dose oral contraceptive. A 70% higher area-under-the-plasma-concentration-time-curve was observed in the 12 women who were receiving oral contraceptives in addition to metoprolol. Further studies need to examine the effect of chronic metoprolol treatment to determine if there is an increased metoprolol response.

Mechanism
Not established.

Clinical Implications
The clinical significance has not yet been established, although clinicians should be alert for increased metoprolol response in women taking oral contraceptives.

Phenylpropanolamine

Evidence of Interaction
There is a case report in the medical literature of a patient treated for hypertension with oxprenolol and methyldopa (McLaren 1976). Two days after beginning therapy with cold tablets containing phenylpropanolamine and acetaminophen, the patient experienced a severe hypertensive reaction (200/150 mm Hg). The day after the cold tablets were stopped the patient's blood pressure decreased to 140/110 mm Hg and later to 140/90 mm Hg.

In 7 hypertensive men treated with β-blockers, O'Connell and Gross (1991) studied the effect of multiple phenylpropanolamine

(PPA) doses. Previously, each patient displayed a mean increase in blood pressure after PPA 25 mg compared with placebo. The patients were given PPA 25 mg 3 times a day for 6.3 days. The PPA caused a small but statistically significant increase in the peak measured systolic and diastolic pressures in the 5 subjects who completed the study. There were no significant differences in the maximum blood pressure change or area-under-the-blood-pressure-time-curves between days 1 and 7 of therapy and placebo.

Mechanism

The interaction may be dependent on the specific drug combination and β-blocker serum concentration (O'Connell 1991).

Clinical Implications

Patients receiving β-blocker therapy should be advised to use cold tablets that do not contain phenylpropanolamine.

Phosphodiesterase Inhibitor

Evidence of Interaction

Boldt and colleagues (1990) studied the effects of enoximone compared to dobutamine in 20 acutely β-adrenoceptor blocked patients. The patients were scheduled for aortocoronary bypass grafting and all suffered from tachycardia. All of the patients were treated with an infusion of esmolol followed 20 minutes later with either enoximone or dobutamine. Enoximone increased myocardial contractility in spite of the effective blockade of β-adrenoreceptors by esmolol, whereas esmolol blocked the β1-adrenoreceptor effects of dobutamine leading to a marked increase in peripheral resistance without accompanying cardiac stimulation.

Mechanism

Not established.

Clinical Implications

Dobutamine may not be the drug of choice for inotropic support in patients pretreated with β-blockers, as enoximone appears to improve hemodynamic status even in patients who are β-blocked (Boldt 1990).

Theophylline

Evidence of Interaction

Propranolol (40 mg every 6 hours) and, to a lesser extent metoprolol (50 mg every 6 hours), were found to reduce the clearance of theophylline in nine healthy subjects (Conrad et al. 1980). Corsi and colleagues (1990) examined the effects of atenolol (150 mg/day) or nadolol (89 mg/day) on the metabolism of theophylline in 6 men who smoked. Smokers were studied because they have relatively high theophylline clearances and would thus be more sensitive to a lowering of clearance by β-adrenoceptor antagonists. In keeping with previous work (Cerasa et al. 1988), atenolol did not affect the clearance of theophylline. In addition, nadolol did not demonstrate an effect on the metabolism of theophylline. Corsi and colleagues (1990) suggest that lipophilicity may be the important factor in determining inhibition of theophylline metabolism by β-blockers.

Mechanism

The reduction of theophylline clearance by propranolol and metoprolol may be due to inhibition of hepatic microsomal drug metabolism.

Clinical Implications

Caution should be conducted during joint administration of β-blockers and theophylline. In patients being treated for asthma, concomitant administration of propranolol and theophylline should be avoided due to the possibility of propranolol-induced bronchoconstriction.

REFERENCES

Abate MA et al.: Interaction of indomethacin and sulindac with labetalol. Br J Clin Pharmacol 31: 363, 1991.

Abdelraham A et al.: Effects of anaesthetic agents on pressor response to beta-blockers in the rat. J Pharm Pharmacol 44: 34, 1992.

Alexander HE et al.: Hypotension and cardiopulmonary arrest associated with concurrent haloperidol and propranolol therapy. JAMA 252: 87, 1984.

Alvan G et al.: Effect of pentobarbital on the disposition of alprenolol. Clin Pharmacol Ther 22: 316, 1977.

Anastassiades CJ: Nifedipine and beta-blocker drugs. Br Med J 281: 1251, 1980.

Anastassiades CJ: Nifedipine and beta-blockade as a cause of cardiac failure. Br Med J 284: 506, 1982.

Angelo-Nelsen K et al.: Timolol topically and diabetes mellitus. JAMA 244: 2263, 1980.

Bailey DG et al.: Interaction between oral verapamil and beta-blockers during submaximal exercise: relevance of ancillary properties. Clin Pharmacol Ther 49: 370, 1991.

Bauer LA et al.: Influence of nifedipine therapy on indocyanine green and oral propranolol pharmacokinetics. Eur J Clin Pharmacol 37: 257, 1989.

Baumrucker JF: Drug interaction—propranolol and cafergot. N Engl J Med 288: 916, 1973.

Blum I et al.: Prevention of hypoglycemic attacks by propranolol in patient suffering from insulinoma. Diabetes 24: 535, 1975.

Blum I et al.: Suppression of hypoglycemia by dl-propranolol in malignant insulinoma. N Engl J Med 299: 487, 1978.

Boldt J et al.: Haemodynamic effects of the phosphodiesterase inhibitor enoximone in comparison with dobutamine in esmolol-treated cardiac surgery patients. Br J Anaesth 64: 611, 1990.

Bruce DL et al.: Preoperative clonidine withdrawal syndrome. Anesthesiology 51: 90, 1979.

Brummett RE.: Warning to otolaryngologists using local anesthetics containing epinephrine. Arch Otolaryngol 110: 561, 1984.

Cairns SA, Marshall AJ.: Clonidine withdrawal (letter). Lancet 1: 368, 1976.

Camanni F, Massara F.: Enhancement of levodopa-induced growth-hormone stimulation by propranolol. Lancet 1: 942, 1974.

Cerasa LA et al.: Lack of effect of atenolol on the pharmacokinetics of theophylline. Br J Clin Pharmacol 26: 800, 1988.

Chiariello M et al.: Effect of furosemide on plasma concentration and b-blockade by propranolol. Clin Pharmacol Ther 26: 433, 1979.

Christensen CK et al.: Renal effects of acute calcium blockade with nifedipine in hypertensive patients receiving beta-adrenoceptor-blocking drugs. Clin Pharmacol Ther 32: 572, 1982.

Collste P et al.: Influence of pentobarbital on effect and plasma levels of alprenolol and 4-hydroxy-alprenolol. Clin Pharmacol Ther 25: 423, 1979.

Conrad KA, Nyman DW: Effects of metoprolol and propranolol on theophylline elimination. Clin Pharmacol Ther 28: 463, 1980.

Corsi CM et al.: Lack of effect of atenolol and nadolol on the metabolism of theophylline. Br J Clin Pharmacol 29: 265, 1990.

Daly K et al.: Beneficial effect of adding nifedipine to beta-adrenergic blocking therapy in angina pectoris. Eur Heart J 3: 42, 1982.

Daneshmend TK et al.: Cimetidine and bioavailability of labetalol. Lancet 1: 565, 1981.

Dargie JH et al.: Nifedipine and propranolol: a beneficial drug interaction. Am J Med 71: 6476, 1981.

Davidson J et al.: Practical aspects of MAO inhibitor therapy. J Clin Psychiatry 45: 81, 1984.

Deacon S et al.: Comparison of atenolol and propranolol during insulin-induced hypoglycaemia. Br Med J 2: 272, 1976.

Deacon S et al.: Acebutolol, atenolol and propranolol and metabolic responses to acute hypoglycaemia in diabetics. Br Med J 2: 1255, 1977.

Dean S, Kendall MJ: Adverse interaction between nifedipine and beta-blockade. Br Med J 282: 1322, 1981.

DePonti C et al.: Effects of nifedipine, acebutolol, and their association on exercise tolerance in patients with effort angina. Cardiology 68: 195, 1981.

Dobbs JH et al.: Effects of aluminum hydroxide on the absorption of propranolol. Curr Ther Res 21: 887, 1977.

Durao V et al.: Modification of antihypertensive effect of β-adrenoceptor-blocking agents by inhibition of endogenous prostaglandin synthesis. Lancet 2: 1005, 1977.

Eggertsen R, Hansson L: Effects of treatment with nifedipine and metoprolol in essential hypertension. Eur J Clin Pharmacol 21: 389, 1982.

Ekberg G, Hansson B-G: Glucose tolerance and insulin release in hypertensive patients treated with the cardioselective beta-receptor blocking agent metoprolol. Acta Med Scand 202: 393, 1977.

Elliott HL et al.: Immediate cardiovascular responses to oral prazosin-effects of concurrent beta-blockers. Clin Pharmacol Ther 29: 303, 1981.

Elliott HL et al.: The interactions between nisoldipine and two beta-adrenoceptor antagonists—atenolol and propranolol. Br J Clin Pharmacol 32: 379, 1991.

Feely J et al.: Reduction of liver blood flow and propranolol metabolism by cimetidine. N Engl J Med 304: 692, 1981.

Filipek B et al.: The effect of ethanol on the antiarrhythmic action of atenolol. Polish Pharmacol Pharm 41: 207–211, 1989.

Formgren H, Eriksson NE: Effects of practolol in combination with terbutaline in the treatment of hypertension and arrhythmias in asthmatic patients. Scand J Resp Dis 56: 217, 1975.

Foster CA, Aston SJ: Propranolol-epinephrine interaction. Clin Pharm 2: 461, 1983.

Gandy W: Severe epinephrine-propranolol interaction. Ann Emerg Med 18: 98, 1989.

Gandy W et al.: Dihydroergotamine interaction with propranolol (letter). Ann Emerg Med 19: 221, 1990.

Goodman A, Gilman L (eds): *Pharmacologic Basis of Therapeutics,* 7th ed., New York, Macmillan, 1986.

Graham RM et al.: Prazosin: the first-dose phenomenon. Br Med J 4: 1293, 1976.

Grajower MM et al.: Hypoglycemia in chronic hemodialysis patients: association with propranolol use. Nephron 26: 126, 1980.

Greendyke RM, Gulya A: Effect of pindolol administration on serum levels of thiordazine, haloperidol, phenytoin, and phenobarbital. J Clin Psychiatry 49: 105, 1988.

Greendyke RM, Kanter DR: Plasma propranolol levels and their effect on plasma thioridazine and haloperidol concentrations. J Clin Psychopharmacol 7: 178, 1987.

Groop L et al.: Influence of beta-blocking drugs on glucose metabolism in patients with non-insulin dependent diabetes mellitus. Acta Med Scand 211: 7, 1982.

Gugler R, Allgayer H: Effects of antacids on the clinical pharmacokinetics of drugs: An update. Clin Pharmacokin 18: 210, 1990.

Haglund K et al.: Influence of pentobarbital on metoprolol plasma levels. Clin Pharmacol Ther 26: 326, 1979.

Hall ST et al.: The pharmacokinetic and pharmacodynamic interaction between lacidipine and propranolol in healthy volunteers. J Cardiovasc Pharmacol 18 (suppl 11): S13, 1991.

Hansbrough JF, Near A: Propranolol-epinephrine antagonism with hypertension and stroke. Ann Intern Med 92: 717, 1980.

Hansten PD: Beta-blocking agents and antidiabetic drugs. Drug Intell Clin Pharmacol 14: 46, 1980.

Hansten PD, Horn JR: *Drug Interactions.* Vancouver, Applied Therapeutics, 1993.

Harris AL et al.: Clonidine withdrawal and blockade (letter). Lancet 1: 596, 1976.

Hesse B, Pedersen JT: Hypoglycaemia after propranolol in children. Acta Med Scand 193: 551, 1973.

Heagerty AM et al.: Influence of cimetidine on pharmacokinetics of propranolol. Br Med J 282: 1917, 1981.

Heagerty AM et al.: Failure of ranitidine to interact with propranolol. Br Med J 284: 1304, 1982.

Hermann DJ et al.: Comparison of verapamil, diltiazem, and labetalol on the bioavailability and metabolism of imipramine. J Clin Pharmacol 32: 176, 1992.

Holm G et al.: Severe hypoglycaemia during physical exercise and treatment with beta-blockers. Br Med J 282: 1360, 1981.

Houben H et al.: Influence of selective and non-selective beta-adrenoreceptor blockade on the haemodynamic effect of adrenalin during combined antihypertensive drug therapy. Clin Science 57: 397s, 1979.

Houben H et al.: Effect of lose-dose epinephrine infusion on hemodynamics after selective and nonselective beta-blockade in hypertension. Clin Pharmacol Ther 31: 685, 1982.

Houtzagers JJR et al.: The effect of pretreatment with cimetidine on the bioavailability and disposition of atenolol and metoprolol. Br J Clin Pharmacol 14: 647, 1982.

Husted SE et al.: Long-term therapy and arterial hypertension with nifedipine given alone or in combination with a beta-adrenoceptor blocking agent. Eur J Clin Pharmacol 22: 101, 1982.

Jacobs RL et al.: Potentiated anaphylaxis in patients with drug-induced beta-adrenergic blockade. J Allergy Clin Immunol 68: 125, 1981.

Johnson G et al.: Effects of intravenous propranolol and metoprolol and their interaction with isoprenaline on pulmonary function, heart rate, and blood pressure in asthmatics. Eur J Clin Pharmacol 8: 175, 1975.

Joshi PI et al.: Nifedipine and left ventricular function in beta-blocked patients. Br Heart J 45: 457, 1981.

Kallen RJ et al.: A complication of treatment of hypertension with propranolol. Clin Pediatr 99: 567, 1980.

Kendall MJ, et al.: Metoprolol pharmacokinetics and the oral contraceptive pill. Br J Clin Pharmacol 14: 120, 1982.

Kieval J et al.: The effects of intravenous verapamil on hemodynamic status of patients with coronary artery disease receiving propranolol. Circulation 65: 653, 1982.

Kirch W et al.: Interaction of atenolol with furosemide and calcium and aluminum salts. Clin Pharmacol Therap 30: 429, 1981.

Kirch W et al.: Interaction of metoprolol, propranolol and atenolol with concurrent administration of cimetidine. Klin Wochenschr 60: 1401, 1982.

Kissel P et al.: Levodopa-propranolol therapy in parkinsonian tremor (letter). Lancet 1: 403, 1974.

Kowey PR et al.: Interaction between propranolol and propafenone in healthy volunteers. J Clin Pharmacol 29: 512, 1989.

Kram J et al.: Propranolol (letter). Ann Intern Med 80: 282, 1974.

Krikler DM et al.: Calcium-channel blockers and beta-blockers: advantages and disadvantages of combination therapy in chronic stable angina pectoris. Am Heart J 104: 702, 1982.

Lager I et al.: Effect of cardioselective and nonselective beta-blockade on the hypoglycemic response in insulin-dependent diabetics. Lancet 1: 458–462, 1979.

Lampman RM et al.: Cardiac arrhythmias during epinephrine-propranolol infusions for measurement of in vivo insulin resistance. Diabetes 30: 618, 1981.

Lilja M et al.: Interaction of clonidine and beta-blockers. Acta Med Scand 207: 173, 1980.

Lotti G et al.: Enhancement of levodopa-induced growth-hormone stimulation by practolol (letter). Lancet 2: 1329, 1974.

McLaren EH: Severe hypertension produced by interaction of phenylpropanolamine with methyldopa and oxprenolol. Br Med J 3: 283, 1976.

Melander A et al.: Enhancement of the bioavailability of propranolol and metoprolol by food. Clin Pharmacol Ther 22: 108, 1977.

Messerli FH et al.: Effects of β-adrenergic blockade on plasma cyclic AMP and blood sugar responses to glucagon and isoproterenol in man. Int J Clin Pharmacol 14: 189, 1976.

Meyers MG, Hope-Gill HF: Effect of d- and dl-propranolol on glucose-stimulated insulin release. Clin Pharmacol Ther 25: 303, 1979.

Miller FA, Rampling D: Adverse effects of combined propranolol and chlorpromazine therapy. Am J Psychiatry 139: 1198, 1982.

Mohler H et al.: Glucose intolerance during chronic β-adrenergic blockade in man. Clin Pharmacol Ther 25: 237, 1979.

Murdoch DL et al.: Evaluation of potential pharmacodynamic and pharmacokinetic interactions between verapamil and propranolol in normal subjects. Br J Clin Pharmacol 31: 323, 1991.

Murthy SS et al.: Pharmacokinetic interaction between verapamil and metoprolol in the dog. Drug Metab Dispos 19: 1093, 1991.

Nardone DA, Bouma DJ: Hyperglycemia and diabetic coma: possible relationship to diuretic-propranolol therapy. South Med J 72: 1607, 1979.

Newman BR, Schultz LK: Epinephrine resistant anaphylaxis in a patient taking propranolol hydrochloride. Ann Allergy 47: 35, 1981.

Newman RJ et al.: Comparison of propranolol, metoprolol, and acebutolol on insulin-induced hypoglycaemia. Br Med J 2: 447, 1976.

Nies AS et al.: Hypertensive response to propranolol in a patient treated with methyldopa—a proposed mechanism. Clin Pharmacol Ther 14: 823, 1973.

O'Connell MB, Gross CR: The effect of multiple doses of phenylpropranolamine on the blood pressure of patients whose hypertension was controlled with beta blockers. Pharmacotherapy 11: 376, 1991.

Ostman J et al.: Effect of metoprolol and alprenolol on the metabolic, hormonal, and hemodynamic response to insulin-induced hypoglycaemia in hypertensive, insulin-dependent diabetics. Acta Med Scand 211: 381, 1982.

Packer M et al.: Hemodynamic and clinical effects of combined verapamil and propranolol therapy in angina pectoris. Am J Cardiology 50: 903, 1982a.

Packer M et al.: Hemodynamic consequences of combined beta-adrenergic and slow calcium channel blockade in man. Circulation 65: 660, 1982b.

Palmer RF: Pharmacological autopsy of anesthetic death for aortography for aortic dissection (question and answer). JAMA 232: 1281, 1975.

Pan HY et al.: Pharmacokinetic interaction between propranolol and the HMG-CoA reductase inhibitors pravastatin and lovastatin. Br J Clin Pharmacol 31: 665, 1991.

Patwardhan RV et al.: Effects of caffeine on plasma free fatty acids, urinary catecholamine, and drug binding. Clin Pharmacol Ther 28: 398, 1980.

Peet M et al.: Pharmacokinetic interaction between propranolol and chlorpromazine in schizophrenic patients. Lancet 2: 978, 1980.

Pelsor DA et al.: Propranolol-induced hypoglycemia during growth hormone testing. J Pediatr 99: 157, 1981.

Perruca E et al.: Effect of atenolol, metoprolol, and propranolol on isoproterenol-induced tremor and tachycardia in normal subjects. Clin Pharmacol Ther 29: 425, 1981.

Pfisterer M et al.: Combined acebutolol/nifedipine therapy in patients with chronic coronary artery disease: additional improvement of ischemia-induced left ventricular dysfunction. Am J Cardiol 49: 1259, 1982.

Ponten J et al.: Bupivacaine for intercostal nerve blockade in patients on long-term b-receptor blocking therapy. Acta Anaesth Scand 76 (suppl): 70, 1982a.

Ponten J et al.: β-Receptor blockade and spinal anaesthesia: withdrawal versus continuation of long-term therapy. Acta Anaesth Scand 76 (suppl): 62, 1982b.

Popp DA et al.: Role of epinephrine mediated beta-adrenergic mechanisms in hypoglycemic glucose counterregulation and post-hypoglycemic hyperglycemia in insulin-dependent diabetes mellitus. J Clin Invest 69: 315, 1982.

Raskin NH: Repetitive intravenous DHE as therapy for migraine. Neurology 36: 995–997, 1986.

Reeves RL, Sen SB: The effect of metoprolol and propranolol on pancreatic insulin release. Clin Pharmacol Therap 31: 262, 1982.

Regardh CG et al.: The effect of antacid, metoclopramide, and propantheline on the bioavailability of metoprolol and atenolol. Biopharm Drug Dispos 2: 79, 1981.

Reggev A, Vollhardt BR: Bradycardia induced by an interaction between phenelzine and beta blockers. Psychosomatics 30: 106, 1989.

Reimann IW et al.: Effects of cimetidine and ranitidine on steady-state propranolol kinetics and dynamics. Clin Pharmacol Ther 32: 749, 1982.

Richards DA et al.: Circulatory effects of noradrenalin and adrenalin before and after labetalol. Br J Clin Pharmacol 7: 371, 1979.

Risch SC et al.: The effects of psychotropic drugs on the cardiovascular system. J Clin Psychiatry 43: 16, 1982.

Robson RH, Vishwanath MC: Nifedipine and beta-blockade as a cause of cardiac failure. Br Med J 284: 104, 1982.

Roerig DL et al.: Effect of propranolol on the first pass uptake of fentanyl in the human and rat lung. Anesthesiology 71: 62, 1989.

Roitman K et al.: Enhancement of bupivacaine cardiotoxicity with cardiac glycosides and beta-adrenergic blockers: a case report. Anesth Analg 76: 658, 1993.

Rosenthal T et al.: Use of labetalol in hypertensive patients during discontinuation of clonidine therapy. Eur J Clin Pharmacol 20: 237, 1981.

Ryan JR et al.: Response of diabetics treated with atenolol or propranolol to insulin-induced hypoglycaemia (abstract). Clin Pharmacol Ther 31: 266, 1982.

Saarimaa H: Combination of clonidine and sotalol in hypertension. Br Med J 1: 810, 1976.

Sagie A et al.: Symptomatic bradycardia induced by the combination of oral diltiazem and beta blockers. Clin Cardiol 14: 314, 1991.

Salvetti A et al.: Interaction between oxprenolol and indomethacin on blood pressure in essential hypertensive patients. Eur J Clin Pharmacol 22: 197, 1982.

Sandler M et al.: Oxprenolol and levodopa in parkinsonian patients (letter). Lancet 1: 168, 1975.

Santiago JV et al.: Epinephrine, norepinephrine, glucagon, and growth hormone release in association with physiological decrements in the plasma glucose concentration in normal and diabetic man. J Clin Endocrinol Metab 51: 877, 1980.

Scandellari C et al.: The effect of propranolol on hypoglycaemia. Diabetologia 15: 297, 1978.

Schafer-Korting M et al.: Atenolol interaction with aspirin, allopurinol and ampicillin. Clin Pharmacol Ther 33: 283, 1983.

Schmeling WT et al.: Negative chronotropic actions of sufentanil and vecuronium in chronically instrumented dogs pretreated with propranolol and/or diltiazem. Anesth Analg 69: 4, 1989.

Schuna AA et al.: Lack of interaction between sulindac or naproxen and propranolol in hypertensive patients. J Clin Pharmacol 29: 524, 1989.

Seideman P et al.: Prazosin first dose phenomenon during combined treatment with a beta-adrenoceptor in hypertensive patients. Br J Clin Pharmacol 13: 865, 1982.

Shand DG et al.: Plasma propranolol levels in adults: with observations in four children. Clin Pharmacol Ther 22: 18, 1970.

Sharma SD et al.: Comparison of penbutolol and propranolol during insulin-induced hypoglycaemia. Curr Ther Res 26: 252, 1979.

Shepherd AMM et al.: Hypoglycemia-induced hypertension in a diabetic patient on metoprolol. Ann Intern Med 94: 357, 1981.

Silver JM et al.: Elevation of thioridazine plasma levels by propranolol. Am J Psychiatry 143: 1290, 1986.

Smits P et al.: Hemodynamic and humoral effects of coffee after b1-selective and nonselective b-blockade. Clin Pharmacol Ther 34: 153, 1983.

Sotaniemi EA et al.: Propranolol and sotalol metabolism after a drinking party. Clin Pharmacol Ther 29: 705, 1981.

Souich P et al.: Enhancement of nadolol elimination by activated charcoal and antibiotics. Clin Pharmacol Ther 33: 585, 1983.

Spahn H et al.: Influence of ranitidine on plasma metoprolol and atenolol concentrations. Br Med J 286: 1546, 1983.

Staffurth JS, Emery P: Adverse interaction between nifedipine and beta-blockade (letter). Br Med J 282: 225, 1981.

Strauss FG et al.: Withdrawal of antihypertensive therapy. JAMA 238: 1734, 1977.

Sulkowski A et al.: Propranolol effects on acute marijuana intoxication in man. Psychopharmacology 52: 47, 1977.

Tabrizchi R, Pang CC: Propranolol antagonizes hypotension induced by alpha-blockers but not by sodium nitroprusside or methacholine. Can J Physiol Pharmacol 67: 83, 1989.

Thringer G, Svedmyr N: Interaction of orally administered metoprolol, practolol and propranolol in asthmatics. Eur J Clin Pharmacol 10: 163, 1976.

Tilstone WJ et al.: Effects of furosemide on glomerular filtration rate and clearance of practolol, digoxin, cephaloridine and gentamicin. Clin Pharmacol Ther 22: 389, 1977.

Timour Q et al.: Possible role of drug interactions in bupivacaine-induced problems related to intraventricular conduction disorders. Reg Anesth 15: 180, 1990.

Tiula E, Neuvonen PJ: Antiepileptic drugs and alpha-1-acid glycoprotein. N Engl J Med 307: 1448, 1982.

Tobias JD et al.: Pulmonary reactivity to methacholine during beta-adrenergic blockade: propranolol versus esmolol. Anesthesiology 73: 132, 1990.

VanHerwaarden CLA et al.: Effects of adrenalin during treatment with propranolol and metoprolol (letter). Br Med J 2: 1029, 1977a.

VanHerwaarden CLA et al.: Haemodynamic effects of adrenalin during treatment of hypertensive patients with propranolol and metoprolol. Eur J Clin Pharmacol 12: 397, 1977b.

Varma DR et al.: Response to adrenalin and propranolol in hyperthyroidism (letter). Lancet 1: 260, 1976.

Venter CP: Severe peripheral ischaemia during concomitant use of beta-blockers and ergot alkaloids. Br Med J 289: 288, 1984.

Vernon C, Sakula A: Fatal rebound hypertension after abrupt withdrawal of clonidine and propranolol. Br J Clin Pract 33: 112, 1979.

Vestal RE et al.: Inhibition of propranolol metabolism by chlorpromazine. Clin Pharmacol Ther 25: 19, 1979.

Waal-Manning HJ: Metabolic effects of beta-adrenoreceptor blockers. Drugs 11: 121, 1976.

Waal-Manning HJ: Can beta-blockers be used in diabetic patients? Drugs 17: 157, 1979.

Wagner F et al.: Drug interaction between propafenone and metoprolol. Br J Clin Pharmacol 24: 213, 1987.

Warren SE et al.: Clonidine and propranolol paradoxical hypertension. Arch Intern Med 139: 253, 1979.

Watkins J et al.: Attenuation of hypotensive effect of propranolol and thiazide diuretics by indomethacin. Br Med J 281: 702, 1980.

Wayne VS et al.: Adverse interaction between beta-adrenergic blocking drugs and verapamil—report of three cases. Aust NZ J Med 12: 285, 1982.

Wiesfeld AC et al.: Acute hemodynamic and electrophysiologic effects and safety of high-dose intravenous diltiazem in patients receiving metoprolol. Am J Cardiol 70: 997, 1992.

Williams DT et al.: The effect of propranolol on uncontrolled rage outbursts in children and adolescents with organic brain dysfunction. J Am Acad Child Psychiatry 2: 125, 1982.

Winniford MD et al.: Hemodynamic and electrophysiologic effects of verapamil and nifedipine in patients on propranolol. Am J Cardiol 50: 704, 1982.

Winniford MD et al.: Randomized, double-blind comparison of propranolol alone and a propranolol-verapamil combination in patients with severe angina of effort. J Am Coll Cardiol 1: 492, 1983.

Wood AJJ: How the beta-blockers differ: a pharmacologic comparison. Drug Ther 13: 59, 1983.

Wray R, Sutcliffe SBJ: Propranolol-induced hypoglycaemia and myocardial infarction (letter). Br Med J 2: 592, 1972.

Yasue H et al.: Prinzmetal's variant form of angina as a manifestation of alpha-adrenergic receptor-mediated coronary artery spasm: documentation by coronary arteriography. Am Heart J 91: 148, 1976.

Yorkston NJ et al.: Propranolol as an adjunct to the treatment of schizophrenia. Lancet 2: 575, 1977.

Young KD, MacDonald G: Treatment of angina pectoris in general practice with a combination of nifedipine and beta-blocker. Br J Clin Pract 26: 103, 1982.

Yudofsky S et al.: Propranolol in the treatment of rage and violent behavior in patients with chronic brain syndrome. Am J Psychiatry 138: 218, 1981.

Yudkin JS: Withdrawal of clonidine. Lancet 1: 546, 1977.

Yust I et al.: Life-threatening bradycardic reactions due to beta blocker-diltiazem interactions. Israel J Med Sci 28: 292, 1992.

Zhou HH et al.: Quinidine reduces clearance of ⟨PM⟩ propranolol more than ⟨MM⟩ propranolol through marked reduction in 4-hydroxylation. Clin Pharmacol Ther 47: 686, 1990.

8

Interactions of Importance in Chemical Dependence

JAMIE G. BARNHILL, ANN MARIE CIRAULO, DOMENIC A. CIRAULO and JOHN A. GREENE

The comorbidity of psychoactive substance dependence and psychiatric illness is common. Psychiatrists are often in the position of prescribing psychotropic medications to patients who may relapse to substance use, making potential interactions of psychotropics with alcohol and drugs of abuse an important clinical consideration. In this chapter we present a brief overview of the most commonly encountered drug-drug interactions among drugs of abuse, ethanol, and therapeutic agents. We also present an overview of disulfiram interactions.

Amphetamines

AMPHETAMINES AND ANTIDEPRESSANTS

MAOIs

Fatal hypertensive reactions have been described between tranylcypromine and methylamphetamine (Mason 1962) and between phenelzine and dextroamphetamine (Lloyd and Walker 1965). An interaction was reported (Devabhaktuni and Jampala 1987) between the monoamine oxidase inhibitor (MAOI) phenelzine and the amphetamine/dextroamphetamine resin complex known on the street as "black beauty." The patient experienced severe hypertension, tachycardia, and a grand mal seizure but survived due to rapid emergency room treatment. The mechanism of the interaction involves increases by the MAOI in the pressor responses of indirectly acting sympathomimetic amines such as the amphetamines (*see also* Chap. 2).

Smilkstein and associates (1987) reported a case of an interaction between MDMA (3,4-methylene-dioxy-methamphetamine) and an MAOI. A 50-year-old man ingested MDMA 1 hour after his usual dose of phenelzine sulfate 15 mg (Nardil). Over the next hour the patient experienced symptoms of palpitations, a sense of uneasiness, difficulty with controlling speech and movement, and abnormal movements. The patient was transported to the emergency room and shortly after was unable to respond to questions. The patient at this time was also profusely diaphoretic with profound toxic movements and opisthotonic arching. Blood pressure was 208/80 mm Hg, heart rate 64 beats/min, respirations 28 breaths/min, temperature 36.9°C (rectal), and trismus was noted. The presence of MDMA was confirmed by gas chromatographic and mass spectographic analyses. The patient was treated with intravenous diphenhydramine, activated charcoal, magnesium sulfate, and supportive care and monitoring. Following treatment the patient normalized 7.5 hours after taking MDMA and 6.5 hours after taking phenelzine sulfate.

Ondansetron

A controlled clinical study (Silverstone et al. 1992) examining the interaction of amphetamine with the 5-HT 3 antagonist, ondansetron, found that pretreatment with ondansetron decreased the effects of amphetamine on hunger and overall subjective state, with no effect on the blood pressure or psychomotor skill changes seen with amphetamine alone. The authors speculated that the interaction is due to altered neurotransmission within the mesolimbic brain regions.

Barbiturates

The greatest number of barbiturate-induced drug interactions result from induction of hepatic microsomal enzymes. This can result in increased drug clearances, decreased plasma levels of drug, and decreased elimination half-lives. Barbiturates also interact pharmacokinetically with other drugs by competitive inhibition of hepatic metabolism. Pharmacodynamically, the barbiturates combine with other central nervous system (CNS) depressants to produce enhanced CNS depression, which may be life threatening in its extreme (*see also* Chap. 6).

BARBITURATES AND ANTIDEPRESSANTS

Tricyclics

The metabolism of tricyclic antidepressants, such as desipramine, nortriptyline, amitriptyline, and protriptyline, is increased in patients receiving barbiturates (Alexanderson et al. 1969, Burrows and Davies 1971, Hammer et al. 1966, Moody et al. 1977). Steady-state plasma levels of nortriptyline were compared in twins when one of the twin pair also received a barbiturate (Alexanderson et al. 1969). The serum levels were reduced by 14 to 60% in the twins receiving barbiturates. The combination of tricylic antidepressants with barbiturates could result in inadequate treatment of depressive symptoms if therapeutic levels of the tricyclic are not achieved.

MAOIs. A possible interaction between barbiturates and MAOIs has been reported (Domino et al. 1962) involving tranylcypromine 30 mg daily by mouth and amobarbital 250 mg intramuscularly. The patient became ataxic, complained of nausea and dizziness, and became semicomatose for 36 hours. It was suggested that the tranylcypromine inhibited the metabolism of the barbiturate. Evidence for this inhibitory action on hepatic enzymes has been further documented in animal studies (Kline 1959, Lechat and Lemergnan 1961, Wulfsohn and Politzer 1962).

BARBITURATES AND ANTIPSYCHOTICS

In a double-blind crossover design experiment, Linnoila and colleagues (1980) examined the effects of phenobarbital (or placebo) on plasma haloperidol and thioridazine levels. After 6 weeks of combined therapy, the phenobarbital plasma levels were within the normal therapeutic range and were unaffected by haloperidol or thioridazine. In contrast, the haloperidol plasma concentrations were significantly lower in the group receiving phenobarbital as compared with placebo. Although the plasma levels of thioridazine were not significantly different between groups, the plasma concentrations of the active metabolite mesoridazine were signficantly reduced. To sustain therapeutic plasma neuroleptic levels in patients taking phenobarbital, dosage increases of 2 to 3 times the dose necessary for patients not taking phenobarbital may be required.

Barbiturates and Benzodiazepines

The influence of phenobarbital on the single-dose pharmacokinetics of clonazepam were studied in 8 subjects by Khoo and associates

(1980). Subjects were studied prior to and following 19 days of phenobarbital treatment. Clonazepam clearance was increased by 19 to 24% when phenobarbital was added. Steady-state levels were approximately 20% lower in patients taking both drugs. The clinical significance of this interaction is difficult to assess, since clonazepam has been shown to have anticonvulsant efficacy over a wide range of plasma concentrations.

BARBITURATES AND ETHANOL

The interaction between barbiturates and ethanol can involve metabolic interactions as well as pharmacodynamic interactions, due to the fact that both compounds exert at least part of their activity at the γ-aminobutyric receptor-ionophore complex (Miller et al. 1988a). Chronic ethanol consumption induces the enzymatic pathways necessary for the metabolism of barbiturates (Lieber 1982), resulting in decreased plasma concentrations. This effect, along with cross-tolerance, results in the need for high doses of barbiturates in many alcoholics. Lower plasma levels of phenobarbital can be clinically significant if they fall below the minimum therapeutic level for seizure control. On the other hand, acute doses of ethanol inhibit the enzymatic metabolism of barbiturates, resulting in elevated plasma levels and/or toxicity (Rubin et al. 1970). The CNS depression can be severe and life threatening. Ethanol levels are reduced by acute ethanol administration (*see* under Ethanol, this chapter).

In one study (Saario and Linnoila 1976) of psychomotor skill changes following ethanol 0.5 g/kg, subjects who had received amobarbital on the previous night demonstrated greater impairment in coordination than was found following ethanol or amobarbital alone.

BARBITURATES AND OPIOIDS

The CNS effects of opioids (Jaffe and Martin 1985) may combine with the effects of barbiturates on the CNS to produce enhanced depression.

Codeine and Secobarbital

The combination of codeine and secobarbital was examined in 65 hospitalized patients (Bellville et al. 1971). Secobarbital combined with codeine produced a greater sedative effect than secobarbital alone. The authors attributed this to a synergistic rather than additive process, since codeine alone was shown to shorten the duration of sleep and interfere with the quality of sleep.

MEPERIDINE AND PHENOBARBITAL

The interaction between phenobarbital and the analgesic meperidine was reported by Stambaugh and associates in 1977 and further studied and described in 1978. Enhanced sedation was found in subjects who received the drug combination. Renal excretion of meperidine was significantly decreased, while excretion of the demethylated metabolite of meperidine was significantly increased as compared with control subjects who received only meperidine. The authors suggest that the enhanced sedation is a result of CNS depression secondary to phenobarbital induction of the hepatic enzyme pathways responsible for demethylation of meperidine and thus the production of greater amounts of the more toxic demethylated metabolite.

Propoxyphene and Phenobarbital

Propoxyphene inhibited hepatic metabolism of phenobarbital in a study reported by Hansen and associates (1980).

Benzodiazepines

As CNS depressants, benzodiazepines may interact with other depressants to produce increased and potentially life-threatening CNS depression.

BENZODIAZEPINES AND BUPRENORPHINE

Reports from Scotland during the 1980s indicated that intravenous temazepam and buprenorphine were used by drug abusers to enhance euphoria (Forsyth et al. 1993). At that time temazepam was marketed as a liquid-filled capsule, which was drawn into a syringe and mixed with buprenorphine. Vasculitis and thrombosis were common complications of the combination.

BENZODIAZEPINES AND ETHANOL

Acute Ethanol

The effects of acute ethanol ingestion on the pharmacokinetics and pharmacodynamics of benzodiazepines have been extensively studied but with conflicting results, often due to such variables as study design, dose of drug, dose of ethanol, route of administration, and duration of testing.

Concomitant administration of benzodiazepines with acute ethanol has been shown to decrease (Greenblatt et al. 1978) or increase

(Hayes et al. 1977) the apparent absorption rate and peak concentrations of diazepam. Ethanol can slow gastric emptying and may be the cause of a delay or slowing in absorption (Cooke 1972). On the other hand, because acute ethanol can inhibit the enzymatic pathway responsible for the metabolism of diazepam, it is also possible that an increase in apparent absorption rate could be the result of decreased hepatic metabolism in the first pass through the liver after absorption and prior to entry into the systemic circulation. Acute ethanol was reported to slow the absorption rate of oxazepam (Mallach et al. 1975).

In a study involving the combination of intravenous diazepam with and without orally administered ethanol (Sellers et al. 1980), diazepam clearance was significantly decreased in the group receiving ethanol. Plasma levels of the major active metabolite of diazepam, n-desmethyldiazepam, were significantly lower in the group receiving ethanol. The authors attributed these findings to ethanol inhibition of the hepatic enzymes responsible for n-demethylation. Not surprisingly, the combination of ethanol and diazepam produced greater impairment on tests of psychomotor skills due to increased CNS depression than did diazepam alone. Using a similar study design, these same investigators (Sellers and Busto 1982) demonstrated significant memory impairment (determined by word recall tests) with the combination. The combination of intravenous diazepam and oral ethanol had previously been reported to produce significant impairment in visual flicker fusion tests (Gander 1979). Desmond and co-workers (1980) found that oral ethanol decreased the clearance of intravenously administered chlordiazepoxide by 50%. This was explained by inhibition of the hepatic enzymes responsible for the conversion of chlordiazepoxide to its demethylated metabolite.

As far back as 1965, the combination of oral diazepam with concomitant oral ethanol was found to impair mental and psychomotor performance due to increased CNS depression (Hughes 1965). Linnoila and Mattila (1973) found significant impairment in coordination when a single dose of diazepam was combined with oral ethanol. Increased impairment in coordination following the combination of oral diazepam and ethanol was also reported by Morland and associates (1974) and by MacLeod et al. (1977). Curry and Smith (1979) demonstrated significant impairment on the Digital Symbol Substitution test when diazepam 5 mg was combined with an oral ethanol dose. This impairment was greater than that seen with either drug alone. Measurements of hand to eye coordination was significantly impaired in a study by Laisi and co-workers (1979) combining diazepam 10 mg with oral ethanol. Aranko and associates (1985) found pronounced psychomotor impairment when oral ethanol was administered 1 hour after a 10-mg oral dose of diazepam. These same investigators compared the effects of this interaction with the effects found following administration of ethanol and lorazepam 2.5 mg. When impairment was ranked, the lorazepam-ethanol interaction-effects were greater than those seen with diazepam and ethanol. The authors did point out that the psychomotor effects of the two drugs were not equipotent at the two doses. There was no tendency toward tolerance to impairment from either interaction when the same subjects were retested with the combinations after 4 days of receiving the drugs. Lister and File in 1983 had previously shown performance impairment resulting from the interaction between ethanol and a 1.0 mg dose of lorazepam. Self-rated sedation scale scores were significantly increased following both ethanol and lorazepam and the combination of the two resulted in an additive effect on sedation.

Palva and Linnoila (1978) examined the effects of ethanol in combination with the main metabolites of chlordiazepoxide and diazepam on psychomotor skills in a double-blind crossover experiment with 40 healthy volunteers. The metabolites that were studied included chlordiazepoxide lactam, n-desmethyldiazepam, oxazepam, and methyloxazepam. All metabolites except n-desmethyldiazepam significantly enhanced alcohol-induced impairment of psychomotor skills measured by choice reaction time, eye-hand coordination, divided attention, proprioception, and flicker fusion test. From this data it was concluded that effects on psychomotor skills from the interaction of ethanol with diazepam are due mainly to the parent compound, whereas metabolites play a part in the psychomotor skill effects of the interaction between ethanol and chlordiazepoxide.

Linnoila and associates (1990) examined the psychomotor and cognitive performance effects of the newer benzodiazepine agent, adinazolam, when given in conjunction with oral ethanol. Both ethanol and adinazolam alone decreased psychomotor and cognitive performance. The combination of the two agents indicated that the resulting decrements in performance were produced by the additive effects of the two agents with no indication of a synergistic effect.

Chronic Ethanol

The combination of chronic ethanol consumption and acute benzodiazepine dosing has not been as extensively studied. The reported data are difficult to compare because of methodologic differences in the studies with respect to duration of ethanol abuse, time since withdrawal, and general physical health of the study population. Little work has been conducted in actively drinking alcoholics. The half-life of chlordiazepoxide was examined in intoxicated chronic alcoholics and normal volunteers by Whiting and associates (1979). The half-life was significantly prolonged in the alcoholics; however, the groups were not matched for age or smoking habits, and acute ethanol intoxication may have inhibited the hepatic metabolism of chlordiazepoxide.

Over a 6-day period of ethanol withdrawal, Sellers et al. (1978a,b) studied the pharmacokinetics of chlordiazepoxide in chronic alcoholics (without evidence of liver disease). Plasma levels of chlordiazepoxide and one of its metabolites, desmethylchlordiazepoxide, were signficantly lower on the 6th day of dosing compared with the 2nd day of dosing. Possible explanations include altered absorption (which is unlikely), the decline of acute ethanol-induced enzyme inhibition, and the unmasking of chronic ethanol induction of enzymes.

Sellman and colleagues (1975a,b) examined diazepam plasma levels following intravenous and oral doses in recently abstinent alcoholics. When compared with normal volunteers, the alcoholics had lower plasma concentrations and lower area-under-the-plasma-concentration-versus-time-curves, suggesting increased total body clearance. The data were, however, very erratic, indicating possible technical problems in sampling or assay. Additionally, the alcoholics all received other medications, making further interpretation difficult. Pond and associates (1979) studied intravenous diazepam in chronic alcoholics on the 1st day of withdrawal and 6 to 8 days later. Alcoholics did not show a significant change in elimination half-life or clearance, although interindividual variation was substantial. In 3 patients, diazepam clearance increased 2- to 4-fold from early to late withdrawal, and in 1 patient it decreased to one-fourth over the study period. Sellers and colleagues (1980) studied diazepam pharmacokinetics following an intravenous infusion in alcoholics undergoing withdrawal and found that calculated parameters were within the range for normal subjects from other studies. The data were once again quite variable with terminal elimination half-lives ranging from 14.7 to 67.5 hours. The alcoholics also varied between "moderate" and "severe" withdrawal. The authors did note that 2 alcoholics had unbound drug clearances in excess of 2500 ml/min, suggesting enzyme induction.

Single oral dose pharmacokinetics of alprazolam were studied in recently abstinent alcoholics and normal control subjects (Ciraulo et al. 1988a). Alcoholics showed no significant difference in any pharmacokinetic parameter but demonstrated significant increases in measures of drug liking and drug-induced euphoria over those seen in control subjects. These data suggest that special care must be used in prescribing chronic treatment with alprazolam in this population.

Cocaine

The abuse of cocaine in all its forms, including rapid delivery methods such as free-basing, injection, crack, rock, and bazooka cocaine, has been widely documented (Chitwood 1985, Gold et al. 1985). In recent years there has been a significant increase in reports of cocaine abuse with secondary drug usage. In 1982 a Client Oriented Data Acquisition Process (CODAP) study indicated that 82% of all primary cocaine admissions reported having at least one secondary drug problem. Chitwood in 1985 concluded that polydrug abusers, whose drug of choice was cocaine, frequently combined cocaine with CNS depressants. The data indicated that 53% used marijuana, 35% used ethanol, 20% used methaqualone, and 11% used heroin at least 75% of the time in conjunction with cocaine use. It is clear that drug interactions in cocaine abusers can be of significant clinical importance.

COCAINE AND ANTIDEPRESSANTS (*See also* THERAPEUTIC INTERACTIONS WITH COCAINE, *this chapter*)

Trazodone

The interaction between cocaine and trazodone was studied in 8 cocaine-using subjects (Rowbotham et al. 1984). Physiologic and subjective effects of a 2-mg/kg oral dose of cocaine were compared following pretreatment with a 100-mg dose of trazodone and with placebo. Trazodone treatment diminished the cocaine-induced effects of increased blood pressure, increased pupil size, and decreased skin temperature. The increase in plasma epinephrine levels after cocaine use was not altered with trazodone, but the increase in norepinephrine levels was larger. Trazodone did not effect cocaine-induced euphoria, although subjects reported diminished feelings of tension and shakiness. The authors reported no evidence of a pharmacokinetic interaction between the two drugs.

Tordoff and colleagues (1991) presented a case report of a 66-year-old patient who experienced a delayed excitatory reaction following ingestion of cocaine and MAOI (phenelzine). The patient was being treated for depression with phenelzine 15 mg twice a day and underwent vocal cord surgery where he received topical cocaine spray 1 ml of 10% solution. The surgery proceeded without incident. After the patient returned to the ward, staff discovered him unconscious, with generalized coarse tremors and marked muscle rigidity. Rectal temperature was 41.5°C. Emergency treatment was started and within 7 hours the patient's condition resolved. The authors proposed that the patient had experienced an excitatory reaction due to increased concentrations of 5-HT following interaction of phenelzine and cocaine.

COCAINE AND ANTIHISTAMINE/DECONGESTANTS

The interaction of cocaine with an over-the-counter cold medicine (Alka-Seltzer Plus®) containing the antihistamine, chlorpheniramine, and the decongestant, phenylpropanolamine, has been reported (Strauss 1989). The patient experienced a psychotic episode with hallucinations and homicidal psychosis. Phenylpropanolamine, an indirect-acting sympathomimetic amine, has induced psychotic episodes in high doses even when administered alone.

COCAINE AND β-ADRENERGIC BLOCKERS

Lange and associates (1990) reported in a clinical trial of 30 stable patient volunteers the occurrence of cocaine-induced coronary vasoconstriction potentiated by a β-adrenergic blocker. This was a randomized, double-blind, placebo-controlled trial. The subjects were randomly assigned to receive either intranasal saline or a 10% cocaine hydrochloride solution 2 mg/kg of body weight. Fifteen minutes following the administration of the intranasal agent a 5-minute intracoronary infusion of saline or propranolol 0.4 mg/min with a total of 2 mg total was given. The results indicated that in the propranolol-treated group following cocaine administration, there was an increase in arterial pressure (systolic mean), rate-pressure product, and transcardiac oxygen content. The authors concluded that at the time of the cardiac catheterization cocaine increased myocardial oxygen supply and decreased coronary sinus blood flow and coronary arterial diameter. They further stated that β-adrenergic blockage may increase the magnitude of cocaine-induced myocardial ischemia.

COCAINE AND ETHANOL

Lundberg and associates (1977) documented a case report of a 21-year-old woman who after several ethanol-containing cocktails snorted a white powder reported to be cocaine and soon experienced convulsions and death. Autopsy showed pulmonary edema with pleural petechiae. Toxicologic analysis revealed cocaine and lidocaine, and a blood ethanol level of 0.05% with no other drugs detectable. The same investigators reported a second case of a 24-year-old man who was found dead with cocaine levels measurable in blood, liver, and gastric contents, and a blood alcohol concentration of 0.12%. Tests were negative for other drugs. The lungs showed edema and congestion. It is not known if ethanol potentiates cocaine toxicity.

Finkle and McCloskey (1977), in a forensic report on the toxicology of cocaine obtained from cocaine deaths reported between 1971 and 1976, found measurable blood ethanol levels, with a mean value of 0.1%, in 22 of 86 cases. The authors drew no conclusions from this combination but speculated that the CNS depression of the pharmacologically effective concentration of ethanol might add to the adverse CNS effects of cocaine.

In a controlled clinical study, Foltin and Fischman (1988) found that when oral ethanol was coadministered with intravenous cocaine, there was a greater elevation in heart rate and blood pressure than was observed with either substance alone. A similar study of the interaction of intranasally administered cocaine and oral ethanol produced only subtle effects on subjective psychological measures (Foltin et al. 1993). The interaction of intranasally administered cocaine and oral ethanol was examined for possible effects on learning and performance in human volunteers (Higgins et al. 1992). On the whole, ethanol was found to be more disruptive to learning and performance than cocaine or ethanol combined with cocaine. Cocaine attenuated the disruptive effects of ethanol on learning and performance more than ethanol attenuated the effects of cocaine on these measures.

Perez-Reyes and Jeffcoat (1992) examined the effects of oral ethanol on intranasally administered cocaine and its resulting metabolite, cocaethylene, in male volunteers. While cocaine exerted no effect on ethanol's pharmacokinetics, ethanol significantly increased the plasma concentrations of cocaine, as well as heart rate and subjective ratings of being "high." When cocaine was administered with ethanol, the metabolite cocaethylene was slower to form and reached lower levels in the plasma. The issues of positive reinforcing and toxic effects of cocaethylene are areas of active research (Sands et al. 1992a).

COCAINE AND MARIJUANA

In a study by Foltin and colleagues (1987), 7 adult male volunteers were administered intravenous cocaine and smoked marijuana alone or in combination. Intravenous doses of cocaine alone (doses 16 mg or 32 mg) produced increases (from baseline) in heart rate that were dose-dependent. The tetrahydrocannabinol (THC) blood levels (0–2.7% THC) also produced elevation in heart rates. The heart rate for those subjects on the combination of cocaine and marijuana was significantly increased over the rate for either drug alone. The heart rate rose by nearly 50 beats/min before plateauing at that rate. Cocaine and marijuana showed increases in arterial pressure equivalent to those seen with the administration of cocaine alone.

COCAINE AND OPIOIDS

Cocaine has been combined with heroin ("speedballing") in an attempt to potentiate the effects of heroin and reduce the jitteriness associated with cocaine (Chitwood 1985). This combination carries more risk than either drug alone, because at high doses both cocaine and opioids depress the respiratory center. The surreptitious injection of a "speedball" by a hospital patient into his own intravenous line was reported to be the cause of tachycardia and hypertension during an elective surgery procedure (Samuels et al. 1991).

In a controlled clinical study, Foltin and Fischman (1992) found that when intravenous cocaine and intravenous morphine were coadministered, neither drug caused any changes in the disposition of the other. Although both intravenous cocaine and morphine alone can significantly increase heart rate and diastolic and systolic blood pressure, the effects of the combination did not indicate a strong additive effect. In a Phase I safety evaluation study of the partial opioid agonist, buprenorphine, there was no apparent interactions involving cardiovascular, respiratory or temperature changes when buprenorphine was combined with intravenous cocaine (Teoh et al. 1993).

THERAPEUTIC INTERACTIONS WITH COCAINE

Several psychotropic medications have been used in the treatment of cocaine dependence. Most rely on a theoretical rationale in which the pharmacologic agent is thought to induce neurotransmitters and/or receptor effects opposite to that of cocaine.

Tricyclic antidepressants, most commonly desipramine (Gawin and Kleber 1984, Gawin et al. 1985a, Tennant and Rawson 1983) and imipramine in combination with L-tryptophan and L-tyrosine (Rosecan 1983, Rosecan and Klein 1986) have been used in the treatment of cocaine dependence. While some early studies found that desipramine was more effective than placebo in decreasing cocaine craving and inducing abstinence, better controlled studies have been less positive (Arndt et al. 1992). For example, Kosten et al. (1992) found a significant effect with placebo at 4 weeks but not after 8 weeks of treatment with imipramine or desipramine. Similarly, another study found that desipramine was more effective than placebo in reducing cocaine use after 6 but not 12 weeks of treatment (Carroll et al. 1984). Some clinicians have suggested that imipramine plus amino acids reduce craving and blocks cocaine euphoria. Doses are typically the same as antidepressant doses (150–300 mg daily) and onset of effect is 2 to 4 weeks.

The mechanism by which cocaine euphoria is blocked by antidepressants is unknown, but hypotheses include blockade of a cocaine receptor or displacement of cocaine from its receptor site. Cocaine also has the potential to interact with tricyclics in an additive or synergistic fashion because both block reuptake of dopamine, norepinephrine, and serotonin. Postsynaptically, tricyclics downregulate receptors while cocaine upregulates receptors.

In a small study of 6 subjects, bupropion, a second-generation antidepressant, was shown to reduce the desire for cocaine in methadone-maintained cocaine users (Margolin et al. 1991). The authors interpreted this modification of cocaine desire as a result of direct influences on dopaminergic transmission by the bupropion (Nomikos et al. 1989). Placebo-controlled double-blind studies await completion on this issue.

Rosen (1992) raised the issue of seizures with the combination of cocaine and antidepressants. He reported the case of a woman who used six lines of cocaine approximately 3 weeks after despramine was started (164 ng/ml) in whom a grand mal seizure developed. It is not clear whether antidepressants and cocaine have additive or synergistic convulsant effects. Even though both reduce seizure threshold, the underlying mechanisms of this action differ greatly (Sands et al. 1992b).

The anticonvulsant, carbamazepine, was studied in cocaine-dependent individuals as a method of reducing cocaine craving (Halikas et al. 1989). Patients reported a significant reduction in cocaine craving even when they found themselves in high-risk situations. In a case study of a single individual, carbamazepine reduced the feeling of a "rush" when cocaine was administered. This individual did not, however, report any change in cocaine craving.

Bromocriptine reduces cocaine craving perhaps by downregulating postsynaptic dopamine receptors (Dackis and Gold 1985). Stimulants such as methylphenidate are probably only useful in cocaine abusers with attention deficit disorder (Gawin et al. 1985b, Khantzian et al. 1983, 1984).

Although amantadine, an indirect dopamine agonist, has been reported to be helpful in preliminary clinical trials, controlled studies do not support its efficacy (Kosten et al. 1992) and animal experiments do not suggest that it decreases cocaine self-injection.

In open trials, buprenorphine reduces cocaine use in methadone patients (Kosten et al. 1988); however, a double-blind controlled study did not replicate this finding (Fudala et al. 1990).

Cocaine and Stimulants

Jaffe and associates (1989) reported a possible interaction of cocaine and mazindol (Sanorex, Mazanor) after Berger and colleagues (1989) found that mazindol decreased cocaine-induced euphoria and reduced cocaine use. Jaffe and associates (1989) reported potentiation of convulsant effects of cocaine in rodents pretreated with mazindol, and suggest caution with the use of mazindol treatment to attenuate craving in the cocaine abuser.

Disulfiram (*See* Table 8.1)

Disulfiram inhibits the activity of many enzyme systems including aldehyde dehydrogenase, dopamine-β-hydroxylase, ethylmorphine *N*-demethylase, and xanthine oxidase. The following section provides a brief overview of interactions of clinical importance.

DISULFIRAM AND ETHANOL

The primary importance of the disulfiram-ethanol interaction is its use for therapeutic purposes (Jaffe and Ciraulo 1984, Kitson 1977). The deterrence to drinking ethanol is created by the anticipation of an unpleasant response to alcohol in patients taking disulfiram. This toxic interaction consists of flushing, palpitations, hypotension, breathlessness, tachycardia, nausea, vomiting, vertigo, blurred vision, and headache. The duration and severity of the drug-induced effect will vary according to the amount of ethanol ingested,

Table 8.1.
Disulfiram Drug Interactions

Drug	Effect of Disulfiram
Ethanol	Flushing, hypotension, nausea, tachycardia, vertigo, dyspnea, blurred vision
Oral anticoagulants	Increases hypoprothrombinemic effects and plasma concentrations of warfarin
Antidepressants (tricyclic)	Inhibits hepatic metabolism, decreasing the clearance of antidepressants
Barbiturates	No effect
Benzodiazepines	Reduces clearance and prolongs half-life of chlordiazepoxide and diazepam (Librium® and Valium®), possibly other benzodiazepines. Oxazepam and lorazepam which undergo glucuronidation are probably not affected
Isoniazid	Change in affect, behavior, and coordination possible, little information available but potentially serious interaction
Metronidazole (Flagyl®)	Psychotic and confusional states documented, potentially serious interaction
Omeprazole (Prilosec®)	One case report of confusion. Muscle rigidity, and catatonic state on drug combinations
Oral hypoglycemics	Does not alter tolbutamide clearance
Paraldehyde	Impairs disposition of acetaldehyde by inhibition of acetaldehyde dehydrogenase. This is a potentially serious interaction
Phenytoin	Inhibits hepatic metabolism of phenytoin, rapidly increasing phenytoin blood levels. Phenytoin toxicity documented

daily dosage of disulfiram, and the individual's sensitivity to this interaction.

In severe cases, the disulfiram-ethanol interaction can progress to disruption of the cardiovascular system, respiratory depression, cardiac arrhythmias, convulsions, coma, and death (Jaffe and Ciraulo 1984).

The pharmacologic basis for this interaction is inhibition of aldehyde dehydrogenase, which prevents metabolism of acetaldehyde to acetic acid.

The management of this interaction is best addressed by prevention in the form of patient education and careful supervision when prescribing disulfiram as an adjunct to the treatment of alcoholism. The patient should be fully informed of potential disulfiram-ethanol interaction. In addition, the patient should be warned about exposure to ethanol in (1) over-the-counter cough and cold medications,

(2) food preparations such as sauces, gravies or flaming desserts, and (3) topical products such as shaving lotions. The degree of severity of the disulfiram-ethanol reaction will dictate the course of treatment. In mild cases of the reaction, treatment should consist of placing the patient in the Trendelenburg position for control of hypotension, administration of oxygen, and careful monitoring for further symptoms. In the case of severe interactions, supportive measures including oxygen and intravenous therapy should be taken immediately. Some clinicians suggest the use of ephedrine to maintain blood pressure (McNichol et al. 1987). Intravenous doses of ascorbic acid (1 g) can provide relief although it is essential to continue monitoring the patient as the symptoms can recur and require further doses of ascorbic acid. In severe cases, gastric lavage may be indicated. A drug not yet marketed in the United States, 4-methylpyrazole, has proven useful in inhibiting the liver metabolism of ethanol to counteract the disulfiram-ethanol interaction.

DISULFIRAM AND ANTIDEPRESSANTS

Maany and associates (1982) described 2 cases of patients who developed acute organic brain syndrome while receiving disulfiram in combination with amitriptyline. The symptoms included confusion, hallucinations, disorientation, and memory loss. MacCallum (1969) reported that in his experience amitriptyline potentiated the effect of disulfiram allowing one to use smaller dosages of the latter drug. The effects of amitriptyline on disulfiram metabolism have not been studied but it has been suggested that the increase of the effects of disulfiram may be due to the increase in the rate of buildup of acetaldehyde. Alternatively, amitriptyline may potentiate the actions of ethanol, which could result in a more severe disulfiram interaction.

Disulfiram markedly inhibited the metabolism of imipramine and desipramine (Ciraulo et al. 1985). Two subjects who had been detoxified from ethanol within 2 weeks received imipramine alone (12.5 mg intravenously) and again following 4 weeks of disulfiram treatment (500 mg daily). One of the subjects also received desipramine (12.5 mg intravenously) under the same conditions. For imipramine, the total area-under-the-plasma-concentration-time-curve increased 32.5 and 26.8% after disulfiram administration. The elimination half-lives were also increased 18.3 and 13.6%. Disulfiram resulted in a decrease of 24.5 and 21.3% in total body clearance of imipramine. Similar findings were found in the desipramine subject, in whom disulfiram treatment resulted in a 32.3% larger area under the curve, an increase of 19.8% in elimination half-life, and a decrease in total body clearance of 24.3%. This interaction could lead to toxicity due to increased systemic availability of the antidepressant after oral administration, an increase in the time required to reach steady-state, and an increase in plasma levels above the therapeutic range. This may explain the toxicity described by Maany and associates (1982).

DISULFIRAM AND BENZODIAZEPINES

The effects of chlordiazepoxide and diazepam are increased and prolonged when administered with disulfiram (MacLeod et al. 1978). This is due to inhibition of the hepatic enzymes responsible for the metabolism of these two benzodiazepines. Patients receiving the combination may require a dosage reduction for the benzodiazepines.

Other drugs whose metabolism is inhibited by disulfiram include oral anticoagulants, such as warfarin (O'Reilly 1972, Rothstein 1968) and metronidazole (Rothstein and Clancy 1969).

Calcium carbamide, an alcohol deterrent not available in the United States, does not inhibit the metabolism of these drugs (Table 8.1).

Ethanol (*See* Table 8.2)

In today's society the use of alcoholic beverages is commonplace. With 29% of women and 13% of men in the United States taking prescribed psychotropic drugs (Parry et al. 1973), and 13.8 % of the population having alcohol dependence or abuse at some time in their life (Helzer et al. 1991), the interaction of ethanol with psychoactive agents is particularly important. In addition, a large number of individuals take nonprescribed psychotropics with ethanol, adding to the magnitude of the interaction (Ciraulo et al. 1986).

Psychotropic drugs and ethanol can interact in the clinical situation in several different ways. They may interact as (1) acute ethanol with acute drug use, (2) chronic ethanol with acute drug use, (3) acute ethanol with chronic drug use, and (4) chronic ethanol with chronic drug use. Other factors to consider include types of drugs taken, dosage combinations, routes of administration, and the presence of organic and/or psychiatric illness.

In general, chronic ethanol consumption induces hepatic metabolic enzymes, thereby increasing first-pass effects and decreasing

Table 8.2.
Ethanol Drug Interactions

Acetaminophen	Chronic excessive alcohol consumption increases susceptibility to acetaminophen-induced hepatotoxicity. Acute intoxication theoretically protects against acetaminophen toxicity because less hepatotoxic metabolite is generated
Aminosalicylic acid	Ethanol reduces hypolipidemic effect
Anticoagulants (oral)	Chronic ethanol consumption induces hepatic metabolism of warfarin, decreasing hypoprothrombinemic effect. Very large acute ethanol doses (more than 3 drinks/day) may impair metabolism of warfarin and increase hypo-thrombinemic effect. Vitamin K dependent clotting factors may be reduced in alcoholics with liver disease, also affecting coagulation
Antidepressants (*see* Chap. 2)	Enhanced sedative effects of alcohol and psychomotor impairment. Acute ethanol impairs metabolism of antidepressants; chronic ethanol enhances metabolism. Fluoxetine, paroxetine, fluovoxamine and probably other SSRIs do not interfere with psychomotor or subjective effects of ethanol
Antipyrine	Chronic ethanol consumption (>1 ml/kg/day) enhances antipyrine metabolism
Ascorbic acid	Ascorbic acid increases ethanol clearance and serum triglyceride levels and improves motor coordination and color discrimination after ethanol consumption
Barbiturates	Phenobarbital decreases blood ethanol concentration; acute intoxication inhibits pentobarbital metabolism; chronic intoxication enhances hepatic pentobarbital metabolism. Combined central nervous system depression
Benzodiazepines	Psychomotor impairment increased with the combination
Bromocriptine	Ethanol increases gastrointestinal side effects of bromocriptine
Caffeine	Caffeine has no effect on ethanol-induced psychomotor impairment
Calcium channel blockers	Verapamil (Calan®) inhibits ethanol metabolism and increases intoxication
Cephalosporin antibiotics	Ethanol produces flushing, nausea, headaches, tachycardia, and hypotension. Cephalosporin antibiotics that have a methyltetrazolethiol side chain produce this disulfiram-like reaction (e.g., cefoperazone (Cefobid®), cefamandole (Mandol®), cefotetan (Cefotan®), and moxalactam
Chloral hydrate	Elevation of plasma trichloroethanol (a chloral hydrate metabolite) and blood ethanol. Combined central nervous system depression. Vasodilation, tachycardia, headache
Chloroform	Ethanol increases chloroform hepatotoxicity
Cromolyn	No interaction
Doxycycline	Chronic consumption of ethanol induces hepatic metabolism of doxycycline and may lower serum concentrations of the antibiotic

Table 8.2.
Ethanol Drug Interactions (continued)

Erythromycin	Ethanol may interfere with absorption of the ethylsuccinate salt. Effects on other formulations unknown
Furazolidone (Furoxone®)	When ethanol is ingested, nausea, flushing, lightheadedness, and dyspnea may occur (ie., a disulfiram-like reaction)
Glutethimide	Blood ethanol concentration increases while plasma glutethimide concentration decreases
H^2-Antagonists	Cimetidine (Tagamet®) potentiates ethanol effects. Increases peak plasma ethanol concentrations and area under the plasma ethanol concentration time curve. Central nervous system toxicity from increased cimetidine serum concentration. Nizatidine (Axid®), and ranitidine (Zantac®), may also increase blood alcohol levels slightly by inhibiting gastric alcohol dehydrogenase. Famotidine (Pepcid®) does not affect blood alcohol levels
Isoniazid (INH)	Consumption of ethanol with INH increases risk of hepatotoxicity. Tyramine containing alcoholic beverages may cause hypertensive reaction
Ketoconazole (Nizoral®) and metronidazole (Flagyl®)	When ethanol is ingested, nausea, flushing, lightheadedness, and dyspnea may occur (i.e., a disulfiram-like reaction may occur with metronidazole). A sunburn-like rash has been reported with ethanol consumption and ketoconazole. A similar reaction may occur with itraconazole (Sporanox®), although no reports exist
Meprobamate	Synergistic central nervous system depression
Metoclopramide (Reglan®)	Enhances sedative effects of ethanol
Milk	Reduces ethanol absorption by delaying gastric emptying
Monoamine oxidase inhibitors	Tyramine containing alcoholic beverages may cause a hypertensive crisis. Pargyline may inhibit aldehyde dehydrogenase and cause a disulfiram-like interaction with ethanol
Narcotic analgesics	Volume of distribution of intravenous meperidine increases with increasing ethanol consumption. Clinical significance unknown. Potential for enhanced CNS depression
Oral hypoglycemic agents	Chlorpropamide (Diabinese®) tolbutamide and tolazamide may cause flushing, lightheadedness, nausea, and dyspnea if alcohol is ingested (i.e., a disulfiram-like reaction)
Paraldehyde	Possible metabolic acidosis
Phenothiazines	Potentiates psychomotor effects of ethanol
Phenytoin	Chronic ethanol ingestion induces phenytoin metabolism
Quinacrine	Possibly inhibits acetaldehyde oxidation
Salicylates	Increases gastric bleeding associated with aspirin, may increase chance of gastrointestinal hemorrhage
Tetrachloroethylene	Combined central nervous system depression
Trichloroethylene	Flushing, lacrimation, blurred vision, tachypnea may occur when patients exposed to trichloroethylene drink alcohol

the amount of drug available to the systemic circulation (Lieber 1982). Acute ethanol consumption, on the other hand, inhibits the hepatic microsomal enzymes responsible for the clearance of many drugs and would thus increase the amount of drug available to the systemic circulation (Hoyumpa et al. 1980, Lieber 1982, Rubin et al. 1970).

ETHANOL AND ANTIDEPRESSANTS

Tricyclic Antidepressants (See also Chapter 2)

The interaction of ethanol with tricyclic antidepressants can produce CNS depression resulting in adverse effects of psychomotor performance (Landauer et al. 1969, Milner and Landauer 1973, Seppala et al. 1975). Anticholinergic effects of tricyclic antidepressants cause a delay in gastric emptying and increased gastric irritation. In several studies, amitriptyline and doxepin (Seppala et al. 1975) have had adverse effects on the motor skills important in driving. Milner and Landauer (1973), however, demonstrated that doxepin is less likely to interact with ethanol to produce increased sedation or adversely effect driving skills. Hyatt and Bird (1987) described 3 cases of amitriptyline augmenting ethanol-induced euphoria in ethanol-abusing and/or -dependent men. These patients used amitriptyline in doses of 200 to 500 mg in combination with ethanol to "stay high cheaply." These patients also reported that they required less ethanol than they were previously accustomed to in order to achieve a desired state of intoxication.

The major route of elimination for tricyclic antidepressants is hepatic metabolism. Ethanol, with its ability to alter hepatic metabolism, would be expected to cause interactions on a metabolic level with antidepressants.

Dorian and associates (1983) evaluated the effect of acute ethanol administration on amitriptyline using a crossover design and found significant increases in the area-under-the-plasma-concentration-time-curve for the combination of ethanol with amitriptyline. This translates to a decreased clearance of amitriptyline when administered with acute ethanol, which is consistent with hepatic enzymatic inhibition. Pharmacodynamic measures such as postural sway and difficulty in word recall were greatly increased over baseline values. The psychomotor skills needed for driving a car were tested in 10 healthy female subjects and were found to be significantly impaired at 1.5 and 4 hours following single doses of amitriptyline 50 mg combined with a 0.5-g/kg dose of ethanol (Hindmarch and Harrison

1989). This same study demonstrated similar impairment with mianserin 20 mg and trazodone 50 mg when combined with ethanol.

In a controlled clinical study of the effects of acute ethanol on the psychomotor and cognitive skills of imipramine and nefazodone (Frewer and Lader 1993), normal volunteers were tested after 8 days of the antidepressants. Imipramine enhanced the psychomotor and memory impairment of ethanol, while nefazodone failed to potentiate the depressant effects of the ethanol.

Fluoxetine in single or multiple doses (30 or 60 mg) did not affect ethanol pharmacokinetics, the subjective response, or psychomotor activity after ethanol administration (Lemberger et al. 1985).

The acute effects of ethanol in combination with single doses of paroxetine has been investigated in a controlled clinical trial of normal volunteers (Cooper et al. 1989). Oral doses of ethanol 50 g were taken alone and 3 hours after an oral dose of paroxetine 30 mg. Although both ethanol and paroxetine alone made subjects feel less alert and less attentive, the combination caused no potentiation of sedative or psychomotor impairment. Others have examined the possible impairment of psychomotor activity related to driving skills in subjects receiving both acute doses of paroxetine and ethanol (Hindmarch and Harrison 1989). The authors concluded that there was little impairment when paroxetine is combined with "social" doses of ethanol (0.5 g/kg of body weight).

The possible interactions of acute ethanol with the antidepressant, fluvoxamine, were examined in normal volunteers (Van Harten et al. 1992). No clinically significant pharmacodynamic effects were demonstrated.

The effects of chronic ethanol consumption on the metabolism and pharmacokinetics of tricyclic antidepressants have been systematically investigated in groups of recently abstinent (10–14 days) chronic alcoholics (with no clinical signs of cirrhosis) and age- and weight-matched controls (Ciraulo et al. 1988b). Imipramine, desipramine, and the primary hydroxylated metabolite of imipramine, 2-hydroxyimipramine, were found to have significantly increased clearances in chronic alcoholics. This is consistent with induced hepatic metabolism following chronic ethanol consumption. Significantly lower peak concentrations following oral imipramine were found in the alcoholic group compared with the control group. Free fractions of drug in plasma were lower in alcoholics, possibly due to the increased levels of the important binding protein, α_1-acid glycoprotein, in the alcoholic group. Since it is that fraction of drug unbound in plasma that is considered active, the lower free fraction of tricyclic antidepressant represents less active drug available to the receptor site of action for a given dose. In a further study of antidepressant pharmacokinetics in abstinent alcoholics, the major hydroxylated metabolite of imipramine, 2-hydroxyimipramine, was administered by intravenous infusion (Ciraulo et al. 1990). The alcoholic group had a greater total body clearance of the metabolite, as compared to age- and weight- matched controls, indicating that higher levels of this metabolite would not be expected after oral dosing with imipramine in alcoholics. Multiple dose imipramine administration was also investigated (Ciraulo et al. 1982) in abstinent alcoholics. Alcoholics had significantly lower imipramine and 2-hydroxyimipramine trough levels than did control subjects, indicating that an interaction of tricyclic antidepressants with chronic ethanol abuse can still occur following an extended period of abstinence. This may also be the case for other classes of drugs cleared by the hepatic microsomal enzyme systems.

The clinician should caution the patient who is beginning tricylic antidepressant therapy that ingestion of ethanol may produce a greater than expected impairment of psychomotor skills, particularly in the first several weeks of therapy when sedation side-effects are most pronounced. The clinician should also be aware of the abuse potential of the euphoria-producing combination of amitriptyline (and perhaps all tricyclics) with ethanol. Monitoring of antidepressant levels is often necessary in recently abstinent alcoholics. The selected serotonin reuptake inhibitors (SSRIs) do not enhance the intoxicating effects of ethanol, nor do they produce additive or synergistic psychomotor impairment.

MAOIs.   Ethanol-containing beverages with high tyramine contents may lead to hypertensive reactions when patients are taking monoamine oxidase inhibitors (MAOIs). Some types of chianti may have a tyramine content as high as 25 mg/ml, beer 2 to 4 mg/ml, ale 8 mg/ml, sherry 3 to 4 mg/ml, and champagne and white wines less than 1 mg/ml (Horwitz et al. 1964) (see Chap. 2).

Clinicians should warn against the use of ethanol-containing beverages with moderate to high tyramine content in those patients receiving a MAOI.

ETHANOL AND LITHIUM (*See* Chapter 4)

ETHANOL AND ANTIPSYCHOTICS (*See* Chapter 3)

When acute ethanol is administered with phenothiazine derivatives, such as chlorpromazine or thioridazine, drugs that are metabolized by hepatic microsomal pathways, there is the potential for serious adverse effects from elevated phenothiazine serum concentrations and potentiation of CNS depressant effects (Milner and Landauer 1971, Saario 1976, Zirkle et al. 1959). These effects may include hypotension, impaired coordination, and severe respiratory depression. Some information has indicated that in patients maintained on phenothiazines there is an inhibition of alcohol dehydrogenase, which could produce increases in the intensity and duration of ethanol intoxication (Domino 1965). This combination is also of serious concern in the case of ethanol withdrawal states since these drugs can lower the threshold for seizures (Jaffe and Ciraulo 1984).

The acute effects of ethanol on the single-dose pharmacokinetics of the newer antipsychotic agent, remoxipride, a dopamine D_2-receptor antagonist, was studied in a controlled clinical trial (Yisak et al. 1990). Healthy male volunteers took single 100-mg doses of remoxipride with and without 0.8-gm/kg doses of ethanol. Ethanol had no effect on the single dose pharmacokinetics of remoxipride. This study does not, however, speak to any possible changes that might occur with chronic dosing of either substance.

Ethanol and Barbiturates

(*See* Barbiturate section in this chapter for effects of ethanol on barbiturates.)

The interaction between ethanol and barbiturates as it relates to the effect on barbiturate metabolism or activity has been described in detail previously. The interaction between ethanol and barbiturates also involves effects on ethanol clearance. In a study combining 50-ml doses of vodka with 30-mg doses of phenobarbital (Mould et al. 1972), blood ethanol concentrations were reduced at 30 and 90 minutes postdose, as compared with those values found with ethanol alone. The hepatic-metabolizing enzymes for ethanol can be induced by barbiturates (Mezey and Robles 1974), but it is unclear why this effect would be seen with acute doses rather than chronic.

ETHANOL AND BENZODIAZEPINES

(*See* Benzodiazepines in this chapter and chapter on benzodiazepines.)

ETHANOL AND NONBARBITURATE SEDATIVE HYPNOTICS

CHLORAL HYDRATE

The interaction between ethanol and chloral hydrate was investigated because both substances share the same hepatic metabolic enzyme pathway (Kaplan et al. 1967, Sellers et al. 1972a,b). Coadministration of ethanol and chloral hydrate resulted in significantly higher and more prolonged trichloroethanol plasma levels. In turn, the chloral hydrate caused an increase in the peak plasma ethanol levels over those found with ethanol alone. The investigators determined that these data, along with reported *in vitro* data, indicated competitive inhibition of alcohol dehydrogenase. Clinically, the combination ("Mickey Finn," "knockout drops") produces an increased CNS depression over that found with either compound alone.

Glutethimide

In a comparison study of the impairment of psychomotor skills following glutethimide alone and in combination with ethanol (Saario and Linnoila 1976), the combination produced greater impairment. However, Mould and associates (1972) demonstrated that glutethimide blood levels were reduced and ethanol levels increased when glutethimide was taken in combination with ethanol.

Enhanced CNS depression is of clinical significance with the concurrent use of glutethimide and ethanol.

Meprobamate

The interaction of ethanol and meprobamate has shown that concurrent use impaired performance on tests of coordination and judgment more than either compound alone (Carpenter et al. 1975, Zirkle et al. 1960). Acute ethanol caused enzyme inhibition and higher circulating levels of meprobamate (Rubin et al. 1970), while chronic ethanol induced the metabolism of meprobamate and lowered circulating levels of meprobamate (Misra et al. 1971).

The clinician should inform patients that the combination of meprobamate and ethanol can seriously depress the CNS, thereby impairing psychomotor performance.

Ethanol and Opioids

Many studies suggest that alcohol abuse by opiate and opiate-derivative addicts is a significant problem (Belenko 1979, Bihari 1973, Gearing 1970, Stimmel et al. 1982). Jackson and Richman (1973) surveyed 471 admissions for heroin detoxification and found that 27% reported daily ethanol use. Bihari in 1973 reported that 50% of methadone patients admitted for inpatient detoxification were also addicted to ethanol.

Linnoila and Hakkinen (1974) demonstrated in a double-blind

study that codeine and ethanol caused increased impairment in driving ability.

The concomitant use of two CNS depressants such as ethanol and opioids (morphine, heroin, codeine, methadone) may be expected to result in enhanced CNS depression. The cumulative effects of the combination of the CNS depressants may range from mild drowsiness to stupor, coma, and potentially fatal respiratory depression.

Perhaps the most clinically important interaction between ethanol and opioids is the ability of naltrexone (Revia®) to block the reinforcing properties of ethanol and decrease the desire to drink (O'Malley et al. 1992, Volpicelli et al. 1992). The findings of O'Malley et al. (1992) suggest that the drinking behavior in those alcoholics treated with naltrexone alone or combined with coping skills training were more successful in preventing relapse than those taking placebo. If a drinking episode did occur it was of shorter duration and less intense.

Hallucinogens

A single case report described a 16-year-old boy who ingested 2 doses of lysergic acid diethylamide (LSD) while taking fluoxetine 20 mg/day. Stupor and a grand mal convulsion developed 3 hours after the initial LSD dose (Picker et al. 1992). There are no other case reports of LSD or other hallucinogens interacting with fluoxetine. On occasion, we have seen some patients with extensive histories of "bad trips" have dysphoric responses to SSRIs (Picker et al. 1992).

Inhalants

Solvent and aerosol inhalation may interact with other drugs by both pharmacokinetic and pharmacodynamic mechanisms. The long-term abuse of volatile chemicals such as aliphatic and aromatic hydrocarbons (toluene, benzene, petroleum distillates, etc.) and trichloroethylenes (halothane, Freon®, chloroform, etc.) can cause toxic damage to the liver and kidneys (Blum 1984) potentially resulting in altered metabolism and excretion of other drugs.

Because inhalants, like other CNS depressants, can impair judgment and distort the perception of reality, the use of inhalants with other CNS depressants could result in further impairment. Although well-established facts are available concerning the dangers of inhalant use and abuse, drug interactions with inhaled solvents have not been well studied. The reader is directed to an excellent review of inhalants (Blum 1984, Sharp et al. 1991) for further information.

Marijuana

The physiologic and psychological impairment caused by marijuana abuse predisposes to drug interactions with CNS depressants. The impairment of motor skills (Casswell and Marks 1973, Moskowitz and McGlothin 1974, Moskowitz et al. 1972, Smiley et al. 1981) as well as the production of adverse psychological effects (Dornbush 1974, Ferraro 1980, Institute of Medicine 1982, Vachon et al. 1974) during marijuana intoxication has been well documented. In addition, the overestimation of elapsed time intervals caused by altered time perception (Ferraro 1980), when combined with the high degree of polydrug abuse found among marijuana users (Tinklenberg et al. 1981) increases the likelihood of drug overdose.

MARIJUANA AND ANTIPSYCHOTICS

Knudsen and Vilmar (1984) described 10 schizophrenic patients maintained on antipsychotic medications (fluphenazine, clopenthixol, perphenazine) whose conditions were acutely exacerbated following abuse of cannabis. The symptoms included mental confusion, impairment of memory, impulsive behavior, hallucinations, and disturbances of perception. This interaction may be due to the anticholinergic effects of cannabis, which decreases the release and turnover of acetylcholine in the hippocampus (Domino 1981, Drew and Miller 1974, Miller 1979). On this basis, cannabis use constitutes a risk factor for patients maintained on antipsychotic medications.

Marijuana and Barbiturates

The major active component of marijuana, THC, was found to produce hallucinations and anxiety in 5 of 7 subjects receiving pretreatment with pentobarbital in a controlled clinical study (Johnstone et al. 1975). This same additive effect was also demonstrated in another study with secobarbital (Lemberger et al. 1976).

MARIJUANA AND COCAINE

(*See* Cocaine in this chapter.)

MARIJUANA AND DISULFIRAM

There is 1 case report of a patient who was taking disulfiram in whom hypomania developed while the patient was smoking marijuana (Lacoursiere et al. 1983). When disulfiram therapy was discontinued, marijuana did not lead to manic symptoms. Rechallenge with marijuana and disulfiram again produced hypomania. On the other hand, many patients taking disulfiram smoke marijuana without adverse consequences, suggesting that the case report reflects an idiosyncratic response (Lacoursiere et al. 1983).

MARIJUANA AND ETHANOL

The combination of marijuana and ethanol produces motor performance impairment (Burford et al. 1975, Franks et al. 1975, Hansteen et al. 1976, Manno et al. 1971, Smiley et al. 1981) and mental impairment (Manno et al. 1971, Hollister 1976) greater than the impairment observed with either drug alone. Mendelson and associates (1986) used a controlled clinical study to examine marijuana and ethanol use patterns among a group of subjects who were users of both marijuana and ethanol. They found that when both ethanol and marijuana were available, marijuana affected ethanol use far more dramatically than ethanol influenced marijuana use. The subjects decreased their ethanol consumption as compared to a period when only ethanol was available.

Marijuana and Opioids

In a controlled study, the major active component of marijuana, THC, potentiated the CNS depression of oxymorphone, producing enhanced sedation and respiratory depression (Johnstone et al. 1975).

Opioids

The opioid drugs produce their major effects on the central nervous and gastrointestinal systems (Jaffe and Martin 1985). Any drug capable of CNS depression has the potential for causing enhanced depression, in addition to the interactions reported below.

OPIOIDS AND ANTIBIOTICS

The antibiotic, erythromycin, prolonged the action of the analgesic, alfentanil (Bartkowski and McDonnell 1990). An elderly man, receiving the antibiotic prior to a surgical procedure, required three naloxone doses following administration of alfentanil during surgery before he was responsive and could stay awake.

Rifampin in daily doses of 600 to 900 mg reduced plasma methadone levels and precipitated opiate withdrawal symptoms in 21 of 30 patients (Kreek et al. 1976). Symptoms of an abstinence syndrome usually develop within 5 days after rifampin is started (Bending et al. 1977, Garfield et al. 1975, Holmes 1990, Kreek et al. 1975).

OPIOIDS AND ANTIDEPRESSANTS (See Chapter 2)

OPIOIDS AND ANTIHISTAMINES

Reports on the abuse of the synthetic opioid analgesic, pentazocine, in combination with the antihistamine, tripelennamine, first appeared in 1965 (Burton et al. 1965). The tablets of pentazocine and tripelennamine were crushed together with a small quantity of water and the resulting mixture was injected intravenously. This combination, often called "blue velvet" or "T's and Blues" (tripelennamine was marketed as a blue tablet; pentazocine was marketed under the trade name, Talwin) reportedly produced a "rush" that opioid addicts consider similar to heroin. These first examples were forensic reports on intravenous drug abusers whose deaths resulted from right ventricular dilation and pulmonary edema secondary to profuse disseminated foreign body granulomata. These emboli contained particulates that proved to be talc crystals and starch particles. Starch and talc are present in tripelennamine tablets as fillers.

The euphoria produced by the drug combination, in addition to the decreased expense and increased availability of the two drugs, led to increasing and continued use. The potentiation of the morphine-like effects of pentazocine by tripelennamine is most likely not an interaction at the opioid receptor, but is due, at least in part, to antagonism of the psychotomimetic actions of pentazocine (Shannon and Su 1982). Acute administration of tripelennamine produced significant threshold lowering for rewarding brain stimulation in rats (Unterwald et al. 1984), and although the magnitude of lowering was substantially less than that observed in studies with other highly abused substances (morphine, cocaine, amphetamine), it suggests that tripelennamine may have a moderate abuse liability of its own. Abuse of this combination increased to peak levels in 1982 (Baum et al. 1987, Poklis 1984), and fell dramatically in 1983 when the manufacturers of pentazocine reformulated the commercial tablet to contain 0.5 mg of the opioid antagonist, naloxone. The theory behind this addition is that if the tablet were crushed, dissolved and injected, the antagonist would block the sought after euphoric response. Additionally, a subcutaneous dose of naloxone 0.5 mg can precipitate a moderate withdrawal syndrome in opioid addicts (Zaks et al. 1971), making abuse of this combination less attractive. When the tablet is ingested orally as recommended, the naloxone is rapidly metabolized in the first-pass through the liver after absorption and is only one-fiftieth as potent as it would be by intravenous injection (Nutt and Jasinski 1974). The addition of naloxone to pentazocine tablets does not reliably produce aversive affects (Lahmeyer and Craig 1987), however, and has not extinguished this abusive interaction. As recently as 1992, the interaction was determined to be the cause of a myocardial infarction in a young patient known to be an abuser (McGwier et al. 1992). The incident occurred following the injection of pentazocine 150 mg and triplennamine 50 mg.

Other antihistamines have also shown patterns of abuse in combination with opiates. The antihistamine, cyclizine, which is primarily marketed for the treatment of motion sickness, has been abused intravenously by opiate dependent individuals (Ruben et al. 1989). When taken in large intravenous doses (50–800 mg [1 standard tablet to 16 standard tablets]), at the same time as oral methadone, the initial effects are of intense stimulation, often with hallucinations, aggressive behavior, and seizures. Following this there are depressive mood changes, with a craving for cyclizine. Tolerance to the effects has been observed to occur but with no clearcut withdrawal syndrome. Little has been studied of this interaction, but the possibility exists that cyclizine itself possesses some abuse potential.

OPIOIDS AND ANTIPSYCHOTICS

Antipsychotics such as promethazine, haloperidol, or chlorpromazine been used in combination with analgesics such as meperidine to potentiate the efficacy of the analgesic. Clinically, the pain is still perceived but the emotional reaction is of less distress and discomfort. Although adequate studies of the mechanism behind this interaction are lacking, some authors (Maltbie 1979) have suggested that haloperidol has direct effects on the opiate receptor. In studies with chlorpromazine and placebo in combination with meperidine (Stambaugh and Wainer 1981), no significant differences were found in peak meperidine serum concentration, elimination half-life, or clearance between groups. There was, however, an increase in the mean excretion of the N-demethylated metabolite following the chlorpromazine-meperidine combination, indicating that changes in metabolite patterns may contribute to the altered effects.

Promethazine has been used in combination with analgesics such as morphine, meperidine, oxymorphone, hydromorphone, fentanyl, and pentazocine to potentiate the analgesic action (Keeri-Szanto 1974). This involves a prolongation, rather than deepening, of the opioid effects and often enables a lower dose of opioid to be administered. There is, however, a greater possiblity of side effects, such as respiratory depression, when the drugs are used in combination.

OPIOIDS AND BARBITURATES (*See* BARBITURATES *in this chapter*)

OPIOIDS AND BENZODIAZEPINES

METHADONE AND DIAZEPAM

The possibility of an interaction between methadone and diazepam has been investigated in controlled studies (Pond et al. 1982, Preston et al. 1985). These studies were carried out to examine the subjective, physiologic, and pharmacokinetic effects of the combination because of reports of high diazepam abuse rates among methadone users (Stitzer et al. 1981), possibly in an attempt to "boost" the methadone effects. Pond and associates (1982) found no changes in methadone metabolism nor any increase in methadone-like subjective effects when repeated low doses of diazepam were administered to subjects on methadone maintenance. Preston and associates used higher doses of diazepam in a dosing pattern approximating that pattern reported by patients on methadone maintenance who abused diazepam (Stitzer et al. 1981), and they found increases in subjective opioid effect scores and increases in physiologic measures such as pupil constriction. With a lack of pharmacokinetic changes, these results tend to imply an interaction at the receptor level.

MIDAZOLAM AND MORPHINE

A controlled clinical study (Tverskoy et al. 1989) found that while midazolam and morphine alone produced marked sedation as measured by visual analog scales, the net sedative result of a combination of the two agents was one of summation with no indication of synergism. This study addressed only the sedation-interaction of these two agents.

OPIOIDS AND SEDATIVE-HYPNOTICS

CODEINE AND GLUTETHIMIDE

The combination of codeine (generally 4 oral tablets of codeine and acetaminophen no. 4, 240 mg) and glutethimide (2 oral tablets containing 500 mg) has been used by opioid abusers to induce a euphoric state similar to that produced by heroin (Feuer and French 1984, Havier and Lin 1985, Shamoian 1975, Shamoian and Shapiro 1969,

Sramek and Khajawall 1981). These tablet combinations are sold on the street in packets and are referred to as "packs," "hits," or "loads." This combination is readily available and relatively inexpensive compared with heroin, while offering an equivalent yet prolonged high, and can be ingested orally rather than injected. Opioid abusers have been reported to ingest 3 to 12 "loads" per day (Sramek and Khajawall 1981), corresponding to 3 to 12 g of glutethimide and 720 to 2880 mg of codeine, although others have reported a maximum daily dose of 5 "loads" (Shamoian 1975). Large daily doses of glutethimide can produce an intoxication that involves a difficult, unpredictable, and lengthy detoxification associated with a high degree of mortality (Harvey 1985, Johnson and Van Buren 1962). Epidemiologic data from the Medical Examiner's Office of New Jersey (Feuer and French 1984) reported 36 deaths attributable to loads during the period 1980–1981, while heroin overdose accounted for 126 deaths. Another review of 16 deaths due to the combination of codeine and glutethimide (Havier and Lin 1985) reported that plasma concentrations were in the high therapeutic range and suggested a possible toxic synergistic effect of the combination. A report on 12 fatal and 26 nonfatal intoxications seen at the University of California at San Diego over a 4-year period indicated that glutethimide plasma concentrations in fatal cases (13.9 mg/liter) and in nonfatal cases (10.0 mg/liter) were not appreciably different and were in fact lower than glutethimide concentrations found in cases involving glutethimide toxicity alone (22 mg/liter in nonfatal cases; 42.7 mg/liter in fatal cases) (Bailey 1985). This indicates that the potentiation of the effects of codeine and glutethimide produces serious effects at lower plasma concentrations than would be found with either agent alone. At the present time, glutethimide is not marketed in the United States.

Smoking

Cigarette smoke is capable of affecting metabolism and action of psychotropic drugs. Polycyclic hydrocarbons present in cigarette smoke stimulate hepatic drug metabolism and can thus reduce blood levels of other drugs whose clearance is dependent on hepatic metabolism (Jusko 1978). This enzyme induction can last for several months after cessation of smoking. In addition to induction of drug metabolism, tobacco smoke contains pharmacologically active substances such as nicotine that can affect drug action.

SMOKING AND AMPHETAMINES

Schuster and co-workers (1979) demonstrated that when normal subjects were given doses of dextroamphetamine the number of cigarettes smoked over the period of the study was significantly increased over placebo levels. In a study by Henningfield and Griffiths (1981), increasing doses of dextroamphetamine produced substantial increases in tobacco consumption. The number of cigarettes, the number of puffs per session, the seconds spent smoking, and cigarette duration were all increased. At the higher doses of dextroamphetamine, the smokers reported that their cigarettes "tasted better" and that smoking was "really enjoyable." The authors offered two possible explanations for these effects, namely, that nicotine may play a pharmacologically active role in the smoking increase or that because dextroamphetamine is a general behavioral stimulant it increases the rate of a variety of learned or stereotypical behaviors.

SMOKING AND ANTIDEPRESSANTS

Imipramine

Steady-state plasma levels of imipramine were compared between cigarette smokers and nonsmokers by Perel and associates (1978). Smokers had significantly lower levels of imipramine as compared with nonsmokers (160 vs. 260 ng/ml). Cigarette smokers may require higher doses of imipramine to achieve efficacy. Lower plasma levels of amitriptyline and its major metabolite, nortriptyline, have also been found in patients who smoke cigarettes (Linnoila et al. 1981).

SMOKING AND ANTIPSYCHOTICS

The interaction between smoking and the antipsychotic agent, chlorpromazine, has been examined (Boston Collaborative Drug Surveillance Program 1974, Vinarova et al. 1984). Smokers and nonsmokers were compared for differences in doses of chlorpromazine necessary to achieve comparable therapeutic effect. Male smokers required twice the dosage of chlorpromazine used in nonsmoking males for control of psychosis. The authors attributed this to higher hepatic enzymatic activity in the smoking group. The Boston Collaborative Drug Surveillance Program found decreased drowsiness with chlorpromazine in patients who were cigarette smokers.

Cigarette smoking also affects haloperidol pharmacokinetics (Jann et al. 1986, Miller et al. 1990, Perry et al. 1993). Jann and associates (1986) found that cigarette smokers had an increased clearance of haloperidol, significantly shorter elimination half-lives, and lower plasma concentrations at given doses than those in nonsmoking individuals. The findings reflect hepatic enzyme induction from cigarette smoking. As suggested by Miller and associates (1990), these pharmacokinetic changes may be particularly important when a patient stabilized on haloperidol stops smoking. The potential for drug toxicity then exists as haloperidol clearance decreases to that level seen in nonsmokers. These findings were verified by the work of Perry and associates (1993), who found that smokers required higher doses of haloperidol to achieve similar concentrations in plasma to those found in nonsmokers.

Cigarette smoking significantly increased the clearance of fluphenazine decanoate when administered as a depot injection (Jann et al. 1985). Smokers might require higher depot doses or more frequent injection of these doses than do nonsmokers to achieve the same plasma concentration profile. Once again, a greater problem would exist when a smoking patient maintained at a particular dose of fluphenazine stopped smoking cigarettes.

The pharmacokinetics of the antipsychotic, clozapine, appear to be altered by cigarette smoking (Haring et al. 1989). Clozapine plasma concentrations at a given dose in cigarette smokers were 81% of the levels found in nonsmokers at the same dose.

SMOKING AND BENZODIAZEPINES

Greenblatt and co-workers (1979, 1980) found that cigarette smokers had increased clearances of diazepam and lorazepam over that found in nonsmoking control subjects. Earlier reports by other investigators (Desmond et al. 1979, Klotz et al. 1975) had indicated that smoking did not affect the pharmacokinetics of diazepam or chlordiazepoxide.

Clinicians should be aware that benzodiazepine dosages may have to be adjusted upward in cigarette smokers to achieve efficacy.

SMOKING AND ETHANOL

Griffiths and associates (1976) undertook a series of controlled studies to evaluate the influence of ethanol on human tobacco self-administration. Subjects were male, recently abstinent, chronic alcoholics. Cigarette smoking was increased 26 to 117% in the ethanol-consuming group over that found in the placebo-administered control subjects. This increase has been noted by other investigators (Maletzky and Klotter 1974, Mello and Mendelson 1972) and further confirmed (Henningfield et al. 1983). This increase has also been noted in studies of both male and female social drinkers (Mello et al. 1980a, Mello and Mendelson 1988). The significance of this substantial increase in smoking may be the result of several mechanisms. It has been suggested that ethanol may selectively interact with the reinforcing properties of cigarettes (Goldberg et al. 1971, Thompson and Schuster 1964). Other investigators have proposed that cigarette smoking potentiates the objective and subjective effects of ethanol (Linckint 1972). Griffiths and co-workers (1974) have proposed that ethanol may act as a nonspecific behavioral stimulant. Other hypotheses to explain this finding include aspects of addictive personalities, oral drives, anxiety states, and general neuroticism (Dreher and Fraser 1967, Maletzky and Klotter 1974, McArther et al. 1958).

SMOKING AND NONBARBITURATE SEDATIVE-HYPNOTICS

In a study of normal volunteers, Crow and co-workers (1978) found that glutethimide had a greater detrimental effect on tracking psychomotor skills in cigarette smokers as compared to nonsmokers. Pharmacokinetic studies showed an increase in glutethimide absorption in cigarette smokers.

SMOKING AND OPIOIDS

Heroin

Cigarette smoking increased during heroin self-administration in comparison to drug-free and methadone detoxification conditions in 11 heroin addicts (Mello et al. 1980b). Variations in cigarette smoking observed during heroin self-administration were not related to the specific daily dose of heroin. Those subjects from both the heavy smokers group and the moderate smokers group demonstrated a marked increase in the number of cigarettes smoked during the heroin self-administration.

Methadone

In a controlled clinical study of 5 subjects, the effects of methadone on cigarette smoking were examined (Chait and Griffiths 1984). Methadone produced a dose-related increase in the number of cigarettes smoked per session (over the number smoked under placebo conditions). These data indicate the possibility of a role for endogenous opioids in the smoking process. Stark and Campbell (1993) found that although smoking increased following acute administration of methadone, the maintenance doses of methadone were not correlated with smoking rates, suggesting that the acute effects of methadone administration on cigarette smoking are nullified as patients habituate to dose level.

Pentazocine

In a study by Vaughan and associates (1976), heavy smokers were compared with nonsmokers with regard to cumulative amount of pentazocine excreted in the urine. The researchers found that heavy smokers had 40% less parent drug in urine, indicating more extensive hepatic metabolism. In another study of 41 patients, the amount of pentazocine needed as a supplement to nitrous oxide anesthesia was higher among heavy smokers.

Clinicians should be aware that heavy smokers may require larger doses of pentazocine than nonsmokers to achieve equivalent analgesia.

Propoxyphene

In a study examining the effectiveness of propoxyphene as an analgesic (Boston Collaborative Drug Surveillance Program 1973), heavy smokers rated propoxyphene as ineffective twice as often as nonsmokers. Heavy smokers may require larger doses of propoxyphene to obtain adequate analgesia.

REFERENCES

Alexanderson A et al.: Steady-state plasma levels of nortriptyline in twins: influence of genetic factors and drug therapy. Br Med J 4: 764, 1969.

Aranko K et al.: Interaction of diazepam or lorazepam with alcohol: psychomotor effects and bioassayed serum levels after single and repeated doses. Eur J Clin Pharmacol 28: 559, 1985.

Arndt IO et al.: Desipramine treatment of cocaine dependence in methadone-maintained patients. Arch Gen Psychiatry 49: 888, 1992.

Bailey DN et al.: Blood concentrations and clinical findings in nonfatal and fatal intoxications involving glutethimide and codeine. J Toxicol Clin Toxicol 23: 557, 1985.

Bartkowski R et al.: Prolonged alfentanil effect following erythromycin administration. Anesthesiology 73: 566, 1990.

Baum C et al.: The impact of the addition of naloxone on the use and abuse of pentazocine. Public Health Rep 102: 426, 1987.

Belenko S: Alcohol abuse by heroin addicts: review of research findings and issues. Int J Addict 14: 965, 1979.

Bellville JW et al.: The hypnotic effects of codeine and secobarbital and their interaction in man. Clin Pharmacol Ther 12: 607, 1971.

Bending MR et al.: Rifampin and methadone withdrawal. Lancet 1: 1211, 1977.

Berger P et al.: Treatment of cocaine abuse with mazindol. Lancet 1: 283, 1989.

Bihari B: Alcoholism and methadone maintenance. Am J Drug Alcohol Abuse 1: 79, 1973.

Blum K: Handbook of Abusable Drugs, New York, Gardner, 1984, p. 211.

Boston Collaborative Drug Surveillance Program: Decreased clinical efficacy of propoxyphene in cigarette smokers. Clin Pharmacol Ther 14: 259, 1973.

Boston Collaborative Drug Surveillance Program: Drowsiness due to chlorpromazine in relation to cigarette smoking. Arch Gen Psychiatry 31: 211, 1974.

Burford R et al.: The combined effects of alcohol and common psychoactive drugs: I. Studies on human pursuit tracking capability. In Israelstam S, Lambert F (eds.): *Alcohol, Drugs and Traffic Safety*, Toronto, Addiction Research Foundation, 1975, p.423.

Burrows GD et al.: Antidepressants and barbiturates. Br Med J 4: 113, 1971.

Burton JF: Mainliners and blue velvet. J Forens Sci 10: 466, 1965.

Carpenter JA et al.: Drug interactions: the effects of alcohol and meprobamate applied singly and jointly in human subjects. J Stud Alcohol 7: 54, 1975.

Carroll KM et al.: Psychotherapy and pharmacotherapy for ambulatory cocaine abusers. Arch Gen Psychiatry 51: 177, 1994.

Casswell S et al.: Cannabis induced impairment of performance of a divided attention task. Nature 241: 60, 1973.

Chait LD et al.: Effects of methadone on human cigarette smoking and subjective ratings. J Pharmacol Exp Ther 229: 636, 1984.

Chitwood DD: Patterns and consequences of cocaine use. Nat Inst Drug Abuse Res Monogr Ser 61: 111, 1985.

Ciraulo DA et al.: Imipramine disposition in alcoholics. J Clin Psychopharmacol 2: 2, 1982.

Ciraulo DA et al.: Pharmacokinetic interaction between disulfiram and antidepressants. Am J Psychiatry 142: 1373, 1985.

Ciraulo DA et al.: Pharmacokinetic mechanisms of ethanol-psychotropic drug interactions. Nat Inst Drug Abuse Res Monogr Ser 68: 73, 1986.

Ciraulo DA et al.: Abuse liability and clinical pharmacokinetics of alprazolam in alcoholic men. J Clin Psychiatry 49: 333, 1988a.

Ciraulo DA et al.: Clinical pharmacokinetics of imipramine and desipramine in alcoholics and normal volunteers. Clin Pharmacol Ther 43: 509, 1988b.

Ciraulo DA et al.: Intravenous pharmacokinetics of 2-hydroxyimipramine in alcoholics and normal controls. J Stud Alcohol 51: 366, 1990.

Cooke AR: Ethanol and gastric function. Gastroenterology 62: 501, 1972.

Cooper SM et al.: The psychomotor effects of paroxetine alone and in combination with haloperidol, amylobarbitone, oxazepam, or alcohol. Acta Psychiatr Scand 80(suppl 350): 53, 1989.

Crow JW et al.: Glutethimide and 4-OH-glutethimide: pharmacokinetics and effect on performance in man. Clin Pharmacol Ther 22: 458, 1978.

Curry SH et al.: Diazepam-ethanol interaction in humans: addiction or potentiation? Commun Psychopharmacol 3: 101, 1979.

Dackis CA et al.: Bromocriptine as treatment of cocaine abuse (letter). Lancet 1: 1151, 1985.

Desmond PV et al.: No effect of smoking on metabolism of chlordiazepoxide (letter). N Engl J Med 300: 199, 1979.

Desmond PV et al.: Short-term ethanol administration impairs the elimination of chlordiazepoxide (Librium) in man. Eur J Clin Pharmacol 18: 275, 1980.

Devabhaktuni RV et al.: Using street drugs while on MAOI therapy. J Clin Psychopharmacol 7: 60, 1987.

Domino EF et al.: Barbiturate intoxication in a patient treated with a MAO inhibitor. Am J Psychiatry 118: 941, 1962.

Domino EF: Psychosedative drugs, in: Dipalma JR (ed.): *Drill's Pharmacology in Medicine*, New York, McGraw-Hill, 1965, p. 337.

Domino EF: Neurobiology of phencyclidine-an update, Nat Inst Drug Abuse Res Monogr 21: 44, 1978.

Domino EF: Cannabinoids and the cholinergic system. J Clin Pharmacol 21 Suppl 8-9: 249S, 1981.

Dorian P et al.: Amitriptyline and ethanol: pharmacokinetic and pharmacodynamic interaction. Eur J Clin Pharmacol 25: 325, 1983.

Dornbush RL: Marihuana and memory: effects of smoking on storage. Ann NY Acad Sci 36: 94, 1974.

Dreher K et al.: Smoking habits of alcoholic outpatients. Int J Addict 2: 259, 1967.

Drew WG et al.: Cannabis: neural mechanisms and behavior-a theoretical review. Pharmacology 11: 12, 1974.

Ferraro DP: Acute effects of marijuana on human memory and cognition. Nat Inst Drug Abuse Res Monogr Ser 31: 98, 1980.

Feuer E et al.: Descriptive epidemiology of mortality in New Jersey due to combinations of codeine and glutethimide. Am J Epidemiol 119: 202, 1984.

Finkle BS et al.: The forensic toxicology of cocaine (1971–1976). Nat Inst Drug Abuse Res Monogr Ser 13: 153, 1977.

Foltin RW et al.: Marijuana and cocaine interactions in humans: cardiovascular consequences. Pharmacol Biochem Behav 28: 459, 1987.

Foltin RW et al.: Ethanol and cocaine interactions in humans: Cardiovascular consequences. Pharmacol Biochem Behav 31: 877, 1988.

Foltin RW et al.: The cardiovascular and subjective effects of intravenous cocaine and morphine combinations in humans. J Pharmacol Exp Ther 261: 623, 1992.

Foltin RW et al.: Behavioral effects of cocaine alone and in combination with ethanol or marijuana in humans. Drug Alcohol Dependence 32: 93, 1993.

Forsyth AJ et al.: The dual use of opioids and temazepam drug injectors in Glasgow (Scotland). Drug Alcohol Dependence 32: 277, 1993.

Franks HM et al.: The interaction of alcohol and δ-9-tetrahydrocannabinol in man: effects of psychomotor skills related to driving. In Israelstam S, Lambert F (eds.): *Alcohol, Drugs and Traffic Safety.* Toronto, Addiction Research Foundation, 1975, p. 461.

Frewer LJ et al.: The effects of nefazodone, imipramine and placebo, alone and combined with alcohol, in normal subjects. Int Clin Psychopharmacol 8: 13, 1993.

Fudala PJ et al.: Outpatient comparison of buprenorphine and methadone maintenance, II: effects on cocaine use, retention time in study, and missed clinic visits. Paper: Scientific meeting of the Committee on Problems of Drug Dependence, Richmond VA, June 1990.

Gander RE: Psychoactive drug quantification by visual flicker sensitivity measurement. Ph.D. thesis, Institute of Biomedical Engineering, Department of Electrical Engineering, University of Toronto, 1979.

Garfield JW et al.: Rifampin-methadone relationship, 1: the clinical effects of rifampin-methadone interaction. Am Rev Resp Dis 3: 926, 1975.

Gawin FH et al.: Cocaine abuse treatment: open pilot trial with desipramine and lithium carbonate. Arch Gen Psychiatry 41: 903, 1984.

Gawin FH et al.: Double-blind comparison of desipramine and placebo in cocaine abuse treatment. Presented at the 24th meeting of the American College of Neuropharmacology, Kaanapoli, Hawaii, December 1985a.

Gawin FH et al.: Methylphenidate treatment of cocaine abusers without attention deficit disorder: a negative report. Am J Drug Alcohol Abuse 2: 193, 1985b.

Gearing FR: Evaluation of methadone maintenance programs. Int J Addict 5: 517, 1970.

Gold MS et al.: Cocaine abuse: neurochemistry, phenomenology, and treatment. Nat Inst Drug Abuse Res Monogr Ser 61: 130, 1985.

Goldberg SR et al.: Nalorphine-induced changes in morphine self-administration in rhesus monkeys. J Pharmacol Exp Ther 176: 464, 1971.

Greenblatt DJ et al.: Effect of a cocktail on diazepam absorption. Psychopharmacology 57: 199, 1978.

Greenblatt DJ et al.: Lorazepam kinetics in the elderly. Clin Pharmacol Ther 26: 103, 1979.

Greenblatt DJ et al.: Diazepam disposition determinants. Clin Pharmacol Ther 27: 301, 1980.

Griffiths RR et al.: Assessment of effects of ethanol self-administration on social interactions in alcoholics. Psychopharmacology 38: 105, 1974.

Griffiths RR et al.: Facilitation of human tobacco self-administration by ethanol: a behavioral analysis. J Exper Anal Behav 25: 279, 1976.

Halikas J et al.: Carbamazepine for cocaine addiction? Lancet 1: 623, 1989.

Hammer W et al.: Antidepressant drugs. In Grattini S, Dukes MN (eds.): *Proceedings of the 1st International Symposium, Milan 1966,* International Congress Series No. 122, Excerpta Medica. Amsterdam, Elsevier, p. 301.

Hansen BS et al.: Influence of dextropropoxyphene on steady-state levels and protein binding of three anti-epileptic drugs in man. Acta Neurol Scand 61: 357, 1980.

Hansteen RW et al.: Effects of cannabis and alcohol on automobile driving and psychomotor tracking. Ann NY Acad Sci 282: 240, 1976.

Haring C et al.: Dose-related plasma levels of clozapine: Influence of smoking behaviour, sex and age. Psychopharmacology 99(suppl): s38, 1989.

Havier RG et al.: Deaths as a result of a combination of codeine and glutethimide. J Forens Sci 30: 563, 1985.

Harvey SC: Hypnotics and Sedatives. In: Gilman AG et al. (eds.): *The Pharmacologic Basis of Therapeutics,* New York, Macmillan, 1985, p. 363.

Hayes SL et al.: Ethanol and oral diazepam absorption. N Engl J Med 296: 186, 1977.

Helzer JE et al.: Alcohol Abuse and Dependence. In Robins LN et al. (eds.): *Psychiatric Disorders in America,* New York, Free Press, 1991, p. 81.

Henningfield JE et al.: Cigarette smoking and subjective response: effects of d-amphetamine. Clin Pharmacol Ther 30: 497, 1981.

Henningfield JE et al.: Cigarette smoking and subjective response in alcoholics: effects of pentobarbital. Clin Pharmacol Ther 33: 806, 1983.

Higgins ST et al.: Effects of cocaine and alcohol, alone and in combination, on human learning and performance. J Exper Anal Behav 58: 87, 1992.

Hindmarch I et al.: The effects of paroxetine and other antidepressants in combination with alcohol on psychomotor activity related to car driving. Acta Psychiatr Scand 80(suppl 350): 45, 1989.

Hollister LE: Interactions of δ-9-tetrahydrocannabinol with other drugs. Ann NY Acad Sci 218: 212, 1976.

Holmes VE: Rifampin-induced methadone withdrawal in AIDS (letter). J Clin Psychopharmacol 10: 443, 1990.

Horwitz D et al.: Monoamine oxidase inhibitors, tyramine, and cheese. JAMA 188: 1108, 1964.

Hoyumpa A et al.: Effect of short-term ethanol administration on lorazepam metabolism. Gastroenterology 79: 1027, 1980.

Hughes FW et al.: Comparative effect in human subjects of chlordiazepoxide, diazepam, and placebo on mental and physical performance. Clin Pharmacol Ther 6: 139, 1965.

Hyatt MC et al.: Amitriptyline augments and prolongs ethanol-induced euphoria. J Clin Psychopharmacol 7: 277, 1987.

Institute of Medicine, National Academy of Sciences: Behavioral and psychosocial effects of marijuana use. In: *Marijuana and Health—Report of a Study by a Committee of the Institute of Medicine Division of Health Sciences Policy,* Washington, DC, National Academy Press, 1982.

Jackson GW et al.: Alcohol use among narcotic addicts. Alcohol World 1: 25, 1973.

Jaffe JH et al.: Drugs used in the treatment of alcoholism. In Mendelson JH, Mello NK (eds.): *The Diagnosis and Treatment of Alcoholism,* New York, McGraw-Hill, 1984, p. 355.

Jaffe JH et al.: Opioid analgesics and antagonists. In Gilman AG et al. (eds.): *The Pharmacologic Basis of Therapeutics,* New York, Macmillan, 1985, p. 491.

Jaffe JH et al.: Potential toxic interactions of cocaine and mazindol. Lancet 2: 111, 1989.

Jann MW et al.: Clinical pharmacokinetics of the depot antipsychotics. Clin Pharmacokinet 10: 315, 1985.

Jann MW et al.: Effects of smoking on haloperidol and reduced haloperidol plasma concentrations and haloperidol clearance. Psychopharmacology 90: 468, 1986.

Johnson FA, van Buren HC: Abstinence syndrome following glutethimide intoxication. JAMA 180: 1024, 1962.

Johnstone RE et al.: Combination of δ-9-tetrahydrocannabinol with oxymorphone or pentobarbital: effects on ventilatory control and cardiovascular dynamics. Anesthesiology 42: 674, 1975.

Jusko WJ: Role of tobacco smoking in pharmacokinetics. J Pharmacokinet Biopharm 6: 7, 1978.

Kaplan HL et al.: Chloral hydrate and alcohol metabolism in human subjects. J Forensic Sci 12: 295, 1967.

Keeri-Szanto M: The mode of action of promethazine in potentiating narcotic drugs. Br J Anaesth 46: 918, 1974.

Khantzian EJ et al.: An extreme case of cocaine dependence and marked improvement with methylphenidate treatment. Am J Psychiatry 140: 784, 1983.

Khantzian EJ et al.: Methylphenidate (Ritalin) treatment of cocaine dependence—a preliminary report. J Subst Abuse Treat 1: 107, 1984.

Khoo KC et al.: Influence of phenytoin and phenobarbital on the disposition of a single oral dose of clonazepam. Clin Pharmacol Ther 28: 368, 1980.

Kitson TM: The disulfiram-ethanol reaction: a review. J Stud Alcohol 38: 96, 1977.

Kline NS: Psychopharmaceuticals: effects and side effects. Bull WHO 21: 397, 1959.

Klotz U et al.: The effects of age and liver disease on the disposition and elimination of diazepam in adult man. J Clin Invest 55: 347, 1975.

Knudsen P et al.: Cannabis and neuroleptic agents in schizophrenia. Acta Psychiatr Scand 69: 162, 1984.

Kosten TR et al.: Buprenorphine detoxification from opioid dependence: a pilot study. Life Sci 42: 635, 1988.

Kosten TR et al.: Pharmacotherapy for cocaine-abusing methadone-maintained patients using amantadine or desipramine. Arch Gen Psychiatry 49: 894, 1992.

Kreek MJ et al.: Rifampin-induced methadone withdrawal. N Engl J Med 294: 1104, 1976.

Kreek MJ et al.: Rifampin-methadone relationship, 2: rifampin effects on plasma concentration, metabolism, and excretion of methadone. Am Rev Resp Dis 3: 926, 1975.

Lacoursiere RB et al.: Adverse interaction between disulfiram and marijuana: a case report. Am J Psychiatry 140: 243, 1983.

Lahmeyer HW et al.: Pentazocine-naloxone: another "addiction-proof" drug of abuse. Int J Addict 22: 1163, 1987.

Laisi U et al.: Pharmacokinetic and pharmacodynamic interactions of diazepam with different alcoholic beverages. Eur J Clin Pharmacol 16: 263, 1979.

Landauer AA et al.: Alcohol and amitriptyline effects on skills related to driving behavior. Science 163: 1467, 1969.

Lange RA et al.: Potentiation of cocaine-induced coronary vasoconstriction by beta-adrenergic blockade. Ann Int Med 112: 897, 1990.

Lechat P et al.: Monoamine oxidase inhibitors and the potentiation of experimental sleep. Biochem Pharmacol 8: 1961.

Lemberger L et al.: Clinical studies of the interaction of psychopharmacologic agents with marihuana. Ann NY Acad Sci 281: 219, 1976.

Lemberger L et al.: Effect of fluoxetine on psychomotor performance, physiologic response, and kinetics of ethanol. Clin Pharmacol Ther 37: 658, 1985.

Lieber CS: Interaction of ethanol and drug metabolism. In Smith LH (ed.): Medical Disorders of Alcoholism. Pathogenesis and Treatment. Philadelphia, WB Saunders, 1982, p. 237.

Linckint F: Interaction of alcohol and other drugs. Toronto, Addiction Research Foundation, no. 783, 1972.

Linnoila M et al.: Drug interaction on driving skills as evaluated by laboratory tests and by a driving simulator. Pharmacopsychiatry 6: 127, 1973.

Linnoila M et al.: Effects of diazepam and codeine, alone and in combination with alcohol, on simulated driving. Clin Pharmacol Ther 15: 368, 1974.

Linnoila M et al.: Effect of anticonvulsants on plasma haloperidol and thioridazine levels. Am J Psychiatry 137: 819, 1980.

Linnoila M et al.: Effect of alcohol consumption and cigarette smoking on antidepressant levels of depressed patients. Am J Psychiatry 138: 841, 1981.

Linnoila M et al.: Effects of adinazolam and diazepam, alone and in combination with ethanol, on psychomotor and cognitive performance and on autonomic nervous system reactivity in healthy volunteers. Eur J Clin Pharmacol 38: 371, 1990.

Lister RG et al.: Performance impairment and increased anxiety resulting from the combination of alcohol and lorazepam. J Clin Psychopharmacol 3: 66, 1983.

Lloyd JT et al.: Death after combined dexamphetamine and phenelzine. Br Med J 2: 168, 1965.

Lundberg GD et al.: Cocaine-related death. J Forens Sci 22: 402, 1977.

Maany I et al.: Possible toxic interaction between disulfiram and amitriptyline. Arch Gen Psychiatry 39: 743, 1982.

MacCallum WAG: Drug interactions in alcoholism treatment (letter). Lancet 1: 313, 1969.

MacLeod SM et al.: Diazepam actions and plasma concentrations following ethanol ingestion. Eur J Clin Pharmacol 11: 345, 1977.

MacLeod SM et al.: Interaction of disulfiram with benzodiazepines. Clin Pharmacol Ther 24: 583, 1978.

Maletzky BM et al.: Smoking and alcoholism. Am J Psychiatry 131: 445, 1974.

Mallach HJ et al.: Pharmakokinetische Untersuchungen uber Resorption und Ausscheidung von Oxazepam in Kombination mit alkohol. Arzneim Forsch 25: 1840, 1975.

Maltbie AA et al.: Analgesia and haloperidol-hypothesis. J Clin Psychiatry 40: 323, 1979.

Manno JE et al.: The influence of alcohol and marihuana on motor and mental performance. Clin Pharmacol Ther 12: 202, 1971.

Margolin A et al.: Bupropion reduces cocaine abuse in methadone-maintained patients. Arch Gen Psychiatry 48: 87, 1991.

Mason A: Fatal reaction associated with tranylcypromine and methylamphetamine. Lancet 1: 1073, 1962.

McArther C et al.: The psychology of smoking. J Abnorm Psychol 56: 267, 1958.

McGwier BW et al.: Acute myocardial infarction associated with intravenous injection of pentazocine and tripelennamine. Chest 101: 1730, 1992.

McNichol RW et al.: *Disulfiram (Antabuse), A Unique Medical Aid to Sobriety*, Springfield, IL, Charles C Thomas, 1987, p. 68.

Mello NK et al.: Drinking patterns during work-contingent and noncontingent alcohol acquisition. Psychosom Med 34: 139, 1972.

Mello NK et al.: Effect of alcohol and marihuana on tobacco smoking. Clin Pharmacol Ther 27: 202, 1980a.

Mello NK et al.: Effects of heroin self-administration on cigarette smoking. Psychopharmacol 67: 45, 1980b.

Mello NK et al.: Concurrent alcohol and tobacco use by women. Natl Inst Drug Abuse Res Monogr Ser 81: 26, 1988.

Mendelson JH et al.: Alcohol and marijuana: Concordance of use by men and women. Natl Inst Drug Abuse Res Monogr Ser 68: 117, 1986.

Mezey E et al.: Effects of phenobarbital administration on rates of ethanol clearance and on ethanol-oxidizing enzymes in man. Gastroenterology 66: 248, 1974.

Miller DD et al.: The influence of cigarette smoking on haloperidol pharmacokinetics. Biol Psychiatry 28: 529, 1990.

Miller LG et al.: Differential modulation of benzodiazepine receptor binding by ethanol in LS and SS mice. Pharmacol Biochem Behav 29: 471, 1988a.

Miller LG et al.: Acute barbiturate administration increases benzodiazepine receptor binding *in vivo*. Psychopharmacology 96: 385, 1988b.

Miller LL: Cannabis and the brain with special reference to the limbic system. In Nahas GC, Parton WDM (eds.): *Marihuana: Biological Effects*, New York, Pergamon Press, 1979, p. 539.

Milner G et al.: Alcohol, thioridazine and chlorpromazine effects on skills related to driving behaviour. Br J Psychiatry 118: 351, 1971.

Milner G et al.: The effects of doxepin, alone and together with alcohol, in relation to driving safety. Med J Aust 1: 837, 1973.

Misra PS et al.: Increase of ethanol, meprobamate and pentobarbital metabolism after chronic ethanol administration in man and in rats. Am J Med 41: 346, 1971.

Moody JP et al.: Pharmacokinetic aspects of protriptyline plasma levels. Eur J Clin Pharmacol 11: 51, 1977.

Morland J et al.: Combined effects of diazepam and ethanol on mental and psychomotor functions. Acta Pharmacol Toxicol 34: 5, 1974.

Moskowitz H et al.: A comparison of the effects of marijuana and alcohol on visual functions. In Lewis MI (ed.): *Current Research on Marijuana*, New York, Academic Press, 1972, p. 129.

Moskowitz H et al.: Effects of marijuana on auditory signal detection. Psychopharmacologia 40: 137, 1974.

Mould GP et al.: Interaction of glutethimide and phenobarbitone with ethanol in man. J Pharm Pharmacol 24: 894, 1972.

Nomikos, GG et al.: Acute effects of bupropion on extracellular dopamine concentrations in rat striatum and nucleus accumbens studied by in vivo microdialysis. Neuropsychopharmacology 2: 273, 1989.

Nutt IG et al.: Methadone-naloxone mixtures for use in methadone maintenance programs, I: an evaluation in man of their pharmacological feasibility; II: demonstration of acute physical dependence. Clin Pharmacol Ther 15: 156, 1974.

O'Malley SS et al.: Naltrexone and coping skills therapy for alcohol dependence. Arch Gen Psychiatry 49: 881, 1992.

O'Reilly RA: Interaction of warfarin and disulfiram in man. Fed Proc 19: 180, 1972.

Palva ES et al.: Effect of active metabolites of chlordiazepoxide and diazepam, alone or in combination with alcohol, on psychomotor skills related to driving. Eur J Clin Pharmacol 13: 345, 1978.

Parry HG et al.: National patterns of psychotherapeutic drug use. Arch Gen Psychiatry 28: 760, 1973.

Perel JM et al.: Tricyclic antidepressants: relationships among pharmacokinetics, metabolism and clinical outcome. In Garattini S (ed.): Depressive Disorders, Stuttgart, Schattauer, 1978, p. 325.

Perez-Reyes M et al.: Ethanol/cocaine interaction: cocaine and cocaethylene plasma concentrations and their relationship to subjective and cardiovascular effects. Life Sci 51: 553, 1992.

Perry PJ et al.: Haloperidol dosing requirements: The contribution of smoking and nonlinear pharmacokinetics. J Clin Psychopharmacology 13: 46, 1993.

Picker W et al.: Potential interaction of LSD and fluoxetine. Am J Psychiatry 149: 843, 1992.

Poklis A: Decline in abuse of pentazocine/tripelennamine (T's and Blues) associated with the addition of naloxone to pentazocine tablets. Drug Alcohol Depend 14: 135, 1984.

Pond SM et al.: Diazepam kinetics in acute alcohol withdrawal. Clin Pharmacol Ther 25: 832, 1979.

Pond SM et al.: Lack of effect of diazepam on methadone metabolism in methadone-maintained addicts. Clin Pharmacol Ther 31: 139, 1982.

Preston KL et al.: Diazepam and methadone interactions in methadone maintenance. Clin Pharmacol Ther 36: 534, 1985.

Rosecan JS: The treatment of cocaine abuse with imipramine, L-tyrosine and L-tryptophan. Presented at the 7th World Congress of Psychiatry, Vienna, Austria, July 1983.

Rosecan JS et al.: Imipramine blockade of cocaine euphoria with double-blind challenge. Presented at the 139th Annual Meeting of the American Psychiatric Association, Washington, DC, May 1986.

Rosen EH: Cocaine drug-drug interactions. J Clin Psychopharmacol 12: 445, 1992.

Rothstein E: Warfarin effect enhanced by disulfiram. JAMA 206: 1574, 1968.

Rothstein E et al.: Toxicity of disulfiram combined with metronidazole. New Engl J Med 280: 1482, 1969.

Rowbotham MC et al.: Trazodone-oral cocaine interactions. Arch Gen Psychiatry 41: 895, 1984.

Ruben SM et al.: Cyclizine abuse among a group of opiate dependents receiving methadone. Br J Addict 84: 929, 1989.

Rubin E et al.: Inhibition of drug metabolism by acute ethanol intoxication. Am J Med 49: 801, 1970.

Saario I: Psychomotor skills during subacute treatment with thioridazine and bromazepam, and their combined effects with alcohol. Ann Clin Res 8: 117, 1976.

Saario I et al.: Effect of subacute treatment with hypnotics, alone or in combination with alcohol, on psychomotor skills related to driving. Acta Pharmacol Toxicol 38: 382, 1976.

Samuels J et al.: Speedballs: a new cause of intraoperative tachycardia and hypertension. Anesth Analg 72: 397, 1991.

Sands B et al.: Cocaine drug-drug interactions. J Clin Psychopharmacol 12: 49, 1992a.

Sands B et al.: Reply to Dr. Rosen. J Clin Psychopharm 12: 445, 1992b.

Schuster CR et al.: The effects of d-amphetamine, meprobamate, and lobeline on the cigarette smoking behavior of normal human subjects. Natl Inst Drug Abuse Res Mongr Ser 23: 91, 1979.

Sellers EM et al.: Benzodiazepines and ethanol: assessment of the effects and consequences of psychotropic drug interactions. J Clin Psychopharmacol 2: 249, 1982.

Sellers EM et al.: Interaction of chloral hydrate and ethanol in man, I: metabolism. Clin Pharmacol Ther 13: 37, 1972a.

Sellers EM et al.: Interaction of chloral hydrate and ethanol in man, II: hemodynamics and performance. Clin Pharmacol Ther 13: 50, 1972b.

Sellers EM et al.: Decline in chlordiazepoxide plasma levels during fixed-dose therapy of alcohol withdrawal. Br J Clin Pharmacol 6: 370, 1978a.

Sellers EM et al.: Drug kinetics and alcohol ingestion. Clin Pharmacokinet 3: 440, 1978b.

Sellers EM et al.: Intravenous diazepam and oral ethanol interaction. Clin Pharmacol Ther 28: 638, 1980.

Sellman R et al. : Reduced concentrations of plasma diazepam in chronic alcoholic patients following an oral administration of diazepam. Acta Pharmacol Toxicol 36: 25, 1975a.

Sellman R et al.: Human and animal study on elimination from plasma and metabolism of diazepam after chronic alcohol intake. Acta Pharmacol Toxicol 36: 33, 1975b.

Seppala T et al.: Effect of tricyclic antidepressants and alcohol on psychomotor skills related to driving. Clin Pharmacol Ther 17: 515, 1975.

Seppala T: Psychomotor skills during acute and two-week treatment with mianserin and amitriptyline, and their combined effects with alcohol. Ann Clin Res 9: 66, 1977.

Shamoian CA et al.: Abuse of an euphoric combination. JAMA 207: 1919, 1969.

Shamoian CA: Codeine and glutethimide. NY State J Med 75: 97, 1975.

Shannon HE et al.: Effects of the combination of tripelennamine and pentazocine at the behavioural and molecular levels. Pharmacol Biochem Behav 17: 784, 1982.

Sharp CW et al.: Inhalants. In Ciraulo DA (ed.): *Clinical Manual of Chemical Dependence*, Washington, DC, American Psychiatric Press, 1991, p. 295.

Sherer MA et al.: A case in which carbamazepine attenuated cocaine "rush." Am J Psychiatry 147: 950, 1990.

Silverstone PH et al.: Ondansetron, a 5-HT$_3$ receptor antagonist, partially attenuates the effects of amphetamine: a pilot study in healthy volunteers. Int Clin Psychopharmacology 7: 37, 1992.

Smiley AM et al.: Driving simulator studies of marijuana alone and in combination with alcohol. Proceedings of the 25th Conference of the American Association for Automotive Medicine, San Francisco, CA, 1981. American Association for Automotive Medicine, p. 107.

Smilkstein MJ et al.: A case of MAO inhibitor/MDMA interaction: agony after ecstasy. J Toxicol Clin Toxicol 25: 149, 1987.

Sramek JJ et al.: Loads. N Engl J Med 305: 231, 1981.

Stambaugh JE et al.: Drug interaction: meperidine and chlorpromazine, a toxic combination. J Clin Pharmacol 28: 140, 1981.

Stambaugh JE et al.: A potentially toxic drug interaction between pethidine (meperidine) and phenobarbitone. Lancet 1: 398, 1977.

Stambaugh JE et al.: Effect of phenobarbital on metabolism of meperidine in normal volunteers. J Clin Pharmacol 18: 482, 1978.

Stark MJ et al.: Cigarette smoking and methadone dose levels. Am J Drug Alcohol Abuse 19: 209, 1993.

Stimmel B et al.: Alcoholism as a risk factor in methadone maintenance. Am J Med 73: 631, 1982.

Stitzer ML et al.: Diazepam use among methadone maintenance patients: patterns and dosages. Drug Alcohol Depend 8: 189, 1981.

Strauss A: Homicidal psychosis during the combined use of cocaine and an over-the-counter cold preparation. J Clin Psychiatry 50: 147, 1989.

Tennant FS Jr et al.: Cocaine and amphetamine dependence treated with desipramine. Natl Inst Drug Abuse Res Monogr Ser 43: 351, 1983.

Teoh SK et al.: Acute interactions of buprenorphine and intravenous cocaine and morphine: an investigational new drug Phase I safety evaluation. J Clin Psychopharmacology 13: 87, 1993.

Thompson T et al.: Morphine self-administration food-reinforced and avoidance behaviors in rhesus monkeys. Psychopharmacologia 5: 87, 1964.

Tinklenberg JR et al.: Drugs and criminal assaults by adolescents: a replication study. J Psychoactive Drugs 13: 277, 1981.

Tordoff SG et al.: Delayed excitatory reaction following interaction of cocaine and monamine oxidase inhibitor (phenelzine). Br J Anaesth 66: 516, 1991.

Tverskoy M et al.: Midazolam-morphine sedative interaction in patients. Anesth Analg 68: 282, 1989.

Unterwald EM et al.: Tripelennaime: enhancement of brain-stimulation reward. Life Sci 34: 149, 1984.

Vachon L et al.: Marihuana effects on learning, attention, and time estimation. Psychopharmacologia 39: 1, 1974.

Van Harten J et al.: Fluvoxamine does not interact with alcohol or potentiate alcohol-related impairment of cognitive function. Clin Pharmacol Ther 52: 427, 1992.

Vaughan DP et al.: The influence of smoking on the intersubject variation in pentazocine elimination. Br J Clin Pharmacol 3: 279, 1976.

Vinarova E et al.: Smokers need higher doses of neuroleptic drugs. Biol Psychiatry 19: 1265, 1984.

Volpicelli JR et al.: Naltrexone in the treatment of alcohol dependence. Arch Gen Psychiatry 49: 876, 1992.

Whiting B et al.: Effects of acute alcohol intoxication on the metabolism and plasma kinetics of chlordiazepoxide. Br J Clin Pharmacol 7: 95, 1979.

Wulfsohn NL et al.: 5-Hydroxytryptamine in anaesthesia. Anaesthesia 17: 64, 1962.

Yisak W et al.: Drug interactions studies with remoxipride. Acta Psychiatr Scand 82 (suppl 358): 58, 1990.

Zaks A et al.: Naloxone treatment of opiate dependence: a progress report. JAMA 215: 2108, 1971.

Zirkle GA et al.: Effects of chlorpromazine and alcohol on coordination and judgment. JAMA 168: 1496, 1959.

Zirkle GA et al.: Meprobamate and small amounts of alcohol: effects on human ability, coordination, and judgment. JAMA 173: 1823, 1960.

9

Electroconvulsive Therapy

CHARLES A. WELCH

Anesthetics

ANTICHOLINERGICS

Evidence of Interaction

The effects of atropine have been carefully studied in electroconvulsive therapy (ECT) (Altschule 1950, Anton et al. 1977, Bouckoms et al. 1989, Miller et al. 1987, Perrin 1961). Atropine increases the heart rate, reduces the number of dropped beats, and reduces the number of premature atrial beats. It virtually eliminates poststimulus asystole and bradyarrhythmias. It does not reduce oral secretions. Glycopyrrolate has similar effects (Swartz and Saheba 1989).

Mechanism

Vagal blockade causes the cardiovascular effects of anticholinergic agents. Identical effects are seen after sectioning the vagus in experimental animals.

Clinical Implications

Anticholinergics should not be routinely administered during ECT, but should be reserved for patients who demonstrate bradyarrhythmias or prolonged poststimulus asystole. Elderly patients with coronary artery disease are at risk for cardiac ischemia due to the increase in cardiac rate caused by anticholinergics.

BARBITURATES

Evidence of Interaction

The three agents most commonly used for narcosis during ECT are methohexital, thiopental, and propofol (Swartz 1993). Methohexital and thiopental both shorten the seizure duration by 40 to 50% (Lunn et al. 1981, Mokriski et al. 1992), with methohexital having a slightly less pronounced effect on seizure duration. Higher doses of methohexital are associated with shorter seizures and longer courses of ECT compared with treatment with lower doses (Nettelbladt 1988). Propofol markedly reduces the duration and intensity of seizures (Boey and Lai 1990), although in one study ECT with propofol has been found as effective as ECT with methohexital (Malsch et al. 1992). Propofol has a smoother emergence syndrome than other brief anesthetics. Barbiturate induction with all three drugs is accompanied by a moderate drop in systolic and diastolic pressure. Methohexital and thiopental both induce cardiac arrhythmias, although methohexital is significantly less likely to do so (Mokriski et al. 1992).

Mechanism

The central depressant effects of barbiturates are responsible for their effect on seizure duration. The mechanism of their hypotensive effect is unknown.

Clinical Implications

Methohexital continues to be the rational choice for routine use in ECT. Although propofol is associated with a more benign emergence syndrome, its inhibitory effect on the ictal process is impressive, and there may be individual patients in whom this reduces the effectiveness of the treatment. Alternatively, ketamine offers an interesting alternative for narcosis, since it actually increases the intensity and duration of the ECT seizure (Staton et al. 1986). However, recovery from treatment takes approximately an hour, making this strategy impractical.

SUCCINYLCHOLINE

Evidence of Interaction

Succinylcholine, a depolarizing paralytic agent, provides almost complete paralysis of skeletal muscle at doses averaging 0.75 mg/kg, although doses vary considerably from patient to patient. Typically, the effects of succinylcholine last 5 to 10 minutes, although individuals with pseudocholinesterase deficiency may take 6 to 12 hours to regain ventilatory competency. Although cholinesterase deficiency is usually hereditary, it is also associated with cardiac failure, uremia, malnutrition, hypothyroidism, and hepatic failure. It may also result from exposure to insecticides or neuroleptics (Marco and Randels 1979). Extended apnea with succinylcholine may also be associated with quinidine, kanamycin, gentamicin, or streptomycin. The use of succinylcholine in patients with acute burns (Dwersteg and Avery 1987) and acute upper motor neuron deficit (McCleane and Howe 1989) is contraindicated because of the marked rise in serum potassium which may occur in these circumstances.

Mechanism

Succinylcholine normally induces a slight and transient increase in serum potassium due to its effect of triggering a single firing of skeletal muscle prior to paralysis. In denervated muscle this effect is more pronounced.

Clinical Implications

Patients with cholinesterase deficiency, thermal injury, or recent stroke may be safely treated with mivacurium 0.25 mg/kg, with reversal by edrophonium 0.5 mg/kg and atropine 0.005 mg/kg (McCain et al. 1992).

Anticoagulants

Evidence of Interaction

A total of 6 cases have been reported of patients receiving ECT during anticoagulant therapy (Loo et al. 1985, Tancer and Evans 1989): 3 patients were heparinized, and 3 were receiving warfarin. No complications were associated with anticoagulant therapy.

Mechanism

In the early use of ECT, some deaths were attributed to cerebral hemorrhage (Madow 1956), and postmortem study of ECT patients has demonstrated petechial hemorrhages (Impastato 1957). Theoretically, the use of anticoagulants could predispose patients to these complications.

Clinical Implications

The theoretical concern regarding intracranial hemorrhage in anticoagulated ECT patients appears not to be borne out in clinical practice. Consequently, anticoagulated patients should be treated according to standard contemporary techniques. However, meticulous attention should be given to blood pressure, and, if significant hypertensive responses occur, they should be attenuated with short-acting intravenous β-blockade (i.e. esmolol 100–300 mg intravenously 2 minutes prior to stimulus).

Anticonvulsants

Evidence of Interaction

The principal *in vivo* effect of all anticonvulsants is to antagonize the initiation, proliferation, and duration of ictal events. Carbamazepine has been reported to interfere with the induction of seizure activity during ECT (Roberts and Attah 1988).

Mechanism

Varies with specific agents.

Clinical Implications

Patients who are taking anticonvulsants for clinical implications, such as epilepsy or bipolar disorder, should usually remain on these drugs throughout ECT, since discontinuation often results in an exacerbation of the underlying illness. It is possible to override the anticonvulsant effect with a modest increase in the intensity of the ECT stimulus, and induce seizures that are of adequate duration, generalization, and effectiveness.

Antidepressants

MAOIs

Evidence of Interaction

The concurrent use of ECT and monoamine oxidase inhibitors (MAOIs) appears to be safe. In a controlled prospective study of patients undergoing ECT or elective surgery, no differences in cardiovascular function were noted between patients with or without MAOIs (El-Ganzouri et al. 1985). One flawed study (Monaco and

DelaPlaine 1964) found no augmentation of efficacy with MAOIs, but this question remains to be adequately researched.

Mechanism

Theoretically, the concurrent use of MAOIs would predispose patients either to hypotensive episodes through their antihypertensive effect, or to hypertension and arrhythmias through their interference with the degradation of circulating catecholamines.

Clinical Implications

At this time there is no evidence that patients on MAOIs must be taken off these drugs for a course of ECT (Freese 1985, Remick et al. 1987). MAOIs may enhance the efficacy of ECT, and the empirical use of this combination in treatment-resistant patients is reasonable. The extensive clinical experience with MAOIs and ECT indicate that combining the therapies does not increase the risks of ECT (Dunlop 1960, Imlah et al. 1965, Muller 1961).

TRICYCLICS

Evidence of Interaction

When administered concurrently with a course of ECT, tricyclics have been found to increase neither the incidence of cardiac ectopy (Janowsky et al. 1981), nor the seizure duration (Markowitz and Brown 1987). There is, however, 1 case report of increased cardiac irritability following acute discontinuation of tricyclics prior to ECT (Raskin 1984). The efficacy of ECT appears not to be affected negatively or positively by concurrent tricyclic therapy (Seager and Bird 1962). However, one retrospective study has reported better outcome in patients receiving combination ECT-TCA than ECT alone (Nelson and Benjamin 1989).

Mechanism

Patients on chronic tricyclic therapy appear to derive some cardiac antiarrhythmic effect, which is protective during a course of ECT (Glassman et al. 1987).

Clinical Implications

Patients on chronic tricyclic therapy should not be abruptly withdrawn immediately prior to a course of ECT. At the clinician's discretion, they should either be withdrawn well prior to the initiation of treatment, gradually withdrawn during a course of treatment, or maintained on a tricyclic throughout their course with the intention to continue it after ECT is completed.

The augmentation of ECT with tricyclics is a reasonable and safe strategy in treatment-resistant patients, although the evidence for its effectiveness is equivocal.

SSRIs

Evidence of Interaction

Patients treated with fluoxetine and ECT were compared with patients receiving ECT alone (Gutierrez-Esteinou and Pope 1989). There were no differences in seizure duration, although a trend appeared for shorter seizures to occur as fluoxetine dosage increased. There is no evidence that fluoxetine or other selective serotonin inhibitors (SSRIs) alter the cardiovascular response to ECT, although this is based on fewer than 20 case reports in the literature. There is as yet no evidence that fluoxetine augments the effectiveness of ECT.

Mechanism

The mechanism by which fluoxetine might decrease seizure length is unknown.

Clinical Implications

There appears to be no adverse effect of continuing SSRIs throughout a course of ECT, although the literature on this question is very limited. SSRIs may be continued through a course of ECT when their use is clinically indicated.

Antihypertensives

β-BLOCKERS

Evidence of Interaction

The use of short-acting injectable beta blockers to attenuate the sympathetic discharge during ECT has been extensively studied (Castelli et al. 1995, Foster and Ries 1988, Howie et al. 1990, 1992, Kovac et al, 1990, 1991, McCall et al. 1991, Stoudemire et al. 1990, Weigner et al. 1991a). These studies have all reported a reduction in heart rate and in systolic and diastolic blood pressure relative to placebo in ECT patients. Both esmolol and labetalol have been associated with shortening of seizure duration in some studies (Howie et al. 1990, Weigner et al. 1991a), but in one study no such effect was noted (Kovac et al. 1990). These drugs are not associated with hypotensive crisis, bradyarrhythmia, or an increase in poststimulus asystole (Castelli et al. 1995).

Mechanism

β-Blockers blunt the sympathetic discharge during ECT-induced seizures at the postsynaptic receptor. Esmolol is selective for the β-1-receptor, while labetalol is not (Gilman et al. 1985). In addition, labetalol has some α-1-blocking activity (McCarthy and Bloomfield 1983). Because of the widespread distribution of these receptors, effects are seen on peripheral vascular resistance, cardiac rate, and cardiac contractility. Pretreatment with esmolol reduces the surge in circulating catecholamines (epinephrine and norepinephrine) during ECT, but labetalol does not (Weigner et al. 1991b).

Clinical Implications

Blunting the cardiovascular response to ECT has not been shown to reduce the overall incidence of adverse effects (Kellner 1991). On the other hand, it is clear that specific patients can be more safely treated with the use of these agents. Criteria for use of beta blockers are not yet established, but their use is widespread in patients with preexisting hypertension, coronary artery disease, and ventricular ectopy. These drugs have not been associated with a significant incidence of hypotension or bradycardia during ECT, and they are probably the ideal strategy for protecting the vulnerable cardiac patient from the sympathetic outflow which occurs during ECT.

NITROPRUSSIDE

Evidence of Interaction

Nitroprusside is a potent antihypertensive given by direct intravenous infusion. It has a rapid onset and short duration of action, and blood pressure is controlled by infusion rate.

Mechanism

Nitroprusside is a peripheral vasodilator.

Clinical Implications

Although a potent antihypertensive, nitroprusside has the disadvantage of producing reflex tachycardia, which, in addition to the sympathetic outflow during a seizure, may induce extremely high cardiac rates. In addition, it may decrease cardiac perfusion. Consequently, its use is not recommended during ECT.

NIFEDIPINE

Evidence of Interaction

Nifedipine has been shown to blunt the hypertensive response to ECT (Kalayam and Alexopoulos 1989, Wells et al. 1989). Nifedipine was administered at a dose of 10 mg sublingually 20 minutes before treatment.

Mechanism

Nifedipine selectively inhibits calcium ion influx across the cell membrane of cardiac muscle and vascular smooth muscle. The clinical effects of this mechanism include coronary artery dilation, increased coronary perfusion, and peripheral arterial dilation.

Clinical Implications

In patients whose pressure is inadequately controlled by injectable β-blockers during ECT, nifedipine is an effective and safe means of augmenting the antihypertensive regimen, without significant reflex tachycardia.

Antipsychotics

Evidence of Interaction

The extensive literature on ECT and antipsychotic drugs has been recently reviewed (Klapheke 1993). Both retrospective and prospective studies indicate that for some chronic schizophrenic or acutely psychotic patients, the combination of ECT and antipsychotics results in a faster or more pronounced response to treatment, earlier discharge, and lower subsequent relapse rate, relative to treatment with either agent alone. It is important to note that the improved efficacy is not universal, and some individual patients show a dramatic response, while others show none, from combined therapy. The presence of affective symptoms is not a prerequisite for good response to combined therapy (Brandon et al. 1985, Dodwell and Goldberg 1989, Taylor and Fleminger 1980).

There is no evidence that neuroleptics improve the effectiveness of ECT in the treatment of major depression (Thase 1992).

Hypotensive episodes and cardiopulmonary arrest have been reported with the combination of both reserpine and chlorpromazine and ECT, but not with other neuroleptics (Bracha and Hes 1956,

Weiss 1955). In a review of the literature, Friedel (1986) reported no evidence of this harmful interaction with ECT and high potency neuroleptics.

Mechanism

The therapeutic mechanism of the combined use of ECT and neuroleptics is unknown.

Clinical Implications

Based on the available literature, the combined use of ECT and neuroleptics is indicated in schizophrenic patients who have not responded optimally to neuroleptic treatment alone (Klapheke 1993). Target symptoms are both positive and negative signs of schizophrenia, and patients without depressive symptomatology may derive dramatic benefit from combined therapy. Patients may respond to less than 12 ECTs, although larger numbers of treatments are commonplace. Both unilateral and bilateral ECT have been reported effective in schizophrenia (Gujavarty et al. 1987, Small 1985).

Benzodiazepines

Evidence of Interaction

There is conflicting evidence as to whether benzodiazepines inhibit the efficacy of ECT (Kellner et al. 1991). One prospective trial (Standish-Barry et al. 1985) found that diazepam 10 mg 12 hours prior to ECT significantly shortened seizures, and a second retrospective study (Pettinati et al. 1990) found that ECT patients taking concurrent benzodiazepines had a higher nonresponse to ECT and a higher incidence of missed seizures. On the other hand, Olesen et al. (1989) found no difference in seizure duration between patients given bedtime oxazepam and those given placebo.

Mechanism

A fully generalized grand mal seizure is the essential therapeutic component of ECT. If benzodiazepines reduce the effectiveness of ECT, it is probably through inhibition of the ictal process, by binding to the gamma-aminobutyric acid-benzodiazepine receptor complex (Enna and Mohler 1987). Intravenous benzodiazepines are highly effective in terminating excessively long seizure activity during ECT. It is important to keep in mind that midazolam has potent, but brief, respiratory depressant activity.

Clinical Implications

The evidence regarding antagonistic effects of benzodiazepines on ECT is preliminary and in need of replication. On the other hand, there is enough empirical evidence and theoretical reason for concern to warrant caution in the use of benzodiazepines during the course of ECT.

Digitalis

Evidence of Interaction

There has been no systematic study of the interaction between digitalis and ECT. On the other hand, there is strong theoretical basis for concern regarding postictal bradycardia or even cardiac arrest in digitalized patients. Since the effect of digitalis is dose related, heightened concern is warranted with digitalis levels above the therapeutic range.

Mechanism

Digitalis glycosides have a vagomimetic action, resulting in slowed conduction at the sinoatrial and atrioventricular nodes. By this mechanism, digitalis glycosides exert a dose-related negative chronotropic effect.

Clinical Implications

Any digitalized patient should have blood levels checked prior to ECT. Although routine pretreatment with atropine is probably unwarranted, atropine should be available in the event of postictal bradycardia. Patients with digitalis levels above the therapeutic range must not receive ECT until blood levels are reduced.

Lithium

Evidence of Interaction

In the past two decades, there have been numerous case reports of severe delirium associated with the concurrent use of ECT and lithium (Mukherjee 1993). There has been only one retrospective study (Small et al. 1980) comparing 25 patients receiving ECT and lithium in combination with 25 patients receiving ECT alone. Patients receiving the combined treatment demonstrated more severe memory loss, a lower therapeutic response, and lower scores on neuropsychological testing during and after treatment.

Two prospective studies report no evidence of ECT-lithium interaction. Coppen et al. (1981) found no evidence of increased encephalopathy in patients who were started on lithium during a course of ECT. Martin and Kramer (1982) likewise reported no increased morbidity associated with concurrent lithium during a course of ECT.

Mechanism

The mechanism of interaction between ECT and lithium is hypothetical and unknown.

Clinical Implications

About 10 to 30% of bipolar patients switch from depression to mania during a course of ECT (Angst et al. 1992). Consequently, there is some clinical basis for continuation of lithium during a course of ECT. On the other hand, the case reports in the literature cannot be ignored. Although evidence for an ECT-lithium interaction is weak, and may indeed be attributed to other issues such as lithium toxicity, certain individual patients may indeed be sensitive to the combined regimen. If there are clear indications for continuation of lithium, it may be reasonable and even therapeutically advantageous. On the other hand, the emergence of delirium or encephalopathy during a course of ECT should be grounds for discontinuation of lithium immediately. All patients receiving the combined regimen should be informed of the potential interaction prior to the initiation of treatment.

Sympathomimetics (Methylxanthines)

Evidence of Interaction

Caffeine augmentation of ECT has been extensively studied (Calev et al. 1993, Coffey et al. 1987, 1990). The use of caffeine sodium benzoate in doses of 500 to 2,000 mg intravenously prior to ECT is associated with an increase in seizure duration and a reduction in number of treatments (Calev 1993) and a decrease in seizure threshold (Coffey et al. 1990). Theophylline at a dose of 200 to 400 mg orally the night before treatment is associated with a lengthening of seizure duration (Swartz and Lewis 1991), but theophylline may cause prolonged seizures (Devanand 1988, Peters et al. 1984).

Mechanism

Methylxanthines may act as proconvulsants by acting as a competitive inhibitor of adenosine, an endogenous anticonvulsant, at the adenosine receptor (Snyder and Sklar 1984).

Clinical Implications

The use of methylxanthines may be indicated for patients in whom it is difficult to initiate seizure activity, or in patients who have brief seizures (<20 seconds). On the other hand, these augmentation strategies have occasionally resulted in protracted seizures (Coffey et al. 1987) or an increase in cardiac ectopy. Consequently, if a patient is showing a reasonable clinical response to ECT, adding methylxanthines to the treatment format is probably unwarranted.

Thyroid Hormone

Evidence of Interaction

The combined use of thyroid hormone and ECT was evaluated by Stern et al. (1993). Patients receiving 50 μg/day of triiodothyronine were compared to patients receiving placebo. The patients receiving thyroid hormone had significantly longer seizures than the placebo group and required significantly fewer treatments. In addition, patients receiving thyroid hormone performed better on cognitive testing post-ECT, and reported a higher degree of subjective improvement. There was no increase in cardiovascular complications in the treatment group.

Mechanism

The mechanism of interaction between thyroid hormone and ECT is unknown. One possible mechanism is the suppression of thyrotropin-releasing hormone, which is known to have anticonvulsant activity.

Clinical Implications

The concurrent use of thyroid hormone and ECT is not associated with cardiovascular or central nervous system toxicity, and indeed the combined regimen may be more effective in the treatment of depression than ECT alone. The evidence for potentiation is not strong enough to warrant routine administration of thyroid hormone to patients receiving ECT, but in treatment-resistant patients an empirical trial of thyroid augmentation is a reasonable strategy.

Tryptophan

Evidence of Interaction

The administration of tryptophan does not augment the effectiveness of ECT (Kirkegaard et al. 1978), but it does increase seizure duration (Raotma 1978).

Mechanism

The mechanism of tryptophan's anticonvulsant action is unknown.

Clinical Implications

Tryptophan is contraindicated during ECT.

REFERENCES

Altschule MD: Further observations on vagal influences on the heart during electroshock therapy for mental disease. Am Heart J 39: 88, 1950.

Angst J et al.: ECT-induced and drug-induced hypomania. Convulsive Ther 8: 179, 1992.

Anton AH, Uy DS, Redderson CL: Autonomic blockade and the cardiovascular and catecholamine response to electroshock. Anesth Analg 56: 46, 1977.

Boey WK, Lai FO: Comparison of propofol and thiopentone as anaesthetic agents for electroconvulsive therapy. Anaesthesia 45: 623, 1990

Bouckoms AJ et al.: Atropine in electroconvulsive therapy. 5: 48, 1989.

Bracha S, Hes J: Death occurring during combined reserpine-electroshock treatment. Am J Psychiatry 113: 257, 1956.

Brandon S et al.: Leicester ECT trial: results in schizophrenia. Br J Psychiatry 146: 177, 1985.

Calev A et al.: Caffeine pretreatment enhances clinical efficacy and reduces cognitive effects of electroconvulsive therapy. Convulsive Ther 9: 95, 1993.

Castelli I et al.: Comparative effects of esmolol and labetalol to attenuate hyperdynamic states after electroconvulsive therapy. Anesth Analg 80: 11, 1995.

Coffey CE et al.: Augmentation of ECT seizures with caffeine. Biol Psychiatry 22: 637, 1987.

Coffey CE et al.: Caffeine augmentation of ECT. Am J Psychiatry 147: 579, 1990.

Coppen A, et al.: Lithium continuation therapy following electroconvulsive therapy. Br J Psychiatry 139: 284, 1981.

Devanand DP et al.: Status epilepticus during ECT in a patient receiving theophylline. J Clin Psychopharmacol 8: 153, 1988.

Dodwell D, Goldberg D: A study of factors associated with response to electroconvulsive therapy in patients with schizophrenic symptoms. Br J Psychiatry 154: 635, 1989.

Dunlop E: Electroshock and monoamine oxidase inhibitors in the treatment of depressed reactions. Dis Nerv Syst 21: 130, 1960b.

Dwersteg JF, Avery DH: Atracurium as a muscle relaxant for electroconvulsive therapy in a burned patient. Convulsive Ther 3: 49, 1987.

El-Ganzouri A et al: Monoamine oxidase inhibitors: Should they be discontinued preoperatively? Anesth Analg 64: 592, 1985.

Enna SJ, Mohler H: Gamma-aminobutyric acid (GABA) receptors and their association with benzodiazepine recognition sites In Meltzer HY (ed): *Psychopharmacology: The Third Generation of Progress,* New York, Raven Press, 1987, p. 265.

Foster S, Ries R: Delayed hypertension with electroconvulsive therapy. J Nerv Ment Dis 176: 374, 1988.

Freese KJ: Can patients safely undergo electroconvulsive therapy while receiving monoamine oxidase inhibitors. Convulsive Ther 1: 190, 1985

Friedel RO: The combined use of neuroleptics and ECT in drug resistant schizophrenic patients. Psychopharmacol Bull 22: 928, 1986.

Gilman A et al.: *Pharmacological Basis of Therapeutics,* 7th ed. New York, Macmillan, 1985, p. 693.

Glassman AH et al.: Cardiovascular effects of tricyclic antidepressants. In Meltzer HY (ed): *Psychopharmacology: The Third Generation of Progress,* New York, Raven Press, 1987, p. 1437.

Gujavarty K, Greenberg LB, Fink M: Electroconvulsive therapy and neuroleptic medication in therapy-resistant positive-symptom psychosis. Convulsive Ther 3: 185, 1987.

Gutierrez-Esteinou R, Pope HG: Does fluoxetine prolong electrically induced seizures? Convulsive Ther 5: 344, 1989.

Howie et al.: Esmolol reduces the autonomic hypersensitivity and length of seizures induced by electroconvulsive therapy. Anesth Analg 71: 384, 1990.

Howie et al.: Defining the dose range for esmolol used in electroconvulsive therapy hemodynamic attenuation. Anesth Analg 75: 805, 1992.

Imlah NW, Ryan E, Harrington JA: The influence of antidepressant drugs on the response to electroconvulsive therapy and on subsequent relapse rates. Neuropsychopharmacology 4: 438, 1965.

Impastato D: Prevention of fatalities in electroshock therapy. Dis Nerv Syst 18(suppl): 34, 1957.

Janowsky EC, Risch SC, Janowsky DS: Psychotropic agents. In Smith NT, Miller RD, Corbascio AN (eds.): *Drug Interactions and Anesthesia,* Philadelphia, Lea & Febiger, 1981, p. 177.

Kalayam B, Alexopoulos GS: Nifedipine in the treatment of blood pressure rise after ECT. Convulsive Ther 5: 110, 1989.

Kellner CH: Labetalol and ECT (letter). J Clin Psychiatry 52: 386, 1991.

Kellner CH, Nixon DW, Bernstein HJ: ECT-drug interactions: a review. Psychopharmacol Bull 27: 595, 1991.

Kirkegaard C, Moller SE, Bjorum N: Addition of L-tryptophan to electroconvulsive treatment in endogenous depression: a double-blind study. Acta Psychiatr Scand 58: 457, 1978.

Klapheke MM: Combining ECT and antipsychotic agents: benefits and risks. Convulsive Ther 9: 241, 1993.

Kovac et al.: Esmolol bolus and infusion attenuates increases in blood pressure and heart rate during electroconvulsive therapy. Can J Anaesth 37: 58, 1990.

Kovac et al.: Comparison of two esmolol bolus doses on the haemodynamic response and seizure duration during electroconvulsive therapy. Can J Anaesth 38: 204, 1991.

Loo H, Cuche H, Benkelfat C: Electroconvulsive therapy during anticoagulant therapy. Convulsive Ther 1: 258, 1985.

Lunn RJ et al.: Anesthetics and electroconvulsive therapy seizure duration: implications for therapy from a rat model. Biol Psychiatry 16: 1163, 1981.

Madow L: Brain changes in electroshock therapy. Am J Psychiatry 113: 337, 1956.

Malsch E et al.: Efficacy of electroconvulsive therapy after propofol or methohexital anesthesia. Anesth Analg 72: S192, 1992.

Marco LA, Randels PM: Succinylcholine drug interactions during electroconvulsive therapy. Biol Psychiatry 14: 433, 1979.

Markowitz JC, Brown RP: Seizures with neuroleptics and antidepressants. Gen Hosp Psychiatry 9: 135, 1987.

Martin BA, Kramer PM: Clinical significance of the interaction between lithium and a neuromuscular blocker. Am J Psychiatry 139: 1326, 1982.

McCain J, Mitlin M, Jahr JS: Is mivacurium chloride, a new short acting non-depolarizing muscle relaxant, useful in ECT procedures? A report of four cases (abstract). Presented at the Gulf Atlantic Residents Meeting, New Orleans, September 5, 1992.

McCall WV et al.: Effects of labetalol on hemodynamics and seizure duration during ECT. Convulsive Ther 7: 5, 1991.

McCarthy EP, Bloomfield SS: Labetalol: a review of its pharmacology, pharmacokinetics, clinical uses and adverse effects. Pharmacology 3: 193, 1983.

McCleane GJ, Howe JP: Electoconvulsive therapy and serum potassium. Ulster Med J 58: 172, 1989.

Miller ME et al.: Atropine sulfate premedication and cardiac arrhythmia in electroconvulsive therapy (ECT). Convulsive Ther 3: 10, 1987.

Mokriski BK et al.: Electroconvulsive therapy-induced cardiac arrhythmias during anesthesia with methohexital, thiamylal, or thiopental sodium. J Clin Anesthes 4: 208, 1992.

Monaco JT, DelaPlaine RP: Tranylcypromine with ECT. Am J Psychiatry 120: 1003, 1964.

Mukherjee S: Combined ECT and lithium therapy. Convulsive Ther 9: 274, 1993.

Muller D: Nardil (phenelzine) as a potentiator of electroconvulsive therapy. J Ment Sci 107: 994, 1961.

Nelson JP, Benjamin L: Efficacy and safety of combined ECT and tricyclic antidepressant drugs in the treatment of depressed geriatric patients. Convulsive Ther 5: 321, 1989.

Nettelbladt P: Factors influencing number of treatments and seizure duration in ECT: drug treatment, social class. Convulsive Ther 4: 160, 1988.

Olesen AC, Lolk A, Christensen P: Effect of a single nighttime dose of oxazepam on seizure duration in electroconvulsive therapy. Convulsive Ther 5: 3, 1989.

Perrin GM: Cardiovascular aspects of electric shock therapy. Acta Psychiatr Scand 36: 7, 1961.

Peters SG, Wochos DN, Peterson GC: Status epilepticus as a complication of concurrent electroconvulsive and theophylline therapy. Mayo Clin Proc 59: 568, 1984.

Pettinati HM et al.: Evidence for less improvement in depression in patients taking benzodiazepines during unilateral ECT. Am J Psychiatry 147: 1029, 1990.

Raotma H: Has tryptophan any anticonvulsive effect? Acta Psychiatr Scand 57: 253, 1978.

Raskin DA: Cardiac irritability, tricyclic antidepressants, and electroconvulsive therapy. J Clin Psychopharmacol 4: 237, 1984.

Remick RA, Jewesson P, Ford RW: Monoamine oxidase inhibitors in general anesthesia: a reevaluation. Convulsive Ther 3: 196, 1987.

Roberts MA, Attah JR: Carbamazepine and ECT. Br J Psychiatry 153: 418, 1988.

Seager CP, Bird RL: Imipramine with electrical treatment in depression—a controlled trial. J Ment Sci 108: 704, 1962.

Small JG et al.: Complications with electroconvulsive treatment combined with lithium. Biol Psychiatry 15: 103, 1980.

Small JG: Efficacy of electroconvulsive therapy in schizophrenia, mania, and other disorders, I: schizophrenia. Convulsive Ther 1: 263, 1985.

Snyder SH, Sklar P: Behavioral and molecular actions of caffeine: focus on adenosine. J Psychiatr Res 18: 91, 1984.

Standish-Barry HMAS, Deacon V, Smith RP: The relationship of concurrent benzodiazepine administration to seizure duration in ECT. Acta Psychiatr Scand 71: 269, 1985.

Staton RD, Enderle JD, Gerst JW: The electroencephalographic pattern during electroconvulsive therapy, IV: spectral energy distributions with methohexital, innovar and ketamine anesthesias. Clin Electroencephal 17: 203, 1986.

Stern RA et al.: Combined use of thyroid hormone and ECT. Convulsive Ther 9: 285, 1993.

Stoudemire A et al.: Labetalol in the control of cardiovascular responses to electroconvulsive therapy in high-risk depressed medical patients. J Clin Psychiatry 51: 508, 1990.

Swartz CM: Anesthesia for ECT. Convulsive Ther 9: 301, 1993.

Swartz CM, Lewis RK: Theophylline reversal of electroconvulsive therapy (ECT) seizure inhibition. Psychosomatics 32: 47, 1991.

Swartz CM, Saheba NC: Comparison of atropine with glycopyrrolate for use in ECT. Convulsive Ther 5: 56, 1989.

Tancer ME, Evans DL: Electroconvulsive therapy in geriatric patients undergoing anticoagulation therapy. Convulsive Ther 5: 102, 1989.

Taylor P, Fleminger JJ: ECT for schizophrenia. Lancet 1: 1380, 1980.

Thase ME: Long-term treatments of recurrent depressive disorders. J Clin Psychiatry 53: 32, 1992.

Weigner MB et al.: Prevention of the cardiovascular and neuroendocrine response to electroconvulsive therapy: I. Effectiveness of pretreatment regimens on hemodynamics. Anesth Analg 73: 556, 1991a.

Weigner MB et al.: Prevention of the cardiovascular and neuroendocrine response to electroconvulsive therapy, II: effects of pretreatment regimens on catecholamines, ACTH, vasopressin, and cortisol. Anesth Analg 73: 563, 1991b.

Weiss DM: Changes in blood pressure with electroshock therapy in a patient receiving chlorpromazine hydrochloride (Thorazine). Am J Psychiatry 111: 617, 1955.

Wells DG, Davies GG, Rosewarne F: Attenuation of electroconvulsive therapy induced hypertension with sublingual nifedipine. Anaesth Intensive Care 17: 31, 1989.

INDEX

Page numbers followed by *f* denote figures; those followed by *t* denote tables.